THE FRAGILE BRAIN

the
Fragile
Brain

The Strange, Hopeful
Science of Dementia

KATHLEEN
TAYLOR

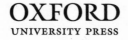

OXFORD
UNIVERSITY PRESS

OXFORD
UNIVERSITY PRESS

Great Clarendon Street, Oxford, OX2 6DP,
United Kingdom

Oxford University Press is a department of the University of Oxford.
It furthers the University's objective of excellence in research, scholarship,
and education by publishing worldwide. Oxford is a registered trade mark of
Oxford University Press in the UK and in certain other countries

© Kathleen Taylor 2016

The moral rights of the author have been asserted

First Edition published in 2016

Impression: 1

Published in the United States of America by Oxford University Press
198 Madison Avenue, New York, NY 10016, United States of America

British Library Cataloguing in Publication Data

Data available

Library of Congress Control Number: 2016942581

ISBN 978–0–19–872608–1

Printed in Great Britain by
Clays Ltd, St Ives plc

Contents

PART 3 Mechanisms

List of Figures

Source: Population data are from the Office of National Statistics Population Estimates for UK, England and Wales, Scotland and Northern Ireland, mid-2013, available from <http://www.ons.gov.uk/ons/rel/pop-estimate/population-estimates-for-uk--england-and-wales--scotland-and-northern-ireland/2013/index.html> licensed under the Open Government Licence v.3.0. Numbers of people with dementia are taken from Table 4.1, 'Number of people with dementia in the UK, by age and sex, 2013', in the 2014 Alzheimer's Society report, Dementia UK: Update. With permission.

List of Tables

Acknowledgements

First, my thanks to some readers and many more writers. The former are the anonymous readers, together with the Delegates of Oxford University Press, who approved *The Fragile Brain* for publication. The latter are all the researchers on whose work I have drawn to write this book. Constraints of space required me to be extremely selective, so my apologies if you are not cited here. (A search for 'dementia' in the open-access research database *PubMed*, as this book went to press early in 2016, produced over 28,000 results.) If you are cited, but my interpretations are not as you would have liked, forgive a fallible fellow mortal. Had I but world enough and time...but I had not, so the imperfections must remain. Any errors are, of course, my own.

I am deeply grateful to John Stein for the interesting and informative discussions we have had about this and related topics. I have learned much from an excellent teacher. I am also indebted to the organizers of the second Oxford Dementia Research Day, 2015, for a fascinating insight into the latest science.

My thanks to my parents—for their kindly if bemused support of their child's vocation—and to my friends, especially to my first reader Gillian Wright. Without her intelligence, literary judgement, and constant good sense there would be many more infelicities in this text. The same is true of my editor at Oxford, Latha Menon, a gem who knows her onions. I am likewise beholden to Jenny Nugée, Kate Farquhar-Thomson, Fiona Barry, and the rest of the excellent OUP team who looked after *The Fragile Brain*.

I would also like to thank the various NHS staff with whom I have had dealings in recent years, especially Julie Pickering at Derby.

Finally, I have drawn not only on research but on the work of charities. Faced with immensely difficult problems and inadequate funding, they are nonetheless doing great work in raising awareness of dementia and other age-related brain disorders. I hope this book will contribute to that project, and I thank them for the resources they provide.

Organizations

If you would like to find out more about participating in research, or obtaining advice or help, about brain disorders discussed in this book, here is a list of relevant organizations offering information, research news, guidance, and searches by local area for clinical services and other support.

UK

- Alzheimer's Research UK.
- Alzheimer's Society.
- Ataxia UK.
- Encephalitis Society.
- Join Dementia Research. This NHS-associated network is designed to put volunteers in touch with researchers.
- Meningitis Research Foundation.
- Mind.
- Stroke Association.
- Young Dementia UK.

US

- Alzheimer's Association.
- Alzheimers.net.

Europe

- Alzheimer Europe.

Australia

- Alzheimer's Australia.
- Alzheimer's Australia Dementia Research Foundation.

Other countries

- Alzheimer's Disease International.

1

Fragile Brains

Boxing Day, 26 December 2013. It's evening, and an elderly lady is climbing her steep stairs to bed.

In her eighties, she is still active, a slim non-smoker who lives alone but knows many of her neighbours. She's had a nice Christmas with friends and she got some lovely presents from her family; she's just been writing thank-you letters. She is in regular touch with people, by letter or phone, when she's not working through a book about science or history. She is a well-liked member of her local church. And she looks after her garden, though not so much at this time of year.

That night she wakes, feeling unwell. She gets out of bed, but something's gone wrong, badly wrong: she can't walk, can't move properly. She falls and can't get up.

And there she lies, for hours ...

She's alive when a worried neighbour finds her. But she'll not be going up her stairs again.

> In patients experiencing a typical large vessel acute ischemic stroke, 120 million neurons, 830 billion synapses, and 714 km (447 miles) of myelinated fibers are lost each hour. In each minute, 1.9 million neurons, 14 billion synapses, and 12 km (7.5 miles) of myelinated fibers are destroyed. Compared with the normal rate of neuron loss in brain aging, the ischemic brain ages 3.6 years each hour without treatment.
>
> Jeffrey L. Saver, 'Time is brain—quantified'[1]

Her older sister, gently told the news, says aghast, 'But strokes don't run in our family!'

Risk factors for stroke include age, smoking, obesity, and too much alcohol. The woman struck down in that last week of 2013 did not live riskily, except by living into her eighties. Nonetheless, from then until her death in May 2014 she was so incapacitated that she needed full-time hospital care. She was apathetic and immobile, and after a while she stopped eating.

Her family is my family. Of my eight closest adult relatives, five have been afflicted with brain disorders in the past few years. (Dementia doesn't run in our family either, yet one of those diagnoses is vascular dementia.) It feels as if fate has turned against us, piling on symptom after symptom: memory loss, speech problems, emotional outbursts, depression and apathy, fatigue, paralysis, even coma. From the slow-progressing atrophy and neurodegeneration of spinocerebellar ataxia—a rare genetic syndrome—to the sudden catastrophe of life-threatening encephalitis—brain inflammation—I'm seeing at close hand the devastation which illnesses affecting our most precious organ can cause to sufferers and to anyone who cares about them.

So this book is about knowing the enemy.

Being diagnosed with any serious disease can be a life-changing shock. The fear and anger, both for patients and their loved ones, can be as strong as in sudden bereavement, the grief as intense and disorienting. When patients are young they may also face the profound existential shock of realizing—as opposed to knowing intellectually—that they are frail and faulty organisms. That sudden awareness ensures that, even if the person survives the illness, nothing will ever be the same again. For better or worse, they will have grown up.

Why is the shock so titanic? Well, many of us who think we've already grown up live lives of steady roles and cosy routines. Perhaps that's true adulthood: the point at which high levels of novelty and excitement become tiresome rather than enjoyable. Unfortunately routine is deceptive. Security tempts us to believe that no matter what chaos infests other parts of the world we've somehow persuaded our corner of the universe to maintain itself just so. It's a necessary illusion—humankind cannot bear very much anxiety—but it's false. The universe goes its own way, and even the most secure of us will be wrong-footed by it now and then. And nothing uproots us quite like bodily failure, because our sense of control and safety is rooted in our bodies.

The sense of control is as much a basic human pleasure as our love of food. We need to feel autonomous; dependency feels both humiliating and alarming. Our desire to control originates in babyhood, when we gain the astonishing power of moving our bodies just by wishing it so. (How magical that power must seem to toddlers, and how they enjoy it! And why not? Even grown-up neuroscientists find it awe-inspiring.) It's the basis of all our subsequent powers and of many desires—including, of course, the dangerous desire to control others.

This is why the seriously ill hospital patient, motionless in bed, can fill us with unease as well as pity. Serious diseases attack our sense of power at its foundations. A superbly tuned machine, whose phenomenal abilities we often take for granted, has failed, and it feels like a betrayal. Such illnesses remind us that in the end, our powers are limited: life and death control us, not the other way round.

Yet diseases, unlike death, bring an extra torment of uncertainty and helplessness. My family, hearing the news of the stroke, didn't know how long and how much our relative would suffer. We did realize, after the first shock, the first delusory hopes, that she was beyond recovery. We struggled to accept that there was absolutely nothing we could do except wait, grieving without formally grieving. There are no rituals when someone is in this half-life, this slow decline towards extinction. The funeral, when it eventually came, was a relief; people spoke of 'a merciful release'. How sad to be thankful that someone you love has died.

Brain disorders are particularly brutal. Whether they arrive with life-wrecking abruptness, or in the slower form of neurodegenerative disorders like dementia, multiple sclerosis, or motor neuron disease, they can inflict the kinds of deaths that get people campaigning for euthanasia. They destroy a person's human nature while he or she is still alive. Motor neuron disease takes away our most basic freedom: physical movement. Stroke can paralyse, bring depression and listlessness, or cut off communication altogether. Some kinds of dementia can turn a spouse into a violent, or violently distressed, stranger—before they eat away the self completely.

The prospect of decline in chronic and progressive brain conditions is a grim one, and fluctuations in the conditions can make daily life extremely frustrating. It is harder to plan ahead when you may or may not need a wheelchair or be too tired to go shopping. And despite all the recent advances in disability awareness many everyday tasks are still near-impossible, or downright humiliating, for the disabled—especially for wheelchair users, what with steps outside shops, cars parked on pavements, and so on. It's not just shops, either. I needed a wheelchair for a while lately, and during that time I had to speak at three major UK literary festivals. At all three I was made, very kindly and unwittingly, to feel like a Martian. But I'm lucky; so far, I'm recovering. For people with brain disorders humiliation all too often comes with the territory, and stays. No wonder many become isolated, when leaving the house makes such demands on physical and emotional reserves.

Carers also suffer, and so can careers. A diagnosis can break lives into pieces and reassemble them in a very different pattern, because brain disorders place huge strain on everyone close to the patient. Some dementia is diagnosed before retirement, and other disorders like multiple sclerosis can strike much earlier. Fatigue can make work impossible, or limit it severely. Not all employers can accommodate workers whose ability to meet deadlines or remember facts may often be in doubt; nor can they always make allowances for carers with unpredictable and exhausting patients. Career loss risks social isolation and depression. It may also bring the need to claim welfare, and a demoralizing feeling of being, in the ugly Nazi phrase, *eine nutzlose Esser*—a useless eater.

In short, life—and sometimes also other people—can inflict ordeals on patients beyond the disease itself. This is especially true for those with brain conditions in which the damage may not always be obvious and the degree of debility can vary, like dementia.[2]

And, of course, many brain conditions offer no hope of recovery. While we are sometimes successful in treating cancer and heart disease, diabetes, and infectious diseases, we can do little for stroke unless the patient is lucky enough to be taken to hospital almost immediately. As for motor neuron disease, dementia, and many other degenerative conditions, there is currently no cure. We are left to watch the slow disintegration, pick up the pieces as best we can, and pray it won't happen to us.

The Fragile Brain is about how scientific research is working to add other options to the last resort of prayer. It is also about what we can all do, here and now, to lower our risk of getting age-related brain disorders. As we shall see, there is a lot we can do, whatever our age. To make the changes, we need to break with the traditional view of brains as halfway to immaterial—sources of selfhood, dreamers of dreams, and drivers of cognition. They may give us minds, but they are material objects: parts of bodies made of proteins, fats, carbohydrates, and other chemicals. To see them as such is to realize that brain health, like bodily wellness, needs active management, especially as we grow older. And to understand how best to manage our fragile brains, we need to understand what ageing and illness do to them. That new, still-patchy, rapidly growing knowledge is the topic of this book.

A word of warning: dementia science is not easy. In my book *The Brain Supremacy* I noted how neuroscientific language tends to coagulate into acronym soup, but it's baby food—easy to swallow—in comparison with the biochemistry, immunology, genetics, and cell biology this book requires.[3] These disciplines boast prose so clogged with abbreviations as to be at times almost unreadable, as well as expecting readers to be familiar with the Greek alphabet. I will not be supplying the kind of gruelling detail likely to induce sick headaches in the uninitiated, but you will meet the odd α (alpha), β (beta), and γ (gamma). There is more detail in the notes for those who want to dig deeper, though some of that detail assumes familiarity with the science. Indeed, *The Fragile Brain* is nearly two books in one, depending on whether you read just the main text or the notes as well.

Note too that much of the science I am discussing is extremely recent work. Any one paper should ideally be replicated at least once, independently, before it is trusted; and as we shall see, even after many years trusted results can be overturned by later findings. I have tried to use multiple sources where possible, though space limitations prevent me from listing them in full. Nonetheless, all scientific statements are provisional, not gospel. (That is true of any book about science.)

The Fragile Brain is concerned with three big questions. The first is about risk factors: what dangers, external and internal, threaten the brain's health? The second is:

what biological mechanisms change in dementia—that is, how do the dangers actually do their damage? Finally, I will ask what this knowledge tells us about practical measures: what can we do to lower our risk of a ghastly old age? I will also attempt to set out what we still don't know.

Brain diseases ruin lives. As so often in science and medicine, however, individual tragedy goes along with fruitful and fascinating study. The science is hugely difficult, and the work is of immense ethical value. If you are a student thinking about a career in bioscience, please consider working in this area; there's so much to do, and so much already happening. (If you would like to contribute in another way, please consider participating in a research study by contacting one of the organizations listed at the front of the book, such as the network *Join Dementia Research*.)

Of course, we still don't know enough; yet amid the misery there is, I think, hope for future generations. That is because the story of age-related brain conditions is also the optimistic story of modern science: promising more than it can yet deliver, but nonetheless already delivering much. Our capacity to do that science is one of our brains' great strengths. It is now facing up to our biggest challenge so far: their weaknesses.

PART 1

The Problem

Lilian, whose love made her decide
to check in with her mate who'd had a stroke,
lost all her spryness once her husband died…
He had a beautiful… all made of oak…
silk inside… brass handles… tries to find
alternatives… *that long thing where you lie*
for words like coffin that have slipped her mind
and forgetting, not the funeral, makes her cry.

Tony Harrison, *The Mother of the Muses*[1]

2

Living Well and Growing Old

The baby boom generation is approaching the age of greatest risk for cognitive impairment and dementia.

Tiffany F. Hughes and Mary Ganguli, 'Modifiable midlife risk factors for late-life cognitive impairment and dementia'[1]

With an ageing population in many Western countries, the problem of age-related brain conditions is gaining urgency. The baby boomers, that charmed generation born between 1946 and 1964, are now experiencing the impact of neurodegeneration, as patients or carers. To those of us who followed them, the boomers often seemed to have it all: free education, jobs for life, good pensions, houses cheap to buy which then rocketed in value. But all the luck and money in the world can't—at present—cure dementia.

Worse, the baby boomers face a double whammy. First, as the term implies, there are a lot of them, and brain diseases are extremely costly and difficult to treat. Even before the current age of austerity Western healthcare systems were struggling with the expense. In societies as complex as ours have become, a relatively minor cognitive impairment—slower and less efficient reasoning, memory failings, problems reading or absorbing information, poor decision making or irrational trustfulness—can seriously damage quality of life, as many elderly people learn when some predator cons them out of their life savings.

Brain disorders such as strokes and Alzheimer's disease are strongly associated with ageing. Both can strike earlier in life—even young children can suffer strokes, while rare early-onset forms of dementia can afflict people in their thirties—but the risk soars after the age of 65. As more of us live longer, more of us survive to stress our healthcare systems. The baby boomers are the first generation fully to feel the pinch.

The Links to Lifestyle

The second tragedy of the baby boomers is that research into age-related brain conditions is now beginning to unravel their causes—and those causal threads lead not just to genes but to environmental, including lifestyle, factors. In other words, how you live in your twenties, thirties, and forties appears to have an impact on your chances of a palatable old age. That crucial information comes too late for the baby boomers.

But the message is not one of total gloom. Higher healthcare costs do not necessarily imply worse overall health, because there are more of us living longer, often better lives, with more ways of treating the diseases we still face. In addition, research suggests that there are things we can do to reduce our risk of getting age-related brain conditions, or at least delay their onset, even in our fifties, sixties, and seventies. There are also hints in the literature that the rate of dementia may be reducing, perhaps due to lifestyle changes already made.

However, just because it isn't in your genes doesn't mean you can change it. We tend to think of genes as fixed fate and 'the environment'—that gigantic scientific glory hole which includes everything from the weather to your lunch choice—as something we can alter. Lifestyle factors are used as moral sticks, with which suboptimal members of society are beaten by the smug and lucky, because they are considered changeable. But genes are not so stolid, and your lifestyle is not all under personal control. Many aspects of your environment certainly exceed your powers of adjustment. Where you live as a child, your parents' socioeconomic status (SES), cultural pressures to drink and smoke, or not, what the people who make your food have put in it without telling you…these are not things you can usually do much about. And they matter.

Barriers to Change

For example, if your parents are very poor the chances of you achieving wealth and success—and hence of maintaining good health into old age—are lower from birth. The food you eat may be worse for you, and you may live in an area where many people have unhealthy habits, such as smoking. This not only exposes you to second-hand smoke, it raises the risk that you yourself will smoke, and do other unhealthy things. Furthermore—and this is the part that right-wing politicians tend to ignore—if you have grown up in poverty, exposed to pollutants, and eating junk food, you and the people you live with will almost certainly have been disadvantaged and damaged. The process started long before you reached the age at which politicians can hold you responsible for your choices.

That damage is partly physical. As we shall see, junk food and pollution and bad neighbourhoods are bad for your brain as well as for your body. But the damage is also psychological. Poor people are often regarded with suspicion in a society as driven by money as ours, and they face social signals that imply they are a burden and a nuisance. Sick and disabled people get similar messages, especially when public debate is hostile to the idea of welfare and ignores the distinction between work-related benefits and those related to sickness (as in the UK government's current promotion of a 'universal credit' welfare system). Dismissing all benefits claimants as lazy scroungers is ignorant even when only fit recipients are considered, let alone the seriously ill.

Stigmatizing generalizations are unreasonable, but they are perennially popular, especially when people feel under threat themselves (ask any tabloid newspaper). They are also an excellent destroyer of morale and deterrent of action. As bioethicist Carl Elliott observed, 'Unlike objects, people are conscious of the way they are classified, and they alter their behavior and self-conceptions in response to their classification.'[2] The change, however, may not be in the direction desired by the person doing the classifying. Calling people lazy may spur a few to prove the label wrong, but it has not proved successful in reducing the amounts paid out in benefits.

With respect to health, stigma can likewise make things worse rather than better. Talk of burdens tends to forget the human beings behind the label, who bear rather heavier costs than the average taxpayer. Worse still is the attitude—of which clinicians as well as the rest of us can be guilty—which interprets poorly understood illnesses as not really genuine. Someone with severe depression, for example, is unlikely to be helped by being told that it's 'all in the mind' (it isn't), just as dementia patients aren't helped by being treated as if they're stupid (they're not). Neither are they likely to feel better if they believe society views them as a useless drain on scarce resources. Would you? Undoubtedly there are malingerers, but they are few compared with the innocents caught up in this casual, everyday abuse. Stigmatizing is hugely counter-productive; it continues because of its psychological benefits for those who do it. But victims of stigma, including people with brain disorders, suffer more than perpetrators gain.

So-called lifestyle diseases, like those resulting from extreme obesity, can draw particular venom, yet even supposedly modifiable lifestyle factors can be a tough challenge to modify in practice, as every dieter, heavy drinker, or smoker knows. It's all very well telling people that they need to eat healthily, lose weight, give up the booze and fags, and take more exercise, but there are big gaps between receiving that information, understanding it, and acting on it.

How the message is conveyed can make a difference. Some studies have found that beginning the lecture by encouraging the audience to reflect on values (other than health) which are dear to them—a technique known as self-affirmation—can make them more receptive to health advice.[3]

Even when the message is received, understood, and acted upon, however, the most strong-willed patient may struggle and fail. Conditions like obesity and alcoholism wreak long-term change on the body so that it does not react in the same way that a healthy body would. Thus being told to 'eat less, move more' may work for someone who has recently become mildly overweight, whereas someone who has been obese for years may require more extreme treatment such as drugs or surgery. The body's adaptation to abnormal physiology makes curing chronic diseases extremely difficult. That is one reason why many clinicians would like to see more effort put into prevention.

If you are poor or ill, the effort you'd have to make to better your lot is massive—if such betterment is possible. It is much greater than the effort your luckier fellow-citizens would need to change their bad habits; and they struggle. Add to this the fact that poorer patients must face the double stigma of poverty and illness, and that they tend to be diagnosed with diseases like dementia later than their higher-income compatriots, and it is no surprise that financial stress and pre-existing ill health, including mental illness, are among the larger risk factors for age-related brain conditions.[4]

I use the term 'luckier' deliberately, because where you were born and to whom, and whether your genes will bring you nightmares, are surely as much down to luck as anything is. But I note too that luck's role in personal fate tends to be acknowledged less among those who've benefited more. It's a neat mental trick for justifying inaction and defending the *status quo*: if you believe that character and willpower bring life's rewards, then you're likely to assume that misfortunes such as poverty and illness result from the eternal fecklessness of the poor and sick, rather than from their circumstances—which could be changed.

One of the clearest lessons from the science of dementia is that in only a tiny minority of cases can the blame for this illness be laid fully on inbuilt characteristics—and to blame a genetic fault is not (or should not be) to blame the person. Environmental hazards are major contributors to brain decline.

Changing lifestyles takes a lot of effort; and there is another problem. We humans, although we can predict the future, have not mastered the art of taking it seriously. Future benefits are heavily discounted in comparison to present costs. 'After all', we think, 'we may fall under a bus tomorrow.' Indeed we may; but as we shall see, it is much more probable that we'll escape the bus and live to a ripe old age.[5] For younger people in good health the horrors of dementia can seem distant and unrelated to their current habits—until they or someone they love falls ill.

There is also the fact that vast chunks of society are economically dependent on our not changing our behaviour, and that the companies who sell us junk food and tobacco are acting as good corporations should and pursuing profit. This, unfortunately, means that they are doing their best to ensure we keep on consuming their products, thereby boosting our chances of an appalling old age.

Current science suggests that you can probably reduce your chances of getting dementia by making certain lifestyle changes. This does not mean that if you have—or get—dementia it's somehow your fault. Unless you have a rare genetic mutation (which is certainly not your fault) the disease will have had numerous causes, genetic and environmental, only some of which could have been altered by you, even in principle. That's before you consider the effort involved in practice: if lifestyle factors were easy to change, we'd have changed them. Nonetheless, the consensus is that it is still worth making alterations if you can, and the sooner the better. The benefits extend far beyond better brain health; and the consequences of poor brain health can be dire.

3

Counting the Costs

Quite apart from the personal costs, age-related brain conditions are already costing us all a fortune. In 2007 a study in the United States estimated that 67 in every 1,000 elderly people (over two-and-a-half million citizens) had Alzheimer's disease, the most common form of dementia.[1] For dementia overall, a 2013 report gave a figure of 5 million seniors affected.[2] That's almost four times as many people as die every year in traffic accidents worldwide.[3]

For comparison, the same study found that, per thousand, the rates for autism and cerebral palsy in children were 5.8 and 2.4, respectively; the rate of Parkinson's disease among elderly people was 9.5; and the chances per year of being brain-injured were about 1.83 for stroke and 1.01 for traumatic brain injury.[4]

Dementia Expenses

The forecasts are for things to get much worse. Another 2007 science headline, in the *British Medical Journal*, read, 'Number of people in UK with dementia will more than double by 2050'.[5]

Alzheimer's charities have been saying for some time that dementia and other age-related brain conditions are *the* biggest health crisis we will face in coming years. To see why, consider the economics of dementia. (Throughout this book I use the United Kingdom as the main example; the situation in rich nations with similar life expectancies, such as the United States, Canada, and Australia, is likely to be comparable. Other countries' costs will vary depending on their healthcare systems, how rapidly their population is ageing, etc.)

The Alzheimer's Society, a UK charity, reckons that by 2012 around 800,000 people in the UK were sufferers, costing around £23 billion a year to look after.[6] That gives a figure of nearly £29,000 per person—roughly the cost, in 2012, of keeping one female criminal in an open prison. About 5% of cases, the Society thinks, have early-onset dementia, diagnosed before the age of sixty-five.[7]

Note that these and all other estimates given here should be treated with caution: they are more educated guesses than scientific data. No one has physically counted dementia patients. Nor would that tell us how many people have the disease, because many who have it have not yet been diagnosed. Furthermore, the rates of dementia may differ from region to region, and from time to time, because of variation in risk factors for the disease (of which more later). For example, a 2007 study in the United States found that rates of Alzheimer's may be going up, while a 2009 study in Europe reckoned that they might be coming down slightly.[8] More recently a big comparative analysis of data from four Western European countries (the Netherlands, Spain, Sweden, and the United Kingdom) hints at a similar conclusion.[9] It amalgamated studies which compared the prevalence of dementia—how many people have the disease—in two groups of elderly people born in different years, to look for changes over time. Studies with the oldest participants found no increase, and studies of younger groups found small decreases, suggesting that dementia rates may indeed be stabilizing, in this region of the world at least.

Western countries and others already have a lot of people with dementia, however, and they must be cared for. In the United Kingdom in 2012, two in every three of the 800,000 citizens with dementia lived in the community (half of them were on their own), where they were looked after by 670,000 primary carers. The other third lived in a care home or were in hospital. The Alzheimer's Society states that 'a quarter of hospital beds are occupied by people with dementia over 65 at any one time', and patients admitted to hospital with a primary diagnosis of dementia stay, on average, three weeks, much longer than for most other medical conditions.[10] Yet from 2000 to 2008, 'the number of people in council-supported care homes in England has fallen from 200,000 to 172,000'.[11] Meanwhile, another study suggested that 'well over double the present total places in care homes would be required by 2043 to maintain the present ratio of institutional to community services for dementia'.[12]

Care homes are expensive. A UK study estimated that costs in 2011 averaged around £550 per week. The same study found that one in five patients admitted dies within months, but about one in five survives for four years or longer, and the longest stay was nearly twenty-four years. The average stay was 462 days (about fifteen months), at a cost of £36,000.[13] Again, the costs are comparable with those of prison.[14] And there are more than three times as many institutionalized patients as there are prisoners.

People with dementia, in short, typically require increasing—and very costly—levels of care. In the words of an expert at the UK think-tank the King's Fund,

'They probably have the most complex care and support needs of any members of society.'[15] Many experts support policies to encourage continued home care, under medical supervision, because patients themselves and their families tend to prefer it; but such policies could also ease the economic costs of dementia.

Dementia Spending

Those costs are enormous; yet they are not matched by what we spend on dementia research. Brain disorders are disproportionately underfunded compared with other

Table 1: UK costs and funding for dementia and other major diseases in 2012.

	Cancer	Coronary heart disease	Dementia	Stroke	Total
Number of cases in 2012	2.3 million	2.3 million	0.8 million	1.2 million	6.6 million
Government research spending	45%	21%	21%	12%	£347 million
Charities' research spending	76%	18%	3%	3%	£509 million
Total spending	64%	19%	11%	7%	£856 million
Total research spending per patient	**£241**	**£73**	**£118**	**£48**	
Healthcare costs	£4.4 billion	£2.4 billion	£1.4 billion	£1.8 billion	£10 billion
Social care costs	£0.6 billion	£0.1 billion	£10.2 billion	£1.1 billion	£12 billion
Combined costs	£5.0 billion	£2.5 billion	£11.6 billion	£2.9 billion	£22 billion
Total costs per patient	**£2,174**	**£1,087**	**£14,500**	**£2,417**	
Ratio of costs to funding	9:1	15:1	123:1	50:1	

Table 1 summarizes data from a research study (Luengo-Fernandez *et al.* 2015), which provided estimates of the financial costs to the United Kingdom, and of government and charitable spending, relating to four major diseases: cancer, coronary heart disease, dementia, and stroke (shown in the columns). For each disease, the rows give the numbers of cases in the United Kingdom, the percentages of government, charitable, and total spending, calculated funding per patient, healthcare and social care costs, calculated costs per patient, and the ratio of funding to costs.

major killers, especially when it comes to voluntary giving. A study of UK data from 2012 compared costs and spending for dementia, cancer, coronary heart disease, and stroke, which together took over half the lives lost that year (55%).[16] Table 1 summarizes the study's findings. It shows that, while the costs of all four conditions were higher than the funding given to them, the discrepancies were much greater for stroke and especially for dementia. Table 1 also shows that, compared with charities, government spends comparatively more on dementia (21%) and less on cancer (46%). Three quarters of charitable giving is for cancer (76%); only three pounds in every hundred goes to dementia.

Global Costs

What of the bigger picture? Worldwide, thirteen per cent of people aged sixty or over already require long-term care. About four-fifths of those who end up in care homes have dementia. As of 2013, it is thought there were 44.4 million people with dementia. This number is projected to increase to an estimated 75.6 million in 2030, and 135.5 million in 2050.[17]

If those estimates are anywhere near right, the rise of dementia will put immense strain on societies and their economies. In the United States alone, the estimated total costs of dementia in 2010 were 'between $157 billion and $215 billion'.[18] In 2013, Alzheimer's Disease International (ADI) said that the 'worldwide cost of dementia care is currently over US$600 billion' [about £350 billion].[19] If the world maintained that level of funding per patient, the bill in 2050 would be over £1 *trillion*, just on dementia (about $1.5 trillion in 2015). Some countries, like the United Kingdom, spend much more than others; the global average per person is around a third of what Britain spends on dementia. If every country were to match UK funding levels, the 2050 cost would be nearly £4 trillion, $6.3 trillion.

Between now and 2050 global GDP is predicted to rise by roughly the same rate, according to a report by those boundless market optimists PwC, in which case the proportion of money spent on dementia would remain around one per cent on the lower-spending projection, two per cent if the rest of the world decides to spend like the United Kingdom.[20] But any way you look at them the sums are huge—and still inadequate. And there are many other demands on funding.

All over the world people are looking at their elderly relatives and thinking in dismay, 'Is this my future?' Meanwhile, governments are wondering how on earth they will be able to pay for their ageing populations.

Is Prevention Better than Cure?

Since the *Soylent Green* solution of euthanasia plus recycling is not an option, the obvious alternative is to find a medical quick fix: a cure for dementia. As will become clear, however, no current sufferer should fool themselves with that hope. The track record of Alzheimer's drugs is lamentable. Available treatments such as memantine do no more than stall the decline for a while. The search for new ones has been extensive, yet as a 2013 review observed, 'Over the period from 1998 to 2011, approximately 100 compounds targeted for the treatment of AD have failed.'[21] Even if an effective drug is discovered, it will take some years to become available; its impact may be meagre, and it may have nasty side effects.

Worse still, many researchers now think that any drug might have to be administered years before the signs of dementia become apparent. This may make large-scale treatment unaffordable. As Alzheimer's scientist Sam Gandy notes, 'The annual per-person cost of a typical biologic drug is roughly equivalent to the annual per-person cost for custodial dementia care in nursing homes, but infusion of the biologic drug would begin ten to twenty years sooner than custodial care.'[22] If the treatment for dementia were as expensive as institutional care and started up to two decades earlier, it is hard to see how this could reduce costs unless the treatment were extremely effective and required only a few years to cure the problem—which is unlikely.

This is why so much of the research into Alzheimer's is focusing on prevention. The aim is to identify factors which increase the risk of getting dementia, to prevent the build-up of certain brain proteins such as amyloid-beta and tau—of which more later—and to encourage behaviours such as eating healthily and keeping active, which seem to reduce the risk.

I must confess to a slight conflict of interest here, as despite not drinking, not smoking, and maintaining a healthy diet, waistline, weight, and blood pressure, I have more experience of serious medical conditions than is typical for my age. I infer that either prevention may not work for everyone, or that the standards for what counts as a healthy lifestyle are beyond what most people can achieve. Besides, to quote Dr Gandy again, 'the focus on moving earlier and earlier in intervention threatens to leave behind those already diagnosed with disease'.[23] This is why we still need scientists to look for treatments.

Nonetheless, successful interventions for dementia could reduce the costs—economic, and in human suffering—for future generations.

The costs of poor lifestyle choices are difficult to estimate, but people have tried. In the United Kingdom, a study of NHS finances in the year 2006–2007 reckoned up the medical costs of five major risk factors for ill health. The cheapest was lack of exercise, at £0.9 billion (1% of the net NHS budget). Smoking and alcohol each cost £3.3 billion (3.5%). Excess weight cost £5.1 billion (5.4%). Problems linked to poor diet topped the league at £5.8 billion (6.1%)—about as much as the NHS spent on cancer in 2011.[24]

This is why the government is so keen to tell you to eat your greens—or at least to stop eating as much junk food as we do. (Well, it's one reason why; another is that urging people to change their ways is easier and cheaper than bullying the food industry or fixing problems like poverty and pollution.) A commercial survey in 2014 found that in the UK people spent, on average, a third of their food budget on fast food—around £29.4 billion a year. Young adults are particularly keen on takeaways, adding to concerns about the nation's ability to pay its health bills in the not-too-distant future. Across the world the sources of ill health vary; smoking, for example, is a big problem in Indonesia, pollution in China, obesity in the United States. But every nation must find money for health care, and as people live longer and take up more 'Western' lifestyles the pressure on national budgets will increase.

4

Brain Disorders Affect All of Us

B rain disorders are not just a concern for the elderly and their families. Age is a big risk factor for some of them, but others can strike at any time. Of my five affected relatives, four were past pension age, but the fifth was a teenager. Her infection almost killed her and has left her with a memory so badly damaged that she was forced to give up her hopes of university. To remember something she writes it down, filling notebooks that may one day provide an unparalleled resource for social historians—but are her only link to her recent past. As with many brain disorders, the impact on daily existence is not easy to understand unless you've seen it or lived it; but it is profound. (Some UK higher education institutions have made great progress in accommodating people with dyslexia, anxiety, depression, and so on, but this rare syndrome would pose a formidable challenge to even the friendliest college.)

There are many conditions that can strike a person long before they reach retirement. Apart from developmental disorders such as autism and Down's syndrome, and the rarer nightmares of early-onset stroke or dementia, human brains can succumb to all manner of problems. Abscesses, addictions, aneurysms, atrophy, cancers, chronic fatigue syndrome, coma, depression, epilepsy, Huntington's disease, hydrocephalus, infections, migraine, motor neuron disease, multiple sclerosis, Parkinson's disease, psychosis, and small vessel disease are but a few. All can transform a successful life into one that may feel unbearable, even when they don't directly end that life.

As the list in the previous paragraph makes clear, brain disorders include another huge public health issue: mental illnesses such as depression and schizophrenia. These can be lifelong, or lethal, and their global costs are staggering: the category 'mental illness and substance use' results in more years with disability than any other medical condition.[1] That is a vast amount of wasted productivity, if you're the kind of person who views other people as economic units. If you see them as human beings, it's an unimaginable amount of misery.

The Hope

All in all, brain disorders take a grim toll on us. As I write, we cannot yet fix damaged brains except in the crudest of fashions—by removing a tumour, for instance, or implanting an electrode. We understand very little about the mechanisms that underlie neurodegeneration, that mysterious and dreadful process underlying conditions like dementia, in which a living brain slowly disintegrates, dying before its body does. And we do not know nearly enough about its causes. This book is in part a plea for more attention—and funding—for dementia research, by governments, corporations, and individuals. By describing the fearsome challenges we face in understanding this condition, it will show you why, after all these years, there is not—and realistically never could have been—a cure for dementia.

Yet I hope to persuade you that despair and fear need not be our only reactions to dementia, either on a personal or a societal level. As we shall see, researchers and doctors are better placed than ever before to do something about age-related brain conditions. If you think, as I do, that our best chance lies in grasping the problem, then our understanding of the brain—in sickness as in health—has grown at an astonishing, and accelerating rate in recent years, and continues to do so. We have better tools, from high-throughput DNA sequencing to stem cells, neurosurgery to neuroimaging. We can now, for the first time, see signs of dementia in a living human brain. There is a real hope that one day we will understand enough about neurodegeneration to be able to take some effective action against it. Prevention, perhaps, and then maybe, eventually, cure. There are many exciting new treatment possibilities, although they are in their early stages.

Patients with age-related brain conditions, however, are not simply targets for medical advances. They are people, each unique, each with a valuable life history and identity. That identity may seem to slip away as the disease takes hold, but how much of that is in the mind of the onlooker? Studies looking at self-perception suggest that in fact, aspects of identity are relatively well preserved. The patient feels like the same person, though perhaps some details are not quite up to date (one study found that Alzheimer's patients underestimate their age).[2] My relative with vascular dementia was uncertain of her name last time I talked to her, but she is still, as I write in September 2015, the same beloved friend as ever she was.

If psychology has taught us anything, it is that human identities and behaviours are strongly social—influenced far more than we commonly realize by the behaviours of those around us. So it is for people with dementia. How they behave may be due to the fear, unease, and stigma they sense in others, as well as to the problems of their dying brains. For that reason, it may be of considerable medical benefit to address the social unease around dementia, as is being done for other feared disorders like cancer and depression.

Forced by our ageing populations, we are at last facing up to the problems of age-related brain conditions. That we are finally beginning to take them seriously is itself a great advance; old people have been remarkably invisible to date, despite their growing numbers. If we can do so on both a scientific and a social level, exploring the science while never forgetting the people at its heart, then we have some hope of taking on one of the biggest challenges confronting us in the twenty-first century.

A Roadmap

This book is a guide to the science of neurodegeneration. For reasons of space, and because it is the most common age-related brain condition, I will concentrate on dementia: specifically, Alzheimer's, on which most research has been done. Much of what we are starting to understand about dementia, however, also applies to other age-related brain conditions such as stroke and Parkinson's disease. They share many risk factors, often co-occur, and are likely to involve shared or similar underlying mechanisms.

This book is not a clinical or practical guide to living with an age-related brain condition, either as a sufferer or as a carer. There are many such, but my aim is different: to summarize what is understood of the science. Readers of my previous books have had a wide range of backgrounds, from neuroscience professional to arts graduate to student. For those unfamiliar with the make-up of human brains, therefore, I will begin with a guide to the stuff that is harmed when someone gets an age-related brain condition. I will largely avoid traditionally emphasized areas like the prefrontal cortex; our business lies in less familiar zones, and with less familiar metaphors, because the brain we shall be meeting here is not the dry, abstracted circuitry of a skull-bound computer. Brimming with life and fizzing with chemicals, it is a wet, organic, dazzlingly complicated entity. Even readers familiar with terms like 'prefrontal cortex' can expect to learn something new.

Having introduced the brain in general, I will turn to the specific case of Alzheimer's and the discoveries which drove the creation of what is now the dominant theory of dementia: the amyloid cascade hypothesis. Amyloid is a protein, so we will need to take a look at how proteins are made and used in brain cells—and at the cells themselves. I will introduce key structures and functions, looking at how cells maintain themselves, and how they die. Dementia is, after all, a condition marked by dying cells.

To understand how dementia does its damage, we need to consider risk factors and causes: the factors that trigger neurodegeneration, and the biological mechanisms that implement the death sentence. Brains are born with an excellent capacity for long-term maintenance, so what makes them go wrong? And how do the causes, the suspects in researchers' hunt for brain killers, exert their dire effects?

Part of the answer, it now seems, may involve a population of brain cells of which, until recently, few people had even heard: glia, and particularly the subset known as microglia. (The word means 'little glue cells'; indeed, one might be tempted to call them gluons, but their discoverer didn't, and subatomic physics has since nabbed the term.) Microglia are the brain's immune cells, and like the immune system elsewhere in the body, they are there to protect and serve, like police constantly alert for danger and damage. Immune changes have been implicated in most if not all of the conditions that lie near the murky, yet socially critical border where physical and mental illness merge, from chronic fatigue to depression to dementia. Research on immune dysfunction in neurodegeneration is growing rapidly.

Another part of the answer involves organs quite distinct from the brain, like the heart and the pancreas. To see why, we will again need to venture beyond neuroscience, with its solid structures, easily identifiable blood vessels and nerve tracts, and beautiful brain scans, and venture to approach the shifting sands of physiology and biochemistry, a seething soup of cells and chemicals. One of my aims in this book is to put you at ease with this more fluid vision of human nature, convincing you that cells and chemicals are central to understanding how the brain works. Neuroscientists began by working out anatomical pathways: the tracts of fibres that linked one clump of brain cells to another. Then they modelled the brain as a computer, passing information from input to output. These days the aim is to work out the biochemical pathways by which each brain cell changes itself and the small, wet world around it. From those minuscule adjustments, affecting billions of cells over many years, come the paths by which we approach and experience old age.

We begin with the neuroscience of that archetypal age-related brain disorder: dementia.

5

Discovering Dementia

I feel as if I've had a blackout. I don't know why I'm here. I feel as if I'm not really me. If you asked me my name, I'm not sure I could tell you. I'm just drifting. I don't know whether something happened yesterday, last week, longer ago... I feel that something's out of kilter. Everything's out of my control.

My relative who has vascular dementia, April 2015

Aloysius Alzheimer was a fine clinician-scientist. Hard working, curious, and meticulous, he was also lucky. He was born in Bavaria, in 1864, into a family who valued education and could afford it. He was able to study medicine at top German universities like Tübingen. And he met three people who would help him towards scientific immortality (see Figure 1).

The first of these vital contacts was the great psychiatrist Emil Kraepelin, to whom we owe much of modern psychiatry. His belief that mental disorders had a brain-and-body basis encouraged a medical, systematic approach to mental illness. He distinguished, as we still do today, between psychoses like schizophrenia (which he called dementia prae-cox), personality disorders like psychopathy, mood disorders like depression and man-ic-depression (*aka* bipolar disorder), and dementia. And his emphasis that mental derangement has a physical basis has been hugely influential on society's attitudes to sufferers, as well as on brain science, the law, and the pharmaceutical industry.

Alzheimer began his research career at the state asylum in Frankfurt-am-Main, working with the unusually humane psychiatrist Emil Sioli.[1] He later moved to Munich to work with Kraepelin, at the latter's invitation. There he joined what became one of the great founding centres of modern brain research, with a staff list that 'eventually read like a Who's Who in neuroscience'—including Hans Creutzfeldt and Alfons Jakob (as in the prion disease CJD, Creutzfeldt-Jakob disease) and Korbinian Brodmann, whose beautiful maps of the human brain are still used today.[2] In this illustrious company Alzheimer pursued his studies in histology, the microscopic study of the brain's material and structures.

The second key contact was neuropathologist Franz Nissl, whose brain-staining techniques Alzheimer would use on the collection of human brains he was assembling.[3] When Nissl moved to Frankfurt to work with Sioli he and Alzheimer became friends. They collaborated on a six-volume textbook, and in 1894 Nissl was best man at Alzheimer's marriage.[4]

Alzheimer's third contact was Auguste Deter, whom he met in 1901 when she was admitted, aged fifty-one, to the Frankfurt hospital where he worked. Auguste had a very peculiar set of emotional and cognitive symptoms, ranging from jealousy, panics, screaming and crying fits to memory loss, confusion, and disorientation. She died four-and-a-half years later of what we now call early-onset dementia. Alzheimer writes of her:

> Soon she developed a rapid loss of memory. She was disoriented in her home, carried things from one place to another and hid them, sometimes she thought somebody was trying to kill her and started to cry loudly.
>
> In the institution her behavior showed all the signs of complete helplessness. She is completely disoriented in time and space. Sometimes she says that she does not understand anything and that everything is strange to her. Sometimes she greets the attending physician like company and asks to be excused for not having completed the household chores, sometimes she protests loudly that he intends to cut her, or she rebukes him vehemently with expressions which imply that she suspects him of dishonorable intentions. Then again she is completely delirious, drags around her bedding, calls her husband and daughter and seems to suffer from auditory hallucinations. Often she screamed for many hours.
>
> Unable to understand the situation, she starts screaming as soon as an attempt is made to examine her. [...]
>
> At the end, the patient was lying in bed in a fetal position completely pathetic, incontinent. In spite of all nursing care, she had developed bedsores.[5]

Some things don't change. My relative who suffered the stroke got bedsores.

When 'Auguste D' died her brain was sent to Munich for Alzheimer to dissect and examine. His subsequent conference presentation and papers are now acknowledged as the first discussions of the disease which bears his name, but which he called only 'An unusual illness of the cerebral cortex'.[6] It was Kraepelin, in a textbook, who named it Alzheimer's disease.

The condition of presenile (early-onset) dementia described by Alzheimer was considered tragic but rare, and 'in a textbook' was where his account remained for years. In 1976, however, the great Alzheimer's researcher and activist Robert Katzman published an editorial, in the journal *Archives of Neurology*, which transformed how Alzheimer's disease was understood. What Katzman argued—in 'The prevalence and malignancy of Alzheimer disease: a major killer'—was that presenile and senile dementia were basically the same disease.[7] The timing might differ (and we now

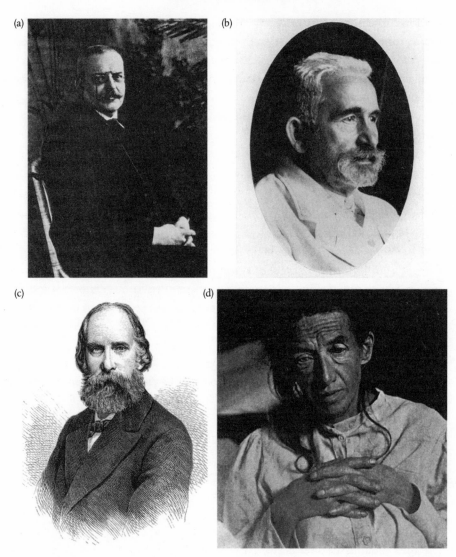

FIGURE 1: Alzheimer and colleagues. Alois Alzheimer (a), his colleague and mentor Emil Kraepelin (b), his colleague and friend Franz Nissl (c), and his most famous patient, Auguste Deter (d).

know that the genetics differ too), but the underlying mechanisms of neurodegeneration, and the symptoms they produced, were similar. This implied that Alzheimer's disease was not a rarity, but a common cause of brain damage in later life.

Alois Alzheimer comes across as a thoroughly likeable man; a colleague described him as someone who 'tried to bring joy to soften suffering'.[8] Yet his name now conjures the nightmare of dementia. What price immortality?

Then again, it may be better than being remembered for writing a doctoral thesis on earwax, as Alzheimer also did.[9]

The Dying Brain

The disease to which Alzheimer's mentor gave Alzheimer's name is the most common of the dementias, estimated to afflict around sixty-two per cent of patients.[10] Other types include vascular dementia, which as the name suggests involves damage to brain blood vessels (17%), mixed forms (10%), and dementia with Lewy bodies (4%, or more, since it is thought to be under-diagnosed). Rarer are Parkinson's dementia (2%), which can have similar symptoms to dementia with Lewy bodies—problems with gait, posture, and movement like those seen in Parkinson's disease. Also uncommon are the various frontotemporal dementias (2% or more, since they too are probably under-diagnosed), which may likewise affect movement more than memory.

Frontotemporal dementias may, furthermore, cause emotional or personality changes, or language problems, depending on exactly where in the brain the disease takes hold. They include conditions such as Pick's disease, first identified as a language problem in 1892 by a doctor, Arnold Pick. Following the chance rediscovery of Alzheimer's original data, it is now thought that Pick's disease may be what Auguste Deter actually had.

Note that the percentages given for the various dementias are not to be taken as final. Estimates vary, especially with respect to Lewy body and frontotemporal dementias.[11] Even in the era of ever-more-helpful neuroimaging techniques, the only guaranteed way to diagnose which form of dementia someone has suffered is to analyse their brain tissue after death. That can produce rather different estimates, as shown by a post-mortem study of 1,050 brains from elderly people with dementia, of whom 660 (62.9%) had been diagnosed with Alzheimer's and 105 (10%) with vascular dementia.[12] Of the 1,050 brains analysed, the pathologist notes that 'At autopsy, 86% revealed Alzheimer-related pathology, but only 42.8% showed "pure" Alzheimer disease, with additional cerebrovascular lesions in 22.6% and Lewy body pathology in 10.8%.' Among the 660 with a clinical Alzheimer's diagnosis, 'Alzheimer pathology was seen in 93%, only 44.7% in "pure" form, and additional vascular lesions and Lewy bodies in 27.7 and 10%, respectively.' In other words, what the doctors say and what the brain says don't always match, which adds to the challenges of researching dementia.

In addition, dementia can be classified as familial (i.e. it runs in families) or sporadic (i.e. there is no obvious family history or medical cause), and as early- or late-onset (the border between early and late is usually either age sixty or sixty-five). Familial cases are often early-onset and due to rare genetic mutations, but some early-onset cases are sporadic, their causes unknown.

Symptoms

Dementia itself is not an illness, but a symptom of numerous illnesses. The Alzheimer's Association defines it as a 'general term for a decline in mental ability severe enough to interfere with daily life'.[13] People think of dementia as memory loss, but that is only one of the cognitive symptoms—and one which may have causes other than dementia.

The search for ways to predict which patients with memory loss or mild cognitive impairment (MCI) will develop dementia is a huge area of dementia research. Yet studies suggest that fewer than half of patients with MCI will get dementia, and a minority will revert to cognitively normal function.[14] Memory loss, and getting lost, are typically the first symptoms that people notice. As the disease progresses, however, faulty reasoning (i.e. significantly worse than the human norm), poor decision making, and failing language abilities can also make communication with dementia patients, and their interactions with the world, increasingly problematic. Confusion and disorientation may also occur, especially in unfamiliar environments.

My elderly relative who was diagnosed with vascular dementia could, I suspect, have been diagnosed long before—and would have been, had the family hurried her into an institution. But she was content and managing at home (sort of, with ever more help), and she had begged her daughter not to put her into care. Then she had a bad fall, was hospitalized, and got her diagnosis. The fall was due to a stroke, which made things much worse—maybe strokes do run in our family after all—and it became clear that living alone was no longer possible. That was in the summer of 2014.

A year later, my relative is in a care home; and now there is no more deluding ourselves that she is simply old and beset by poor short-term memory. The lost look in her eyes, which used to be occasional, is now nearly permanent; the flashes of sharp wit and humour are less and less common. As a result, her family faces the kind of everyday heartbreak familiar to anyone who has a loved one with dementia. The last time we showed her photos of the great-grandchildren I'm not sure she really recognized them, though she was, as always, polite and interested. She still knows me, for now.

Like many families, we deal with this by focusing on the practicalities; and there are plenty of those. One challenge is to know what she herself wants. We can't ask her, because her thoughts are no longer stable enough to be taken as accurate reflections of her settled opinion—if such a thing exists now. Her sense of time has vanished, so she lives in a tiny window of the present, like the famous neurological patient H. M. about whom I learned as an undergraduate.[15] Conversations are instantly forgotten. Unless they are there with her, friends and family might as well not exist, except for a shrinking number of memories. Current events leave no mark, and nor do places; she never asks about her old house. She doesn't know where she is, or why. Sometimes, however, she is clearly aware of, and frustrated by, her memory problems, and by being in a strange place for no reason that she can recall. But that too is fading.

These are cognitive symptoms, the familiar demons of dementia. What I hadn't fully registered from the science is just how much the illness alters the emotional landscape. Alzheimer's original report captures this well, noting how his patient screamed, cried, was jealous, and fearful. My relative's emotions are likewise variable: sometimes when her daughter visits she'll be happy, other times she'll soon be in tears. Which version represents how she really feels? We don't know, and neither do the care home staff.

Dementia is not just memory loss and cognitive weakening. It involves anger at an increasingly incomprehensible world, frustration at personal helplessness, and fear when things happen that—to the sufferer—make no sense. These emotions may be overwhelming, since the person's ability to regulate or repress them is not what it once was. And without the defusing capacity to interpret emotions—to knit them into a coherent story about why one feels this way given what has happened—they can be frighteningly raw.

For families and carers, dementia patients' apparently irrational behaviour may be more comprehensible if we see it as a reaction to stressful events by someone who feels lost and vulnerable and scared. We might not think the events stressful, but we have much higher thresholds. Even so, most of us know the feeling of intolerable suffocation that comes with being overloaded with information, work, demands to act, or even just too many people talking. As dementia takes hold, it takes less and less to reach that point where things become unbearable.

Brain Changes

The cognitive and emotional symptoms of dementia are accompanied by characteristic changes in the brain. These are overlaid, however, on the normal alterations of age; so let us look at those first.

In healthy elderly people brain volume may shrink, and the volume of brain fluid grow, by about 0.2–0.5 per cent per year.[16] A small 1997 study estimated that between the ages of twenty and a hundred, male brains show an average weight loss of twenty-two per cent, occurring gradually, and female brains lose about twenty per cent, especially after age seventy.[17] The rate of atrophy quickens as retirement recedes into the past. For comparison, body weight, as measured by the body mass index (BMI), tends to rise until age sixty-five, then flatten out, then drop sharply after age eighty.

One might expect that brain shrinkage in normal ageing would be due to brain cells dying off. However, it is not at all clear that this is the case. A 2003 study of sixty-two male and thirty-two female brains estimated that the difference in cell numbers across the lifespan from youth (twenty years) to old age (ninety years) was around ten per cent. That is roughly equivalent to losing one neuron for every second of adult life.[18] It sounds dramatic, but we humans have a lot of neurons to lose. The average adult male brain is thought to contain about 86 billion neurons and to lose about one millionth of its total per day.[19] (Female brains are typically somewhat smaller.)

Recall that beyond the familiar conclaves of chattering neurons there is another, 'non-neuronal' brain: the brain of white matter and glial cells. Just as every city is kept alive by largely uncelebrated workers, so every brain survives to fizz with activity because of these other cells, whose healthy functioning is critically important. Glial cells exist in similar or greater numbers to neurons and seem to diminish at similar rates with ageing. Their importance is illustrated by a 2007 study of newborn and adult human brains which counted cells in one particular area of the brain, the thalamus. On average, the researchers found 11.2 million neurons in newborn thalami, and 6.43 million in adults' thalami: that is, the quantity of neurons nearly halved. Glia, by contrast, averaged 10.6 million in newborns and 36.3 million in adults, more than tripling their numbers. So the ratio of neurons to glia in this area changes from roughly 1:1 to roughly 1:5 as we grow up.[20] Glia matter for adult capabilities. (And neuron loss does not begin in old age.)

Brain cells are slowly lost as we grow older. But what other changes alter ageing brains?

Ventricles

Neurons need glia, just as cortex needs white matter and subcortex. If you suffer damage to certain subcortical areas, such as the brainstem, then no matter how thick and well fed your cortex is you won't be doing *any* reasoning, imagining, or making decisions. The old Yiddish saying 'I need this like I need a hole in the head' is especially resonant for these areas, the body's life-support department, where holes can be lethal.

There is, however, one hole, or set of holes, in your head that you do need. These are the fluid-filled chasms called ventricles, the brain's wet core.[21] If grey matter, packed with neurons, is like a city's built environment, and white matter is like its electric cabling, then the ventricles are its parks: refreshing spaces necessary for health. The images in Figure 2 show their location in the brain. To me, they look a bit like the nacelles of *Star Trek*'s starship *Enterprise*, or the inkblots used in Rorschach tests.[22]

Cities are certainly not as efficient as brains, and they are far simpler; but the metaphor has some depth. Both contain much more than their obvious structures. Both require insulation and defence: protection from damage and disease. Both have problems: damaged and derelict areas, poor housing, congested transport links. Brains, like cities, must be maintained and repaired. They need access points for on-going supplies of energy and nutrients, and means of storing and moving objects and information. They need a method of converting energy into useful forms, like heating (or cooling), and they definitely need waste disposal.

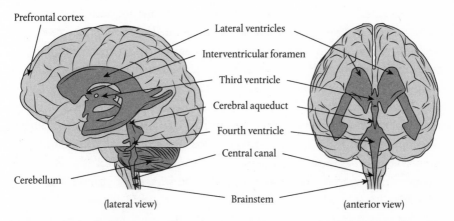

FIGURE 2: The ventricles. The left-hand image is a lateral view of a (stylized) human brain: sideways on with the front of the brain on the left. Cortex is shown in light grey. The right-hand image is from the front of the brain looking back through it, with the brainstem at the bottom. The ventricles, shown in darker grey, comprise the large lateral and smaller third and fourth ventricles and the channels connecting them: the foramen, cerebral aqueduct, and central canal.

Many cities have ornate buildings and green spaces. Brains, tucked away inside a shielding layer of bone, are less concerned with their appearance, or the weather. Evolution needs no fleshy Shard to show off its abilities in neuron building; its preferred form of expression is the network, not the tower. Brains do, however, have internal spaces, of which the most noticeable are the ventricles.

The ventricles are not just holes, however elegant. They are crucial to brain health because they supply essential cerebrospinal fluid. In normal ageing they expand; in neurodegenerative disorders they become severely enlarged. Moreover, nearby regions like the hippocampus, brainstem, and basal forebrain in Alzheimer's, and the cerebellum in spinocerebellar ataxia, often show early signs of neurodegeneration.

Also near the ventricles are major brain pathways containing millions of nerve fibres connecting cortex and subcortex.[23] Damaged or poisoned ventricles can thus quickly affect the brain's information superhighways, its ability to integrate information and trigger coherent reactions, its capacity to form memories, and its control of emotions and moods.

Neurotransmitters and Ion Channels

As well as affecting their structure, ageing also changes the way brains function. To understand the changes, we need to know how healthy brains send signals.

All cells use signalling molecules to communicate, but none is more skilled and subtle than the neuron. Like a squid signalling by changing colour, neurons use their skin—their cell membrane—to communicate. They do this in two ways—one electrical, one chemical—and the tools they use are specialist proteins: neurotransmitters and ion channels. Both require a good deal of infrastructure—and thus energy—to manufacture them, ship them from the nucleus to the synapses, release them on command, and tidy up afterwards ready for next time. Since lack of energy and infrastructure problems are both thought to worsen with age and in Alzheimer's, and since problems with neural communication are thought to underlie the cognitive problems of dementia, understanding how neurons talk to each other is essential for understanding what may be going wrong in the disease.

Figure 3 shows a highly schematic neuron. Its shape is distinctive: the rounded cell body, branching dendrites, and a long protruding axon terminating in synapses. In the centre of the cell is the nucleus, storehouse of DNA, where proteins are produced. Like all the body's cells, neurons are full of cytoplasm. It in turn is full of internal structures—organelles like the nucleus, mitochondria, endoplasmic reticulum, Golgi apparatus, and vesicles—and other material, like sugars and proteins. How is such complexity possible?

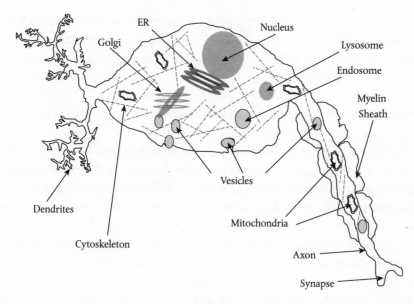

FIGURE 3: A schematic view of a neuron. Major internal structures are shown (not to scale). Dendrites process signals from other cells; the axon transmits signals to the synapse. Internal structures include the nucleus, endoplasmic reticulum (ER), and Golgi apparatus, where proteins are produced, folded, and packaged into vesicles. The diagram also shows vesicles that can be used to secrete material from the cell, ingest material from outside the cell, or transport material within the cell. Vesicles can also be converted to endosomes and lysosomes, which have specialized functions such as breaking down proteins.

The Marvel of Fat

Cells are defined by their membranes, which keep their inner gloop and the universe apart. Cellular membranes utilize an unsung wonder of creation, the lipid bilayer. This remarkable structure owes its existence—and we owe ours—to a substance many people loathe: fat. The fats in question are mainly triglycerides, phospholipids, and cholesterol (of which more later), and they have a very useful chemical property. One end of the molecule, the 'head group', readily dissolves in water, while the other end, the 'hydrocarbon tail', much prefers the company of other fats. The technical term for this double character is 'amphipathic', from the Greek for 'both states', and it is essential for all cellular life. This is because, in a watery environment like the body, fat molecules form pairs whose hydrocarbon tails are attracted to each other and whose water-seeking head groups face outwards. The result is a double layer of molecules, the lipid bilayer.[24]

Cell membranes, internal and external, are lipid bilayers with other molecules stuck in or on them. Thinner than the film of a soap bubble, they allow cells to separate and control their innards.[25] This setting of limits and separation of powers makes everything possible, from the simplest bacteria to the intricacies of your cerebral billions. Membranes also enable a cell to take in material from the outside (endocytosis) or release material through it (exocytosis, *aka* secretion). Endocytosis is done by budding off vesicles—small hollow bubbles of fat—on the inside of the cell membrane, secretion by vesicles fusing with it and releasing their contents into the extracellular space.[26]

As noted earlier, the dominant hypothesis in Alzheimer's research is that dementia results from abnormal proteins; so why dwell on fats? Well, lipid bilayers may let cells compartmentalize their functions, but lipids and proteins themselves are not so tidily separate. Confirmation comes from the genetics of dementia. Gene studies have found many possible links to genes which may be faulty in Alzheimer's, but so far only one has proved scientifically outstanding: repeatedly replicated, greatly increasing disease risk. It is not, as you might expect, the gene for amyloid production, but for a protein called apolipoprotein E (ApoE; the variant is known as ApoE4).[27] What does ApoE do? It transports fats, notably cholesterol, around the body and brain, where they are used to maintain and repair cell membranes. It also binds to and transports amyloid protein.

Lipid membranes form a barrier to watery fluids like cytoplasm. (I was reminded of the principle when my flatmate poured some hot cooking fat down the kitchen sink, creating a fatberg which efficiently stopped any water from passing.) Having this barrier allows cells to set up electrochemical gradients—differences in the amounts of charged material on one side and the other—and to transmit information by varying those gradients. Neurons maintain an electrical gradient across their cell membrane, the membrane potential, by controlling the quantities of charged particles (ions) on either side. Cell cytoplasm is similar to seawater, so it has plenty of ions such as sodium, potassium, and chloride, which can be moved in and out of the cell to change the gradient. Gradients can be huge. The concentration of calcium, another key signalling molecule and one of the causal suspects in dementia, is about 20,000 times higher outside the cell than inside.[28]

Membranes are not pure fat: they are studded with proteins. Some of these serve to announce the cell's identity to other cells. For example, a protein called CD47 is a self-marker, signalling 'Don't eat me' to the hunter-killers of the immune system. Neurons, microglia, and other brain cells have different surface proteins; and rather as we change our appearance during life, so cells' surface proteins vary in different states, places, and stages of development.[29]

Other cell surface proteins are receptors: complex structures that allow cells to monitor their environment. They change their shape when activated by certain molecules, and the change triggers events—intracellular signalling—that alter the cell in complicated ways. Signals from outside may be chemical (like a receptor's activation), electrical (like ion flows across a membrane), or mechanical (like a muscle stretch or a bang on the head). Signalling pathways convert these into a common electrochemical currency.

Neurons communicate by means of extremely rapid signals variously called 'spikes', 'impulses', 'firing', or 'action potentials'. During these events, the membrane potential swings from negative to positive and back again within a few milliseconds. Action potentials are created by the opening and closing of receptors shaped like tiny tubes of protein: ion channels. These let only certain ions in or out of the cell, thereby changing the balance of charges inside and out (i.e. the electrical potential across the membrane).

Some of these channels, like the glutamate receptors, are opened when a particular molecule (glutamate) binds to the receptor protein. Others react to changes in the membrane potential caused by signals received from other cells.[30] Thus a cell which receives a lot of signals is liable to send a lot of signals; but even cells which are not currently firing can be made more or less likely to fire by changes which affect the membrane potential—such as the opening of ion channels or the activation of other receptors by neurotransmitters. Importantly for our purposes, neuron activity can also be altered by damage to the membrane, especially when that damage punches holes in it. One of the proteins most directly implicated in Alzheimer's, amyloid, is thought to do exactly that, as we shall see.

Ion channels are like doors that let molecules through the cell membrane, but there are also numerous proteins called transporters, or pumps, which act like bouncers. Powered by energy from molecules of ATP, these push their target molecules across the membrane. Ion pumps for calcium, sodium, or potassium ions, for example, allow neurons to rebalance their electrical charges between action potentials. One of these pumps is disrupted by amyloid, which in turn disrupts calcium signalling. That can have a big impact on the cell's ability to communicate.

Neurons use chemicals as well as electricity. When an action potential flows along a neuron's cell membrane and reaches a synapse, it reaches an area jammed with vesicles full of signalling molecules. These include neurotransmitters like glutamate, as well as other molecules such as neuropeptides (small proteins) and chemokines (molecules which cells use to move and attach to each other). An action potential, like an online order, can trigger delivery. Calcium ions pour into the synapse and stimulate the release of vesicles: fusing with the cell membrane, these release their contents into the synaptic gap between the cell and its neighbour. The liberated molecules quickly diffuse across the gap to interact with cell surface proteins—receptors—on the other side.

Glutamate and the Power of Calcium

The brain's primary 'excitatory' and 'inhibitory' neurotransmitters are glutamate and GABA; receptors for these two molecules excite or inhibit other neurons, respectively.[31] Most neurons in the cortex use glutamate; a minority uses GABA. Some cells deeper in the brain use other neurotransmitters such as acetylcholine, noradrenaline, serotonin, histamine, and dopamine.[32]

Some receptors for neurotransmitters like glutamate and acetylcholine, as well as some ion channels activated by changes in the membrane potential, allow calcium into cells.[33] When they are over-activated by too much stimulation, calcium can flood into neurons, driven by the massive difference in gradient. Positively charged calcium ions (Ca^{2+}) are one of the most important players in cell signalling, but their functions depend on extremely tight regulation.[34] In excess they can be deadly.

As well as its importance for bones and teeth, calcium regulates many aspects of cell function and development. Among much else, it affects transcription factors like nuclear factor kappa B (NFκB), a regulatory protein vital for the control of inflammation (of this more later). Calcium is an important controller of neurons' shape and of how their axons grow; and hence of the neuronal networks which underlie our ability to learn and our mental lives. It is able to do so many different things in the cell because it interacts with so many proteins, and also because it is—in healthy cells—only allowed to enter the cytoplasm very briefly and at tightly controlled locations.

But calcium ions are dangerous. Other key units of cells' internal currency, such as negatively charged phosphate ions (phosphorus + oxygen, PO_4^{3-}), are normally dissolved in watery solutions like cytoplasm. Calcium, however, can solidify when it binds to other molecules. A famous example is its bond with carbonate ions; calcium carbonate is what seashells are made of. This solidity is fine for sea creatures needing houses, but not for brains. Researchers working on dementia are increasingly of the opinion that many brain problems—including neurodegeneration—may be caused by substances like calcium and amyloid solidifying in the wrong places.[35]

Normally, calcium ions are controlled by squadrons of regulatory proteins, which pounce as soon as the ions enter the cytoplasm, often forming cage-like structures around them. They bind to their target in many different ways, with different affinities (different degrees of enthusiasm).[36] In addition, calcium is stored within the cell, in an organelle called the endoplasmic reticulum. This web-like structure spreads widely through the cytoplasm, allowing calcium signals to access all areas. Its surface membrane contains receptors that are calcium ion channels, and when they are activated by intracellular signals small amounts of calcium are released into the cytoplasm.[37] This release is tightly controlled, and it occurs only in the area where the receptors have been activated. This, together with the many regulatory proteins, makes calcium signalling subtle and nuanced, not just on and off.

When that regulation fails, an inrush of calcium can shock or even kill a cell, a phenomenon known as excitotoxicity. In epileptic seizures, for example, some neurons begin to fire intensely, and the resulting over-stimulation of glutamate receptors causes excitotoxic damage. (Epileptic seizures may be more frequent in dementia sufferers, although a link between the two conditions is not established except in certain rare mutations.[38]) There is evidence from animal models that neurons may also be hyperactive early in Alzheimer's, and that excitotoxicity could help to cause the cell death seen in dementia. Applying drugs that block amyloid production reduces the damage, putting amyloid on the suspects' list as a cause of excitotoxic cell death. And one of the standard treatments for Alzheimer's, memantine, blocks the type of glutamate receptor involved in, and prevents, excitotoxic damage.

GABA

Not all neurons use glutamate. Key to the function of cortex are inhibitory interneurons, which use GABA. They suppress the activity of other neurons, and they are crucial for keeping brain activity under control.

Inhibitory interneurons regulate the coordinated activity of large networks of neurons into synchronized patterns of activity. This synchronization, which increases the energy demand on neurons, can unite cells from across the brain. It forms distinct patterns of brain activity for every combination of stimuli and responses: a near-infinite set of brain states which can represent every experience known to human beings.[39] Inhibitory interneurons help us keep those experiences separate, allowing us to make sense of the world. They are influenced both by cortical glutamatergic neurons and by other neurotransmitters, emitted from cells much deeper in the brain.

Deep Brain Transmitters

Glutamate and GABA may be the main languages of cortical conversation, but they are not the only neurotransmitters. Large-bodied cells in the deep subcortex, clustered into small nuclei, send long-ranging axons over vast tracts of cortex, and they use other molecules: histamine, dopamine, serotonin, noradrenaline, or acetylcholine.[40] Deep neurons are the primary supply of these transmitters to cortex, and they can have a huge influence. This is not just because of their many synapses with cortical neurons, but because they can release neurotransmitters into the brain's interior fluids to ooze where they may, increasing the range of target cells.[41] This allows the subcortical nuclei to control important aspects of brain function like alertness and attention, sleep, mood, and motivation.

These cells are especially vulnerable in neurodegeneration and their failure is an early pathological marker. Why might this be? One possibility is that their nearness to the ventricles makes them more vulnerable to toxins. Another is the immense metabolic demand of maintaining their larger size, exceptionally long axons, and huge numbers of synapses. For example, consider the mid-brain dopamine neurons, which fail in Parkinson's disease. These astonishing cells have been estimated 'to give rise to more than 1 million synapses and have a total length exceeding 4 metres' (counting all their branches).[42] In terms of energy consumption they teeter on the edge of sustainability, so when energy supply becomes a problem, cells like these are likely to suffer first—with severe consequences for people with Parkinson's.

Also vulnerable are neurons in the basal forebrain, which use the neurotransmitter acetylcholine. Just as damage to dopaminergic neurons is a key event in Parkinson's, so damage to acetylcholinergic neurons is one of the earliest signs of Alzheimer's.[43] Abnormal amyloid and tau proteins affect these neurons before they spread into the cortex. Amyloid, for example, inhibits a major acetylcholine receptor on their surface and has been shown to accumulate inside them.[44]

The 'cholinergic hypothesis' of Alzheimer's proposes that it is damage to these neurons that is the key initiating event for the disease. This idea dominated the field before the advent of the amyloid hypothesis, and to date its clinical record is rather better. Of the four drug treatments commonly used for Alzheimer's, three boost acetylcholine levels by inhibiting the enzyme which degrades it, acetylcholinesterase. (The fourth is the glutamate-targeting memantine.[45])

None of the four drugs either cures or prevents Alzheimer's, though they can ease some of the symptoms. This is why neither glutamate nor acetylcholine has to date won the struggle for dementia research supremacy. Besides, science, like any other facet of culture, is subject to fashions, and acetylcholine's current advocates are few compared with amyloid's.[46] Nonetheless, some researchers are keen to reignite interest in acetylcholine. They argue that the failure of acetylcholine-boosting drugs to halt or reverse dementia might have been because the treatment came too late: it was given to people already diagnosed, by which time brain damage is surely well under way. (You will encounter this argument again when we come to look at newer Alzheimer treatments: it is used by amyloid researchers to explain why so many anti-amyloid drugs have failed.) Perhaps giving anticholinesterases much earlier in life might be more helpful; though as ever problems of side effects, costs, etc. apply.

Recent epidemiological research has given the cholinergic hypothesis a boost.[47] Studies looking at senior citizens' use of common medicines which act to suppress acetylcholine cells—anti-cholinergics like the anti-depressant amitriptyline and the allergy treatment Benadryl—found that the more treatments they reported taking or were prescribed, the higher their risk of dementia.[48]

When acetylcholine levels drop, the entire brain feels the lack, as this subcortical transmitter has a wider cortical reach than dopamine, serotonin, histamine, or noradrenaline. Its main subcortical source, the nucleus basalis of Meynert, also gets information from brainstem sources of other neurotransmitters, and from cortex. In response, its neurons stretch their synaptic fingers throughout the cortical carapace.[49] This makes cholinergic signalling very responsive to 'higher-level' events—like thoughts and mood swings.

Acetylcholine improves the brain's ability to process information and can exert fast, global effects on brain function. By stimulating inhibitory interneurons it increases alertness and attention, filtering out weak signals and helping the brain to process what matters most without being distracted by irrelevant stimuli.[50] Because the nucleus basalis is most extensively connected with areas involved in emotion, visceral, and memory processing—areas like the amygdala, hippocampus, and temporal lobe—it is well placed to interpret the body's emotional reactions and link them to what is currently going on in the cortex.[51] When it fails, we would expect to see confusion, disorientation, and emotional disruption. (As Alzheimer showed us, dementia is an emotional as well as a cognitive disorder.)

Synapses

Another noticeable change that comes with ageing affects the links between brain cells: the synapses.[52] Neurons form connections via these minuscule gaps between cells, across which chemicals released by one cell are squirted when the neuron sends a signal.[53] These ligands—e.g. neurotransmitters and neuromodulators; the word 'ligand' is from the Latin for 'things that bind'—transmit signals by binding to and activating receptors. (As so often in physiology, the distinction is not absolute. One cell's ligand can be another cell's receptor.)

On average, cortical neurons are thought to make about 7,000 synapses with other cells.[54] A typical neuron extrudes one long axon and many shorter dendrites (see Figure 3), both of which may sprout many branches with synapses on them.[55] Dendrites gather and process incoming signals. Axons transmit them onwards.

Synapses are titchy: tens of nanometres across.[56] Dendrites extend across millimetres at most, whereas an axon can range across centimetres in the brain, and over a metre in the human body. Human neurons vary in size. The largest—motor neurons in the spinal cord that send axons all the way to the toes—are about a tenth of a millimetre across.[57]

Crucially, synapses show plasticity. That is, their strength—i.e. the likelihood that a signal sent from one cell will trigger a signal in its synaptic partner—can change depending on how many signals flow through them. Generally synaptic strength increases as a synapse is more frequently used and the cellular machinery adjusts accordingly, although abnormally high and sustained neural activity can damage both synapses and cells (as in excitotoxicity). Rarely used synapses may die off altogether, but well-trodden neural pathways become easier, and quicker, to tread. This flexibility is the basis of learning and memory: experience written in proteins. Its loss, as synapses weaken and die, is what makes dementia so devastating.

When it comes to brains, many people think of grey matter as the important bit, despite the fact that neurons make up only around half of brain tissue. After all, both 'grey matter' and 'brains' are used to mean 'intelligence'. Yet white matter—neural cabling—really matters.[58] It is unglamorous but essential, like the electrical systems powering our cities, to which it is often compared.[59] We may think of ageing as damaging our grey matter, but neurons are often preserved even when shrinkage around the edges (cortical atrophy) is clearly visible in a brain scan. What is lost is efficient connectivity. Brain imaging scans which can detect white matter changes find that white matter integrity appears to decline in later life; but it does so unevenly across the brain's pathways.[60] Tracts linking sensory to motor areas are less affected than tracts linking the two hemispheres, or those between areas involved in complex cognitive or emotion-related processing—those near the ventricles. Longer axons may be affected more than shorter, more local connections. Some axons fail completely, others simply slow down.

These changes are seen even in healthy old age. They are much more severe in white matter disorders like multiple sclerosis, and also in dementia.[61]

Myelin

Why is healthy white matter so crucial for effective brain function? To answer this question, we need to venture into the realm of glial cells and consider that odd-sounding beast, the oligodendrocyte.

Oligodendrocytes are the cells that make the white matter white. The term, from Greek sources, means 'few-tree (or few-branched) cell'. Relative to neurons, this is a fair description; but branching is not what these underrated cells are about. Instead, their skills lie in wrapping.

Oligodendrocytes are keen producers of a substance called myelin, a mix of protein and fat which is an electrical insulator. Guided by chemical signals from neurons and from other glia, they wind themselves in spiralling layers around the larger axons of neurons, forming a thick sheath of myelin.[62] Oligodendrocytes talk to neurons (and *vice versa*) and seem to prefer to wrap active ones.[63] They can also provide metabolic support in the form of molecules like lactate, which neurons can use for fuel.

It is the layered myelin sheaths cuddling axons that allow neurons to reach so far so fast, sending their messages across the brain's landscape. Consider that the smallest brain cells may be around five microns—five thousandths of a millimetre—in diameter, while the distances travelled by axons passing from one side of cortex to the other may reach 15 cm (if brain cells were people, that would be a ten-kilometre run).[64] Sustaining the neural signal over such distances, let alone the huge domains covered by spinal neurons, is a remarkable feat, and it is possible thanks to oligodendrocytes.

Furthermore, the signals reach their target far quicker than even the fastest athlete can run 10 km, providing the rapid reactions we humans take for granted. The maximum signalling speed, or conduction velocity, along a myelinated axon is about sixty times faster than that along an unmyelinated one: up to 120 metres per second or just under 270 miles per hour. As the journal *Nature Education* comments, that is 'race car speed'.[65] When myelin weakens, brain signalling slows down.

Oligodendrocytes wrap around multiple axons. Individual sheaths are separated by gaps, about a micron across, called nodes of Ranvier. The myelin makes it much more likely that electrical charges will flow rapidly from one node to the next, rather than oozing out of the axon into the extracellular space. By thus 'jumping' from node to node, the signal can travel further faster, in smaller-diameter axons.[66] This means that more axons can be packed into the space available, creating 'nature's most exquisite work': a tightly packed brain. The phrase is from the seventeenth-century Danish master-anatomist Niels Stenson, who also remarked that 'God and nature do nothing in vain'.[67] That is apposite for neuroscience. Inside the skull there isn't much room for frivolous excess.[68]

Ageing brains lose myelin, sometimes so much that the axon inside cannot survive. When an axon is destroyed, so are its synapses, removing the cell's ability to send messages. Alternatively, axons stripped of myelin may be recoated, but more thinly and with shorter sheaths. This slows down signal transmission from cell to cell.

Without communication neurons are worse than useless, because as dead axons degenerate they produce toxins, damaging or killing the whole cell. Injured neurons may die politely, engulfed by microglia—or they may spew their innards into the extracellular space. Those innards are highly toxic, so the mess must be cleared up quickly to stop it affecting nearby cells. And since one of the systems which works less well as we grow older is the microglial system for mess-clearing, a loss of neuronal communication in ageing brains can have considerable impact beyond the broken circuits themselves.

Wiring Damage

To see the effects of white matter damage independent of other effects of ageing, researchers study demyelinating diseases like multiple sclerosis (MS) and leucodystrophy. They mainly target younger people, and they can be as dreadful as Alzheimer's. About half of patients with MS suffer cognitive impairment, and some end up with dementia.[69] Children born with leucodystrophy may not even reach adulthood.

Our focus is on adults, so let us consider MS. It is an archetypal brain inflammatory disease, an autoimmune disorder—where the immune system mistakenly identifies a native, 'self' protein as foreign, and attacks it. In MS the attack burns holes in white matter. The underlying inflammatory mechanisms of MS have been intensively studied in humans, aided by neuroimaging, and in animals.[70] The initial inflammatory reaction, which attracts immune cells from the body into the brain, damages oligodendrocytes. Areas of damaged myelin form lesions visible on brain scans, then heal as oligodendrocytes replenish the myelin, then form elsewhere. But the regenerative capacity of oligodendrocytes is not infinite; and once the inflammation starts damaging axons, not only they but their neurons may die off, leading to irreversible disease progression.

This is why MS is such a challenge: its symptoms can be extremely unpredictable and variable. They range from fatigue, pain, poor concentration, and memory problems to loss of sensory, sexual, urinary, bowel, or motor function. Most sufferers experience a relapsing-remitting form of the disease—in which symptoms shift as different areas of the brain are affected—followed by a phase of deterioration; a minority faces decline from the point of diagnosis.[71] Certain treatments can help some people with some symptoms, such as fatigue. But as I write, MS has no cure.

Like many immune conditions, and like dementia, MS is affected by the patient's environment. Studies of its prevalence—how many people have the disease—and incidence—how many people get it in a given period—show that it afflicts more people at more northern latitudes. In the United Kingdom, estimates range from 96 per 100,000 in southern Guernsey to over 200 per 100,000 in Scotland and Northern Ireland. Moreover, the disorder, which mainly affects young adults (particularly women) appears to be becoming more common.[72] This pattern—environmentally influenced, hard to diagnose, varying manifestions, and currently undefeatable—is typical of brain disorders.

Many MS researchers focus on identifying risk factors which vary geographically or over time, such as vitamin D deficiency. People in cloudy northern countries are especially prone to this deficiency, as I was reminded by a blood test which showed that I had it. Symptoms, I can confirm, include fatigue and muscle ache; and if you take the pills every day the symptoms stop. If only MS and dementia could be so easily fixed.

The causes of MS are not well understood, although progress is being made. Viruses, low vitamin D, iron, poor diet, problems with cellular energy production, and genes are among the suggestions. As we shall see, these are also suspects for Alzheimer's. There are other links between the two disorders, apart from shared symptoms. Research on human brains has found that less well myelinated areas tend to develop earlier amyloid deposits, a key marker of Alzheimer's.[73] Indeed, it has even been proposed that Alzheimer's pathology may result from attempts to repair damaged myelin.[74]

Other brain disorders can also shed light on the neuroscience of dementia. One such is that common and debilitating condition, schizophrenia. To see how it can contribute, we need to know a little bit more about brain anatomy.

From Birth to Death in the Brain

Consider the cortex, the brain's outer rind, with its two halves curving over and around the brain's core like a pair of cupped hands. Left and right hemispheres are connected by the mighty cabling of the corpus callosum, which is only the most obvious example of the brain's staggeringly complex network of connections. Each hemisphere has its four lobes—frontal and occipital at the front and back, parietal and temporal in between—marked out by deep grooves, and each lobe is distinctively scarred and fissured. Information flows from back to front, from perceptions to decisions to movements, in great transcortical pathways. Neural signals pour from primary sensory areas like visual cortex through the parietal and temporal lobes—areas that help create our understanding of objects, their locations, contexts, and meanings—to the frontal and prefrontal cortex where movements are controlled.

It can be helpful to think of the brain and nervous system as layers of networks, each linking inputs (from world and body) to outputs (which alter both). The oldest, simplest layers involve short chains of neurons linking a sensory input, such as a sharp pain, to a motor output, such as jerking back the burned finger. In humans, the simplest reflexes can be triggered without any need to trouble the central brain: the input reaches the spinal cord and stimulates motor neurons there, which set off the reaction. Longer, more complicated input–output chains—involving brainstem, then other subcortical, cortical, and finally prefrontal cortical areas—are overlaid on this primeval linkage of stimulus to response. In upper levels of the hierarchy, signals take longer to complete the circuit.

Longer neural pathways also mean more branches and junctions where signals from other parts of the brain can blend into the flow. Layers in the brain are heavily interconnected; thus lower-level circuits can influence activity at higher levels and *vice versa*. Brains have often been compared to organizations as well as to cities, with the prefrontal cortex as management and subcortical areas as the workforce.[75] If the brain were an organization, each successive synaptic junction would allow more members to influence decision making. Yet no human collective is as efficient as a brain.

Neuroscientists distinguish primary areas of cortex, which mediate the initial stages of sensory perception and the final cortical stages of motor control, from 'association areas'.[76] The latter, which include large parts of the temporal, parietal, and frontal lobes, are involved in more complex functions such as emotion regulation and the sense of agency which are disrupted in schizophrenia, and dementia. They are where signals from multiple brain areas and senses are brought together. Researchers have long known that certain areas of cortex develop earlier than others: the primary cortices become established before the evolutionarily later association areas. In ageing, and in dementia, the order is reversed: association areas fail first.

In 2014, a multi-centre neuroimaging study of 484 healthy humans aged from eight to eighty-five suggested an intriguing link between schizophrenia and dementia.[77] It has to do with how brains grow and age. The study, by Gwenaëlle Douaud and colleagues, assessed which areas of brain showed most variability across their nearly 500 participants. The researchers were able to identify two trends over time: a gradual shrinkage in size with ageing, which applied to the entire brain, and a trend in which size rose to a maximum around age forty, before declining again. This latter trend, which has also been noted for aspects of cognition such as episodic memory and fluid intelligence, was only seen for some brain regions.[78]

The regions in question form a network of mainly association cortex which develops late—it is still immature in adolescence—and degenerates early.[79] When Douaud and her colleagues looked at data from unhealthy brains, they found that their network looked very similar to the cluster of areas which develop abnormally in schizophrenia and degenerate first in Alzheimer's disease. So perhaps these two frailties are, at least in part, reflections of how human brains are built.

Douaud *et al.* cite a proposal by US researcher George Bartzokis—an untimely loss to science; he died in August 2014, aged fifty-eight—that myelination, which also increases up to midlife and then diminishes, may play a central role.[80] Thus the grey matter changes observed in their neuroimaging scans may result from underlying changes in white matter. They conclude that knowing *what* happens in schizophrenia and Alzheimer's—the mechanisms that go wrong—will not explain everything about them. *When* these processes affect a growing or ageing brain is also crucial.

Dementia: A Problem of Association?

In dementia, patients lose much more cortical tissue than in normal ageing (see Figure 4). As we have seen, different areas of the brain melt away at different rates, with the most complex functions and latest-maturing areas affected first: the earliest signs of damage are typically in the prefrontal cortex and in the parietal and temporal lobes.[81] In Alzheimer's, the worst-affected regions of cortex tend to be in the temporal lobes.[82] These are home to areas involved in language comprehension, speech, object recognition, emotional processing, and episodic and semantic memory. Temporal cortex overlays structures like the amygdala and the hippocampus, which are also involved in emotion and memory.[83] Hippocampal sclerosis, a condition in which the area shrinks due to cell damage, is frequent in dementia (and also in some forms of epilepsy).

One study of post-mortem human brains at various ages found that in healthy people's brains the number of neurons in the superior temporal sulcus, an area of association cortex, was maintained 'across the sixth to ninth decades'. In Alzheimer brains it halved.[84]

As in healthy ageing, however, neuron loss appears to follow white matter damage. A study of brain biopsies taken from temporal and frontal lobes of people a few years into an Alzheimer's diagnosis found a 'greater loss of synapses than that of neurones', with up to a third fewer synapses per neuron.[85] As the distinguished Alzheimer's researcher Dennis Selkoe has noted, 'Even at the end of the disease, quantitative correlations of postmortem cytopathology with premortem cognitive deficits indicate that synapse loss is more robustly correlated than are numbers of plaques or tangles' or other signs of cell damage.[86] Synapse loss is therefore considered a major cause of dementia's problems. Lost connections stop thoughts being linked together.

The extent and location of damage seems to correlate with the degree of functional impairment affecting the patient (as, for example, the term 'frontotemporal dementia' implies).[87] Thus hippocampal damage is associated with memory and navigation problems, prefrontal damage with confusion, personality change, and IQ decline, and so on.

I say 'seems to correlate' because the degree of correlation varies with, among other things, the measurements used to assess both structure and cognition.[88] There

Healthy   Severe
brain   AD

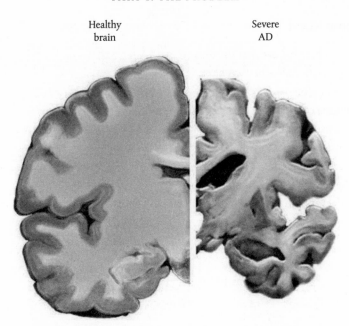

FIGURE 4: Sections through a healthy brain and one with severe Alzheimer's disease. The left-hand image shows a healthy brain, sliced after death. The right-hand image shows a section from a brain of comparable age from a patient with advanced dementia. There is far less tissue and ventricles are enlarged.

are many ways to measure structural brain damage, from local changes of volume or cortical thickness—e.g. in the hippocampus or prefrontal cortex—to measures of global shrinkage such as whole-brain atrophy.

There are also numerous ways of assessing dementia and cognitive impairment psychologically, such as the Mini-Mental State Examination (MMSE) score. Even asking the patient to do a simple, unthreatening task like drawing an analogue clock can highlight whether there is cause for concern.[89] In this test the clinician provides a pre-drawn circle and asks the person to put in the hour numbers—some versions also request that the time be set to ten minutes past eleven. Cognitively impaired patients often place the numbers unevenly or fail to draw the hands correctly. Neither clock drawing, nor the MMSE, nor any of the other methods available have been accepted as the gold standard for diagnosing dementia, however. As noted earlier, that currently requires post-mortem investigation.

Brain and Mind

Most researchers believe that the link between failing brains and failing minds is not merely correlational—the two happen to change in similar ways—but causal. This may seem obvious; surely the immediate cause of Alzheimer's is the pathological accumulation of damage to neural tissue. Yet a 2013 study of 856 post-mortem brains serves as a useful reminder that we do not yet have the full story. It looked at kinds of brain damage commonly linked to Alzheimer's, including protein changes and strokes, and found that they explained less than half of the variation in cognitive decline between the participants.[90]

Other factors must therefore be contributing to the luck that keeps some brains healthy and sends others into the spiral of dementia. Those factors include additional structural changes like synapse loss, which can be seen post-mortem in dementia, as can changes in many brain proteins. Functional changes in how brain regions communicate, how synapses work, levels of neurochemicals, and protein production are also involved.[91]

This reminds us why research into Alzheimer's and other age-related brain conditions is so immensely difficult, slow, and expensive. The number of potential variables is gargantuan, and only a very few are assessed in any one piece of research. When reading an article about Alzheimer's, what was not studied is often as important as what was discovered. Furthermore, many of the variables co-vary, making them harder to tease apart with the statistical methods used in many large-scale studies.[92] For example, blood pressure, environmental wear and tear, and blood sugar all tend to increase with age (they are positive covariates of age) while physical activity and heart efficiency, cardiac output, tend to reduce (they are negative covariates).

Researchers do not yet fully understand how neurodegenerative changes affect cognition in dementia. The theory is that damage affects connections between cells first, reducing the number of synapses; cells themselves die later. That neurodegeneration is responsible for cognitive impairment is widely accepted. But what causes the neurodegeneration? If abnormal proteins are involved, as many people think, what makes them abnormal?

That is the million-, or billion-dollar question, and even a quick glance at the literature shows the vast array of answers that have been proposed. For dementia, (bad) luck is a many-splendoured thing. One almost feels that no potential cause for anything biological should be taken seriously unless it has been linked to neurodegeneration, somehow. This book cannot possibly cover all the contenders, but you will get to know some of the best supported, and many others will be mentioned.

Despite the complexity, great progress has already been made—and it began with Alois Alzheimer.[93] His meticulous dissections not only grounded dementia in the abnormal brain, they identified three characteristic abnormalities still used to define Alzheimer's disease.

The first and most obvious of these hallmarks is brain tissue shrinkage, including white matter damage and cell loss (see Figure 4).[94] The second hallmark is found

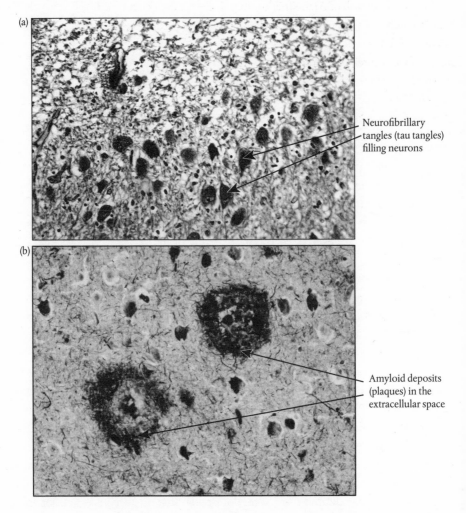

(a)

Neurofibrillary tangles (tau tangles) filling neurons

(b)

Amyloid deposits (plaques) in the extracellular space

FIGURE 5: Tau tangles and amyloid plaques. Brain slices stained (using silver) to reveal the presence of abnormal tau protein which has formed tangles (above, dark teardrop shapes) and amyloid protein which has formed plaques (below, large circular shapes).

inside surviving cells: twisted skeins of material, mostly made of a protein called tau (see Figure 5). Sometimes—no one yet knows exactly why—this forms itself into twisted filaments, which in turn entwine to form tau tangles. When cells die, the tau can be left as a characteristic 'ghost tangle'.[95]

Tau, though a marker for neurodegeneration, is not specific to Alzheimer's. Traumatic brain injury and some degenerative disorders affecting frontal cortex are among the other conditions linked to abnormal tau.[96]

The third hallmark of Alzheimer's grows in the spaces between cells, marring the brain's landscape with clumps of solid matter called plaques (see Figure 5). Vaguely circular, and with a dense core, they look like cortical verrucas.[97] Their main component is also a protein, amyloid-beta.

Amyloid plaques are also not exclusive to dementia, as we shall see. Nonetheless, they were the major clue that scientists followed as they started to hunt for the causes of neurodegeneration. Tau tangles have been much studied, but the main focus of Alzheimer's research has been on amyloid. With amyloid, therefore, we begin.

6

Protein Problems

In May 1984 a very specialist journal called *Biochemical and Biophysical Research Communications* published a short report about protein analysis.[1] The authors George Glenner and Caine Wong were researchers at the University of California, San Diego, and their publication took up only six pages (including all of twelve references). Its impact was to be out of all proportion to its brevity.

The study purified a protein associated with Alzheimer's disease and determined its molecular structure. Variously called beta-amyloid, amyloid-beta, or Aβ, it accumulates in brain tissues and on brain blood vessels, interfering with their function. It is the major constituent of the plaques observed by Alzheimer, although these contain other proteins as well as Aβ.[2] Glenner and Wong's analysis was field-defining, opening up dementia to the fast-developing techniques of molecular biology. As a result, amyloid plaques, once detectable only by staining dead brain tissue, can now be assessed in living brains, using PET neuroimaging.[3]

Amyloid was already known to exist elsewhere in the body, most typically in the liver, kidneys, spleen, intestines, and artery walls. It is not a specific molecule, but rather a name for numerous proteins which all show the same unusual behaviour: they like to stick together. Such proteins can agglomerate into structures known as beta-sheets—hence amyloid-beta—which are extremely tough (the same structure gives silk fibres their great strength). In some cases, called amyloidoses, the resulting build-up of solid protein deposits can damage body organs.[4] Eleven years after his pioneering publication, sixty-seven-year-old George Glenner died from a form of amyloidosis.[5]

Amyloidoses were known in the seventeenth century. One report describes 'the autopsy of a woman whose spleen was so hard that it could scarcely be cut with a knife'.[6] The term 'amyloid', however, is from the nineteenth century. From the Greek word for 'starch', it was first used in the plant sciences. Its medical use is due to a mistake by a great biologist. Rudolf Virchow, among much else, made immense contributions to our understanding of cells, diseases from thrombosis to cancer, and brain anatomy (e.g. Virchow-Robin spaces, of which more later). He thought the deposits found in amyloidoses were made of starch. By the time this was disproved the name had stuck.

Later in 1984 a second study by Glenner and Wong linked Alzheimer's disease to Down's syndrome, finding Aβ in both disorders.[7] People with Down's syndrome usually develop dementia in midlife, much earlier than most Alzheimer's cases; but in both conditions Aβ builds up around brain blood vessels. Linking Alzheimer's to Down's allowed the gene responsible for Aβ to be tracked to chromosome 21, which is duplicated in Down's.[8] Aβ also forms plaques, and these structures, so characteristic of Alzheimer's that they form part of its diagnostic criteria, appear in the brains of patients with Down's syndrome as well.[9]

Writing about Alzheimer's is a sombre business. For light relief I use dark humour, telling friends who ask about the book, 'I've been thinking a lot about amyloid. My head's full of it.' (Smile broadly, wait for the blank look.) In fact, not having been scanned, I don't know the state of my amyloid deposits. But surely people under pension age needn't expect to have amyloid deposits? Not necessarily. Studies on post-mortem brains suggest that protein problems are not confined to the elderly. Amyloid can begin building up years or decades before clinical symptoms of cognitive impairment appear. An analysis of brains from 1,046 people aged between twenty-six and sixty-five found some level of amyloid deposition in 161 of them (around 15%).[10] This is why dementia treatments might have to start much, much earlier to be successful.

Having a mother with Alzheimer's is associated with more likelihood of amyloid deposits, as are environmental stresses such as pollution. Plaques have even been found in a small autopsy study of children exposed to high levels of air pollution in Mexico City, at the time one of the most polluted places in the world.[11] Thus both genes and the environment contribute to your chances of plaque formation, as we shall see.

The Amyloid Cascade

The amyloid cascade hypothesis, first fully set out by John Hardy and Gerald Higgins in 1992, proposes that it is the build-up of Aβ which is the crucial step on the path to Alzheimer's, triggering harmful changes which ultimately lead to the death of brain cells.[12] It is increasingly debated, and it has changed considerably over the years, but it is still the field's leading hypothesis. It is strongly supported by genetic evidence: mutations in genes related to Aβ processing are associated with Alzheimer's, and some cause rarer, early-onset forms of Alzheimer's (although not all early-onset dementias have known genetic causes).

Yet as we shall see, critics have challenged the idea of amyloid plaque deposition as *the* cause of Alzheimer's, or even *a* cause. And there are other dementias in which amyloid does not seem to play a major role. To understand how the amyloid hypothesis works, therefore—and the objections to it—we will need to look more closely at the chief suspect, and how it comes to be in brains at all.

Alzheimer's has a genetic component, yet there is no amyloid gene. Paradoxical? No. Our DNA contains a gene, identified in 1987, for a larger protein, a precursor molecule inside which Aβ lurks.[13] This amyloid precursor protein (APP) is evolutionarily ancient and highly conserved, which implies that it may have important functions.[14] One of those is the production of Aβ, and to understand that we need to know a little more about how cells work with proteins.

A Brief Guide to Protein Production

As every sculptor knows, there's a vast gulf between getting your block of marble and honing it into the vision you imagined. Likewise, a protein hot off the gene press is not yet in its final state, but must be folded into an exquisite sculpture, a process that requires the endoplasmic reticulum (it doesn't just store calcium). Fresh proteins are therefore transported from the cell nucleus to the endoplasmic reticulum, where they are subjected to various chemical processes—collectively known as 'post-translational modification'—to give them their final 3D look. The extra adjustments give cells, in effect, more machinery to play with, since they can greatly alter a protein's function, switching it on or off, or tagging it for transport or destruction.[15]

However, protein folding can go wrong. As we shall see, many scientists think that the abnormal folding of proteins like amyloid and tau is the basic problem leading to neurodegeneration. Misfolding happens all the time, but the endoplasmic reticulum monitors protein quantity and quality. It can tell the nucleus to reduce production if necessary, and it also has quality control procedures, so that wrongly folded proteins can be disposed of before they cause problems. If too much problematic protein builds up, an 'unfolded protein response' can stimulate waste disposal systems, inflammatory responses, or even cell death.[16] Because protein build-up is a feature of neurodegenerative diseases, research into how these systems function—and fail—is on-going and intense.

Once folded, proteins are passed from the endoplasmic reticulum to another intracellular structure, the Golgi apparatus, for packaging and delivery to their destinations: the nucleus, the cell membrane, a distant synapse, or wherever. The packages used are vesicles (see Figure 3). These bud off the Golgi apparatus to enclose finished proteins and are then chemically labelled with addresses and delivery instructions.

Vesicles are essential for cells; they keep innards apart and allow them to be moved about. For example, used proteins can be broken down for recycling—in specialized vesicles called lysosomes—without the entire cell being destroyed (usually). Quarantine is essential; cell activity, and health, depends on where chemicals are as well as their quantities, as we saw with calcium. Vesicles are also used for signalling between cells. In neurons, for instance, they carry molecules of neurotransmitter from the central cell body to its output stations, the synapses. It can be a long trek: motor neurons in the human spinal cord can stretch for a metre.

Vesicles do not float randomly around the cell. They move like trams along internal tracks called microtubules. These link up like bones in a skeleton to give the cell its structure, its 'cytoskeleton'. Neurons' distinctive shapes, with their long axons and spreading tree of dendrites, rely on this network of protein girders, which also provides internal highways along which cell components can be moved.

The cytoskeleton has long been of interest to Alzheimer's researchers because one of its major components is tau protein, which, as we noted earlier, undergoes chemical changes early in the disease.[17] No one is quite sure yet what makes tau the subject of excessive attention from phosphate-bearing enzymes, but the resulting 'hyperphosphorylated' tau becomes excessively fond of other tau and rather less fond of its work on microtubules. And neglected microtubules tend to fall apart, eventually wrecking cells.[18]

Like amyloid, tau can aggregate into strands, called filaments. These form twisted pairs: another, less famous double helix. Over time, dense tangles of protein form, which clog up cells, disrupt their cytoskeletal transport systems, and alter gene expression and other cellular functions. Alzheimer's involves the gradual destruction of synapses, axons, and finally the cells themselves, and many researchers see tau as a major suspect.[19]

Location, Location, Location

For amyloid production, vesicles trundling along the cytoskeleton take APP molecules out to the cell membrane once their post-production editing is complete. APP sits across the membrane, such that its ends stick out on either side. On the end inside the cell is a part of the molecule that binds to an intracellular protein called clathrin. Clathrin, discovered by British scientist Barbara Pearse, is essential for cell transport, and APP's clathrin-binding domain acts like a postage stamp, saying 'Bring me inside' to the cellular machinery.[20] Thus APP is not simply built in the nucleus, shipped out to the cell's frontier, and left to its fate. Instead, like a diplomat, it shuttles back and forth, recalled from the membrane to the interior, and then either recycled or repackaged and sent back to the membrane.

This matters because APP's location has much to do with its cellular fate—and on that fate, some researchers believe, depends the balance between healthy neurons and neurodegeneration.

The Vital Start

APP was labelled 'amyloid precursor' because in 1987 no one knew what it was for, other than providing brains with Aβ. Researchers are still not sure, but the consensus appears to be that APP is a good thing for brain health. It is directly neurotrophic (cell-nourishing) and beneficial for learning and memory. It seems to regulate synapse growth and plasticity, and it may also influence cell adhesion (cells need to stick to each other to grow, develop, and communicate). Mice with lower APP levels have neurons with fewer dendrites and synapses. APP may also regulate other key neurotrophins like BDNF (brain-derived neurotrophic factor) and NGF (nerve growth factor), and it may be important too for brain development.[21]

Neurotrophins are 'neuron-nurses', boosting cells' vitality and increasing the growth of synapses. They also enhance synaptic plasticity, neurons' remarkable ability to alter the strength of the connections between them—in response to the signals they receive—or even to form new connections. Synaptic plasticity is the basis of learning and memory, and BDNF is known to be important for learning and also in stress responses. Its production, and synaptic plasticity, diminish in the elderly.[22] Needless to say, BDNF and other neurotrophins are among the factors scientists are seeking to boost in order to stave off dementia.

In addition, APP may be good for the brain's oxygen supply. A 2012 study of APP knockout mice (animals genetically engineered to lack the gene for APP) found that under normal conditions they were not very different from normal mice; but they were much more likely to die after an ischaemic stroke—in which blood vessels become blocked—and die quickly. Such strokes are increasingly common in old age and dementia. The timing is of interest because much of the harm in ischaemia is done not by the initial blockage—when neurons experience low oxygen levels (hypoxia)—but later, as blood rushes back into vessels. (This 'reperfusion injury', which can have profound long-term effects, increases oxidative stress and inflammation, damages capillary walls, and affects the mechanisms by which brains control their blood flow.) Yet APP-lacking mice feel the consequences of ischaemia early, and they also react badly to hypoxia by itself. APP levels rise after both ischaemic stroke and hypoxia in people as well as rodents. These findings suggest that APP is acting to protect neurons against lack of oxygen, rather than later damage to blood vessels.

APP can bind to numerous chemicals vital for brain function, including iron, copper, and cholesterol. These are on the suspects' list in Alzheimer's, and they give us a hint of what scientists have slowly been uncovering: the fact that APP's biochemical network is immensely complex and influential.[23] Drug developers trying to reduce Aβ production cannot, therefore, simply block APP without risking major side effects. Instead, they have sought to find ways of blocking the process by which Aβ is made.

APP's Butchers

Both ends of APP, inside and outside the cell, are attractive to enzymes called secretases. When these approach the molecule they chop bits off it (cleavage). The liberated segments enter the surrounding fluid, a process known as secretion; hence secretase. It is from APP's dismemberment that Aβ is born. But how it is dismembered is crucial.

Three enzymes are involved, imaginatively called alpha (α), beta (β), and gamma (γ) secretase (see Figure 6). All three cleave APP, but they bite in different places. When α-secretase gets in first it cleaves APP at a point inside the Aβ molecule, splitting the unborn amyloid in two so that Aβ is never produced. When β-secretase acts first, however, it cleaves APP at the outer edge of Aβ. The stump is then cleaved by γ-secretase at the inner edge of Aβ, letting amyloid loose.[24]

The α-secretase pathway is considered the normal, healthy one and its products are usually in the majority.[25] They include a protein called sAPPα—the 's' stands for 'soluble'—which, like APP and other neurotrophins, seems to be good at keeping synapses healthy. (To borrow a friend's exquisite paraphrase, s-A-P-P-α makes you h-A-P-P-y.) sAPPα also inhibits β-secretase, thus reducing amyloid production. So the two pathways, one leading to sAPPα and the other to Aβ, seem to compete; more of one means less of the other.

Again, location matters. The α-secretase mainly acts in the cell membrane, so sAPPα is secreted outside the cell. In neurons, however, much β-secretase—amyloid-producing—activity takes place internally.[26] This secretase works best in acidic environments like those found in lysosomes (specialized vesicles which are the cell's waste disposal sites); and its activity is increased by stressors like hypoxia and oxidative stress (of which more later). Thus in cells under strain, APP shuttled back from the membrane, via clathrin, and sent for recycling may be converted into Aβ. This can then build up inside the cell, or be secreted outside it to form amyloid plaques.

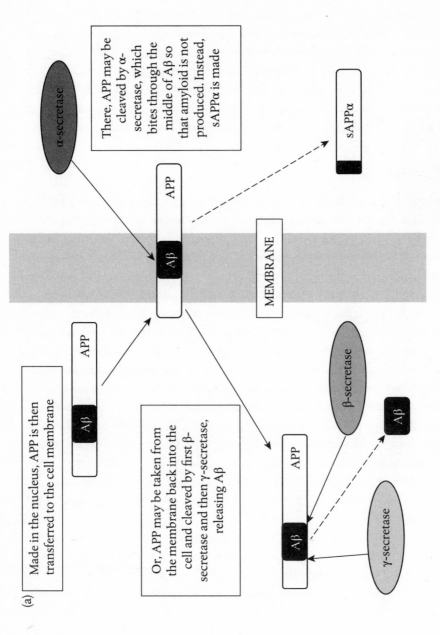

FIGURE 6a: Amyloid processing. Processing of the amyloid protein precursor (APP) molecule (upper left), which contains the Aβ molecule (shown in black).

(a)

Made in the nucleus, APP is then transferred to the cell membrane

There, APP may be cleaved by α-secretase, which bites through the middle of Aβ so that amyloid is not produced. Instead, sAPPα is made

Or, APP may be taken from the membrane back into the cell and cleaved by first β-secretase and then γ-secretase, releasing Aβ

APP

APP

APP

APP

Aβ

Aβ

Aβ

Aβ

sAPPα

MEMBRANE

α-secretase

β-secretase

γ-secretase

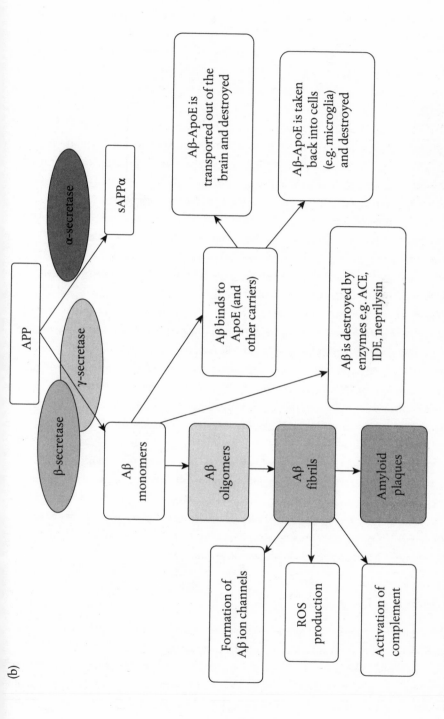

FIGURE 6b: The conversion of APP into either sAPPα (α-secretase pathway) or Aβ (β-, γ-secretase pathway), and what happens to the amyloid thereafter. See Chapter 9 for details.

Note that plaques do not appear all of a sudden. Rather, they are the endpoint of a process that begins with single Aβ proteins (*aka* monomers) uniting to form groups—called oligomers—of varying sizes. Smaller oligomers are soluble, larger ones insoluble; and they can grow to form long strands (inconsistently called fibrils, not polymers). Fibrils congeal into twisted sheets of protein, forming insoluble clumps: amyloid plaques.[27]

The amyloid cascade hypothesis gains much of its strength from genetic studies. Rare early-onset familial Alzheimer's cases have mutations in the APP gene and in genes coding for the secretases, especially γ-secretase, which is built from four proteins. One of these is so clearly linked to dementia that it was called 'presenilin'.[28] Assuming these mutations lead to more Aβ production, they provide strong support for the hypothesis.[29] So does a 2012 study in *Nature* describing a mutation in the APP gene which reduced amyloid production by nearly half: people with this mutation were protected against cognitive decline and dementia.[30] Cell culture experiments and animal studies in which Aβ build-up appears to be harmful to neurons provide additional support for the amyloid hypothesis.

The discovery that the enzyme which lets Aβ loose in the brain is γ-secretase raised hopes that interfering with this protein might reduce amyloid production and hence treat Alzheimer's.[31] Unfortunately, a clinical trial of a γ-secretase inhibitor, semagacestat, found that patients receiving the drug not only failed to improve on cognitive tests but actually worsened. They also 'lost more weight and had more skin cancers and infections, treatment discontinuations due to adverse events, and serious adverse events', as well as considerable immune system abnormalities.[32] The trial was abandoned.

Researchers think the failure might be due to semagacestat targeting other proteins as well as γ-secretase. Multitasking proteins are a common problem in drug trials; the law of unintended consequences is a constant threat in applied biochemistry. Unfortunately for the makers of semagacestat, γ-secretase chews up more than just APP.[33] Thus the enzyme's suppression affected other pathways than amyloid processing, with unpredicted and dangerous results.

Which Amyloid?

Plaques are the endpoint of amyloid formation, and these clogging mats of protein cause all the other problems in dementia, from vascular dysfunction to cell death. Or so it was initially thought. In the mid-2000s, however, scientists developed neuroimaging techniques for detecting amyloid plaques in living brains, and this exposed a problem.[34] The correlation between having lots of plaques and poor cognition was a good deal weaker than would be expected if the plaques were causing the cognitive impairment. Some people survive well into old age with heavy brain amyloid burdens. Others can have dementia with little sign of amyloid. Scientists frequently remind us that correlation is not causation, but causation does rather imply that there should be correlation.

When researchers face findings that seem to contradict their hypothesis … they do some hard thinking. Aβ research has become intense over the past ten years: when I did a database search on the topic of 'amyloid beta' from 2005 to 2014 I found about 55,000 results, more than double the number from the previous decade.[35] As a result of all this hard work it is now thought that amyloid plaques may not be the cause of Alzheimer's, because the amyloid fibrils in plaques are 'mature' and relatively inert. Monomers can also be crossed off the suspect list (probably). Low levels of this single molecule form of Aβ may in fact be beneficial. Like their precursor APP and their alternative sAPPα, Aβ monomers seem to enhance memory and synaptic plasticity and to act as neurotrophins.[36] So perhaps the two amyloid-processing pathways are less antagonistic than they seem, at least when their outputs are low.

However, when levels of Aβ monomers increase they are more likely to combine to form oligomers; and these are another matter. Small, soluble forms of amyloid—oligomers and immature 'protofibrils'—are the top suspects according to revised views of the cascade hypothesis. They have been shown to reduce synaptic plasticity, and to be neurotoxic in cell cultures, rodents, and primates.[37] Like human beings, Aβ molecules can, it seems, be innocuous in isolation but deadly as part of a gang.

That Aβ is such a shape-shifter, from single molecules to strands and clumps and back again, is one reason why unravelling its functions has proved so exceptionally difficult. Different forms behave in varying ways. They prefer to bind with different molecules, and they exert different mechanical as well as chemical forces.[38]

Another reason is that Aβ itself exists in multiple varieties, depending on exactly where the secretases bite through APP. The resulting varying-length proteins fold in different ways, with different consequences for their behaviour. The most dangerous version is thought to have forty-two amino acids; the most plentiful version has forty. Usually about nine times as much $A\beta_{40}$ is made as $A\beta_{42}$, but in Alzheimer's levels of $A\beta_{42}$ seem to rise. The two extra amino acids make a big difference. $A\beta_{42}$ is keener on company than its shorter colleague; when its levels go up, more oligomers form. Changing the ratio of $A\beta_{40}$:$A\beta_{42}$ may thus alter amyloid's toxicity.

APP has between 695 and 770 amino acids (like Aβ, it exists in more than one length).[39] Thus $A\beta_{40}$ and $A\beta_{42}$ are small, in protein terms.

If oligomers are the most damaging form of Aβ, you would think that by the time they have matured into fibrils and plaques the damage has been done. In which case, how can there be people who have developed plaques, but who don't have cognitive symptoms?

One answer is that Aβ's journey from monomer to plaque need not be a one-way trip. Rather, the likelihood of individual molecules moving from one state to another may depend on a delicate set of chemical balances between the different states. High levels of monomers may push oligomer formation, and high levels of oligomers may promote plaques. (An analogy is the way salt crystals can form in salt water exposed to sunshine: as the water evaporates it makes the remaining liquid saltier, tipping the balance towards the solid state.)

However, the amyloid cascade hypothesis proposes that whatever process causes brain Aβ levels to rise is not a one-off, but a continual elevation of amyloid levels. So even if plaques soak up some of the dangerous Aβ oligomers, more are constantly forming.

Furthermore, the process may be reversible, so if levels of soluble amyloid were to drop, plaques might shed oligomers. Some researchers think that this ability of plaques to act as reservoirs for smaller, soluble Aβ fragments could explain why some drugs designed to attack plaques seem to make dementia symptoms worse.

Thus the presence of plaques need not correlate with the extent of cognitive impairment. Some studies do suggest that cognitively normal folk with large amounts of brain amyloid are likely to deteriorate faster than those with low amyloid levels, but they are not as yet conclusive. What is needed is the power to detect smaller, soluble forms of amyloid, and the neuron damage they are thought to cause, in living human brains. As this book went to press in mid-2016 the technology was still a work in progress.

Protein not Wanted

The amyloid cascade hypothesis proposes that too much Aβ is causing neurodegeneration, which in turn causes the cognitive and other problems besetting people with dementia. The next question is: how might too much Aβ come about? There are three obvious ways. The brain could be producing too much protein, for various reasons. Amyloid from elsewhere could be getting into the brain. Or there could be a failure of waste disposal mechanisms, which would normally clear away excess protein. One of these, or some combination of them, must be the case for both familial and sporadic dementia if the amyloid hypothesis is right.

We'll begin at the beginning, with production.

7

Too Much Amyloid?

Why might amyloid be produced in excessive quantities in Alzheimer's patients? Perhaps their genes are different, such that more APP is produced; or there is more β-secretase/less α-secretase around, so more Aβ is made. Alternatively, perhaps something stimulates the production of APP, or tilts the balance towards higher levels of amyloid in some other way. To see what scientists think is going on, we need to know more about how proteins like amyloid are produced. And for that we need to call upon a science that may seem very distant from brain research: atomic physics. Without its help we cannot understand how cells transact their business, how environmental factors like your diet can affect the genes and proteins in your brain, and how a protein like amyloid could fold into a shape deadly to neurons.

A Dip into Physics

Everything in a cell is made of molecules, which are made of atoms (mostly carbon, hydrogen, and oxygen, with smaller amounts of other elements such as iron, nitrogen, chlorine, and sulphur), which are made of neutrons, protons, and electrons. Put another way, everything that happens in a cell or a brain—including neurodegeneration—ultimately depends on the quantities, positions, and movements of electrical charges: negative electrons and positive protons.[1] (Electrons repel each other; protons abhor other protons; electrons and protons are mutually attracted.)

Interactions between atoms involve changes in their distributions of electrical charges, mainly through the movement of those peculiar, shape-shifting subatomic entities, electrons. Good health requires well-shepherded electrons. Cells can tolerate great numbers of not-quite-right interactions, but as they mount up—leaving more and more electrons in the wrong place at the wrong time—the cell's systems struggle to cope.

Atoms can exchange electrons, becoming ions and forming ionic bonds. Or they can share electrons between them, forming covalent bonds.[2] Organic—carbon-based—compounds rely heavily on covalent bonds, which are typically stronger and harder to break than ionic bonds.[3] The type of bond affects how the molecule behaves. Fats, with large numbers of tough covalent bonds, do not dissolve in water. By contrast, the ease with which ions can break free allows them to be used in many important cell-signalling pathways which involve moving electric charges through watery fluids—including those by which neurons communicate.

Many proteins are soluble in watery fluids like blood and cell cytoplasm, but can also interact with fats. Aβ, for example, can diffuse through the extracellular space to spread its havoc, or agglomerate into plaques; but it can also engage with cell membranes, to damaging effect.

Both ionic and covalent molecules can form 'functional groups'. These are units of the currency in which cellular transactions are conducted: components which, when attached to a protein, fat, carbohydrate, or nucleic acid (i.e. DNA or RNA), can significantly alter that molecule's behaviour.[4] Among the most important functional groups are calcium ions, phosphate groups, and sugars. (The process of attaching sugar molecules is called glycosylation.) The careful management of functional groups is crucial to cell function. When it goes wrong brains get problems—as in dementia, when too many phosphate groups become attached to tau.

Chemical bonds between atoms give molecules their basic physical structure and properties. In fats, for example, carbon atoms linked by single bonds form straight chains (as in saturated fats), whereas double bonds kink the chain (as in polyunsaturated fats). Saturated fats, being straighter, can pack more tightly together than kinky polyunsaturated fats.[5] And C=C bonds offer more options for interaction, so unsaturated fats are more reactive: more likely to form links with other molecules.

Where the bonds are also makes a big difference. Omega-3 and omega-6 fatty acids, beloved of fish oil salespeople, are both polyunsaturated, but they have C=C bonds in different positions. Omega-6s such as arachidonic acid tend to boost inflammatory responses, while omega-3s such as EPA and DHA are mainly anti-inflammatory—and the two types tend to inhibit each other's activity.[6] The distinction matters because inflammation is one of the chief suspects in unhealthy ageing and neurodegeneration, and inflammation can be influenced by diet, including the long-term consumption of omega-3s. Humans get omega-3s from fish, nuts, seeds, and green leafy vegetables; omega-6s are in red meat and grain-based products like bread and cereals. Needless to say, given how many of us choose hamburgers rather than cabbage, many people who eat Western-type diets are deficient in omega-3s;

and some researchers think this may put them at greater risk for age-related brain disorders.

'Protein Function is Governed by Shape and Charge'

Fatty acids form chains, but many molecules have more complicated 3D shapes. As a protein folds, for instance, distant regions—in terms of the original genetic sequence—may be brought into close physical proximity.[7] This can have implications for how the protein works: a bulge at one point may block access to another area, or a fold form a cage which can trap a smaller molecule like calcium. Furthermore, the presence of adjacent electrical charges can be enough to affect the neighbours, with or without the formation of chemical bonds.[8]

A protein's 3D shape depends in part on its genetic sequence, since that determines the amino acids in its structure and the types of chemical bonds they contain. However, the shape also depends on how electrical charge is distributed across the molecule. This is why adding a functional group—like a phosphate group—to a protein can change its shape and hence its function, switching a chemical process on or off and ultimately changing a cell's behaviour. It is also why the behaviour of Aβ changes as it gathers into oligomers, fibrils, and plaques.

Gene Control

Proteins, unlike fats and carbohydrates, come from genes. Kids learn in school about DNA, and how it is curled up in two long, paired strands made of nucleotides. Each nucleotide consists of one of four bases (A, T, G, C) to which a compound of sugar and phosphate is attached.[9] If you think of DNA's famous twisted ladder shape, the sugar-phosphate backbone provides the two vertical frames, while pairs of bases (A with T, G with C) form the rungs. On a single strand of DNA, a group of three bases forms a codon. Each codon is the genetic instruction for one amino acid.

To make a protein, the strands of DNA are unwound from each other and one is copied, by a set of processes called transcription, to form another long, stringy molecule called RNA. The copy is not exact: errors may occur, and in RNA the base T is replaced by another, U. Further processes—translation—then 'read off' the RNA to form strings of amino acids: proteins.[10] The overall process is called gene expression.

It was once thought that DNA, changing the cellular world by producing proteins, itself stayed constant, like a library book repeatedly read, but never scribbled on. Now we know that's not true. What happens in cells can affect DNA, silencing some genes, increasing the expression of others, and even changing the genetic code. The young science of epigenetics looks at how DNA can be modified, gene expression altered, and more or less protein produced, by such 'ungenetic' factors as your diet, whether you smoke, and the stresses you experience.[11] Epigenetics is of especial interest in brain disorders like dementia because decades of gene hunting have failed to find obvious culprits (with a few exceptions such as ApoE). Instead, most neurodegenerative disorders seem to be influenced by numerous genes, each having a small effect. They are also greatly affected by environmental factors, as we shall see; and these effects increase with age. This suggests that epigenetic changes during life, triggered by exposure to environmental risks, could be involved.

There are complications. (This is biology; of course there are complications!) Your environment—from air to food to the social whirl that buoys you up or stresses you out—is constantly affecting your genes. That changes you; but research suggests that the process began before you were even conceived, affecting the DNA in your mother's eggs and father's sperm. Some research has even suggested that the children of older parents may be more at risk of Alzheimer's, although the link is by no means proven. Epigenetic changes may affect as-yet-unborn descendants, transmitting the impact of one person's lived experience to their offspring. The doctrine of original sin lives on, with payback for the parents' bad habits visited upon the children. For instance, whether your parents smoked while you were in the womb will have altered your gene expression and risk of disease.

Understanding how genes can be switched on or off is vital because the expression of many genes alters with age. One of the biggest areas of dementia research involves studying gene expression changes in Alzheimer's.

So how can gene expression be silenced, or encouraged? By moving electrons. DNA's shape—how tightly or loosely the double helix twists—is affected by its electrical charges, just as with any other molecule. This is the key to understanding gene control.

DNA does not simply float free in the nucleus. Humans use wood, plastic, or little pieces of cardboard to hold sewing thread or wool tidily; but evolution, stitching and knitting organisms together, came across the same principle long ago. DNA is wrapped around proteins called histones. (The combination is called chromatin.)

Unlike little pieces of cardboard, however, histones are not simply passive carriers but active regulators of gene expression. They form an important part of the interface between DNA and its environment—between nature and nurture, if you like. (If you do like, bear in mind that nature and nurture are more closely bound than any conjoined twins.) Recall that DNA is full of phosphate groups, which make it negatively charged. Gene expression can be controlled by changing the charge on the histone molecules, making them more negative or positive, and thus more repelled by, or attracted to, the DNA.[12] Thus nurture, via the chemical manipulation of electrical charges, has an on-going impact on nature. This is not just theory. Histone-related genes have been implicated in numerous brain disorders, including depression, schizophrenia, multiple sclerosis, stroke, and Alzheimer's.[13]

The cell's ability to control its genetic material is far more sophisticated than we used to think. As well as histone regulation, cells can talk to their DNA in other ways. Intracellular signalling pathways can activate proteins in the cytoplasm called transcription factors. Once triggered, these move into the nucleus—they are also called nuclear factors—and bind directly to DNA molecules, regulating gene expression. Transcription factors include receptors for fat-soluble molecules like thyroid hormone, vitamins A, D, and E, the sex steroids oestrogen and testosterone, glucocorticoids like cortisol (involved in the body's responses to stress), and cholesterol, enabling these chemicals to influence protein production.[14] Transcription factors can affect many genes, and those genes tend to have related functions, so the effect can be to switch on (or off) an entire cellular programme, such as axon growth, cell division, or cell death.

An example already mentioned is nuclear factor kappa B (NFκB), a transcription factor which controls over 150 genes involved in inflammation.[15] NFκB has many roles, but one of particular interest to clinicians is that it acts as an interface between stress responses and the production of pro-inflammatory molecules called cytokines (of which more later). NFκB thus connects two major suspects in neurodegeneration, so it is of great interest to researchers working on dementia, as well as to those studying mental illness, resilience, and trauma.[16]

Linking stress to inflammation is one example of how body chemistry allows cells to respond to their environment by changing their production of proteins (and of RNA, which can independently contribute to cellular signalling). Another example is the link between brain activity and genetic control, which helps keep healthy brain cells supple and responsive to changing stimuli. Within neurons, certain proteins allow levels of activity, and the amounts of certain receptors for the major neurotransmitter glutamate, to regulate, and be regulated by, DNA.[17] This allows the cells to vary their gene expression, and hence how reactive they are to stimuli, depending on what is happening in the networks of which they are a part.

Epigenetics is of great interest because of its implied promise that genes—including faulty genes in neurodegenerative disorders—could one day be switched on or off by clinicians to cure diseases. Such deliberate gene control is already mundane in animal experiments; nowadays it can even be applied merely by shining a particular colour of light onto an animal's (genetically engineered) brain.[18] Extending the techniques to people must be done carefully, however, especially when many genes may be involved, as in sporadic dementia. What scientists need to do is work out which genes to target, and how to do it safely; and that is a gigantic challenge.

Amyloid Production

The end result of gene expression is that cells make more or less of proteins such as APP. These then undergo post-translational modifications before being delivered to their cellular (or extracellular) destinations. There they may undergo further changes, like being chopped up to make amyloid. Theoretically, clinicians could intervene at any or all of these stages to lower amyloid production.

That would help in dementia if too much amyloid is being made in the brains of people who develop the condition. For rare genetic (familial) forms of Alzheimer's, which are typically early-onset, analyses of human brains and animal models suggest that this is the case. The underlying mutations appear to produce excessive amounts of the more toxic $A\beta_{42}$, and amyloid pathology is clear post-mortem.

Most Alzheimer's is late-life and sporadic, however, and here the case—like the genetics—is less clear. For example, a 2007 human study found that the 'total amount of APP mRNA in AD and control brain did not differ' (mRNA levels indicate how much protein is being made).[19] Of course, APP is only part of the story: there might be a shift in how APP is chopped up by secretases. If, for example, α-secretase's activity were diminished, or β- or γ-secretase's enhanced, more Aβ might be produced, or more $A\beta_{42}$ and less $A\beta_{40}$—as seems to happen in familial Alzheimer's.

To address this issue, a 2010 study measured brain amyloid production in sporadic Alzheimer patients and in controls (people of similar ages who died without having dementia), looking at both $A\beta_{42}$ and $A\beta_{40}$.[20] On average, it found no overall difference for either version of the protein.

This does not necessarily rule out changes in amyloid production being a contributing factor to sporadic dementia. More studies, on much larger populations, are needed, since we do not yet know whether sporadic dementia is the same disease across all sufferers. The lack of obvious differences in amyloid production does, however, encourage researchers to consider other options. In Chapter 8 we'll look at one of them: that amyloid might be coming from elsewhere.

8

Transfers In?

Could amyloid be reaching the brain from elsewhere in the body? APP and Aβ are both produced outside the central nervous system, notably in the gut and blood. Getting into the brain, however, is far from easy. To see why, let us take a look at one of the natural wonders of the body's world: the border between the vascular system and the brain.

The cerebral arteries and veins are not simply motorways for blood, along which it roars on its passage through the brain. These are roads that can change their width to regulate traffic flow, under nervous system control. They are also couriers, and at some point the vital supplies must be dropped off: transferred from pulsing vessels to hungry cells. The blood–brain delivery system must be highly efficient, robust, and universal in its reach.

Since blood is a carrier of wastes, poisons, and pathogens as well as nutrients, the system also needs to be choosy about what it delivers. Every organ in the body regulates its interactions with blood, but the brain needs particular protection, due to its unusual chemistry and the intricate and subtle ion balances of neurotransmission. Its normal pH of around 7.2 is close to the neutral point of pure water, 7.0.[1] However, neural activity is extremely sensitive to calcium levels and to ambient pH; so the brain's extraordinary capacity for turning perception into thought and action depends on 'good barriers' as well as on good neurons.[2] Brain activity can also alter both calcium and acidity levels: research suggests that active neurons cause the pH in their vicinity to drop, as do adverse events like strokes. It is thought that this acidification may be one way in which strokes, and excessive neuronal activity, can harm brains. Low pH can damage synapses and affect cell calcium, potentially triggering cell death.

Finally, because the skull is stuffed so full of brain cells that space for the supply chain is at a premium, the system needs to achieve all this with minimal use of building materials.

Travelling Blood

To meet these constraints, evolution has come up with one of the most remarkable structures in existence: the blood–brain barrier.

Arteries branch and narrow, forming arterioles, which eventually become capillaries. If arteries are motorways, capillaries are the local roads where postal workers park and walk to houses. Capillary walls are made up of a single layer of specialized endothelial cells. These are only about 200 nm across (0.2 thousandths of a millimetre); a typical cell would be about 50 times wider.[3] Thus for much of the blood–brain barrier's enormous extent, only one cell's breadth—and a slim cell at that—stands between blood and brain.

The statistics are astonishing, though as so often they are more guess than gospel.[4] The number of capillaries in the human brain is thought to be about 100 billion—comparable to the number of neurons—and the distance a molecule would have to travel from a capillary to reach brain tissue is about 25 μm (25 thousandths of a millimetre) at most. Thus 'every neuron is virtually perfused by its own blood vessel', meaning that substances carried into the capillaries can affect neurons almost immediately.[5] Someone has calculated that the total surface area of human brain endothelial cells is about 20 square metres—one hundred million times greater than its thickness. That makes it about ten times as big as the skin.[6] Stuck end to end, the total length of a brain's capillaries would be about 400 miles or 644 kilometres—roughly the distance from Edinburgh to London, or Boston to Washington. If you were to look at a post-mortem brain, the major blood vessels would be visible, albeit stained an unlovely brown by the preservative. What you wouldn't see is the vascular density: how packed full the tissue is of capillaries. Your organ of reason is a blood-soaked sponge.

For all this colossal coverage, it has also been estimated that the volume occupied by the capillaries is minuscule: 5 millilitres, which would fill an average teaspoon but not a big one. That's well under one per cent of the brain's total volume.[7] Capillaries average only around 8 μm in width, and the minimum width may be half that.[8]

Yet the point at which blood meets brain is not simply a layer of skinny endothelium, across whose frontier anything (comes and) goes. It is much more interesting, and better defended, than that.

Where Blood Meets Brain

If you get hay fever you may well have cursed the small but aggravating molecule histamine, even as you swallowed a pill to suppress it. But histamine has many other uses than ruining a person's summer. One of the less well known is for demonstrating the blood–brain barrier. If you were to inject a mouse with radiolabelled histamine and then scan its body for radioactivity, you would see a remarkable image: the mouse's body dark with histamine except for a pure white brain and spinal cord. Something is keeping the nervous system clean.[9]

The name scientists associate with the discovery of the blood–brain barrier is that of the great German physiologist Paul Ehrlich, who shared the Nobel Prize for physiology or medicine in 1908. Using dyes, he showed that not all substances in blood could access the central nervous system.[10] Ehrlich is best known as a founding father of immunology and chemotherapy, and the man to whom we owe the concept of 'magic bullets'. But his methodical studies with dyes were crucial in establishing haematology, the science of blood.

You can see an image of histamine radiolabelling, with the central nervous system (CNS) clearly spared, in an open-access review by William Pardridge, published in 2005. Pardridge shows how effective a barrier the blood–brain barrier is by considering drug therapies which target the brain. In general, pharmaceuticals come in two sizes: small or large. Small-molecule drugs are chemicals like aspirin or histamine. Large-molecule drugs, also called 'biologics', are based on proteins and include vaccines and antibodies.[11] If you suspect that the bigger molecules may have trouble passing the blood–brain barrier, you are correct: Pardridge noted that 'all large-molecule products of biotechnology' are barred.[12] He added, however, that almost all smaller drugs—about ninety-eight per cent—also fail to cross the barrier.

Only about five per cent of available drugs treat brain or spinal cord disorders, despite the huge toll exacted by failing brains. That the blood–brain barrier is so good at keeping stuff out is a major reason why humans can live so long and retain so many of their faculties. But that same prowess makes brain disorders exceptionally challenging to treat.

Blood–brain barrier research has advanced greatly since 2005. Developments in nanomedicine and the ability to culture model tissues—including blood–brain barrier models—are crucial, but other, older technologies are also being 'repurposed'. In Alzheimer's research a 2015 study in mice used ultrasound to open up the blood–brain barrier. It found that this improved brain signs of the disease as well as the animals' performance on memory tasks.[13]

Setting aside such artificial methods of entry, the brain's defences are not easily conquered. After all, they keep most of us reasonably healthy and *compos mentis* for decades, under constant assault from pathogens, pollutants, unwise dietary choices, and so on. So what makes the barrier so effective? Let's look a little more closely.

Endothelial Cells

Moving from blood to brain, an invader—whether pathogen or protein—must cross the layer of endothelial cells. They are an effective deterrent of water-soluble molecules, including glucose and some vitamins (e.g. B6 and B12). When required, these are ferried across the blood–brain barrier by specialized transporter proteins.[14]

This points towards one way in which pathogens, or drugs, can get across the blood–brain barrier: by acting as ligands for receptors on the endothelial cell's blood-facing membranes. Activating such receptors can trigger their ingestion back into the cell, and with them goes their cargo. Both ligand and receptor may then enter the cell's waste disposal or recycling pathways, but sometimes the ligand can escape across the endothelial cell's brain-facing membrane into brain tissue. Certain bacteria, including those that cause meningitis, use this method to penetrate the blood–brain barrier.[15]

Fat-soluble molecules such as vitamin D can pass through a lipid membrane and thus diffuse across the endothelial cell. Even these, however, face restrictions: more chemically active molecules, like unruly entrants to a nightclub, may be barred.[16] The cells of the blood–brain barrier have proteins called ABC transporters which actively pump out many molecules. They are of interest in dementia because they help to clear the brain of amyloid.

How about slipping between the endothelial cells? This is prevented by their tight junctions. These specialized zones are rich in interlocking proteins, containing more than forty species, many of which are found nowhere else. Names like occludin, the claudins, and the JAMs (junctional adhesion molecules) reflect their functions in binding cells together, shutting out would-be entrants to the brain.

Tight junctions are often compared to Velcro, the fabric fastener made of tiny hooks and loops. Unlike Velcro, however, they are not passive mechanical fixtures but active participants in a sophisticated system of border control which allows only certain molecules through. Unfortunately that system weakens with age. Tight junctions can also be affected by proteins which increase during disease, including Aβ.[17] Thus weaknesses in the blood–brain barrier, which links our cerebral and our vascular systems so directly, have a major role in the deleterious effects of ageing and illness on the brain.

Amyloid Entry

APP and Aβ made elsewhere in the body may be able to cross a weakened blood–brain barrier. But APP is a sizeable protein, so we would not expect it to be able to penetrate a healthy brain. Aβ, however, is small, and experiments on animals have shown that Aβ administered peripherally (injected into the stomach) can build up in brain blood vessels and then gradually accumulate in the brain itself.[18]

How does Aβ slip across the border? Like pathogens, it can take the receptor route, binding to a molecule with the memorable acronym of RAGE.[19] RAGE is of interest in neurodegeneration because it has multiple potentially damaging effects on cells, such as activating NFκB—and hence pro-inflammatory cytokines—and interfering with crucial cell signalling pathways. It is activated not only by Aβ but by certain products of high-temperature cooking processes like frying. Such products build up in healthy ageing brains, but more so in brains undergoing dementia; they have also been linked to diabetes. (Thus not only what we eat, but how we cook it, may be important for cell health.)

Aβ's ability to bind to RAGE could thus both give it access to the brain and allow it to do damage once it gets there. Aβ can also bind to ApoE, whose variant ApoE4 is a major risk factor for Alzheimer's. Research in mice suggests that when Aβ binds to ApoE4, but not to the other ApoE variants, it can then be transported into the brain more effectively by RAGE. Interestingly, the presence of ApoE4 also reduces the clearance of Aβ out of the brain.

A major source of blood Aβ is activated platelets—small blood cells crucial for coagulation and wound healing, among much else. Activation switches cells into a more responsive state in which they produce a different range of proteins: for platelets, those needed for blood clotting and wound healing.[20] Platelet activation is triggered by, among other things, inflammation and infection, certain dietary fats, and Aβ itself.[21] This suggests one way in which external factors like diet and infection could potentially affect neurodegeneration: by activating blood cells which then churn out Aβ.

In Chapter 9, we turn from where amyloid comes from to how brains dispose of it.

9

How to Clean Your Brain

There is evidence that, however amyloid comes to be in the brain, getting rid of it may be a major problem in ageing and dementia. Research in mice has found that some types of amyloid (larger oligomers) may be cleared particularly slowly, and that these therefore build up with age.[1] The same 2010 study which found no difference in Aβ production in Alzheimer's patients did find evidence of reduced brain clearance.[2] People with the risky variant of ApoE also show lower clearance, as do people with early-onset dementia.

How does a healthy brain rid itself of amyloid? By spewing it out, or chewing it up, or both.

To understand how the brain ejects amyloid, we need to know something of brain-washing. Not the coercive psychology which was the topic of my first book, but the flow of liquids through a brain which keeps it operational.[3] That flow involves four interacting systems, all of which use that most useful of molecules: water (if the brain were a city it would get its supplies by sea). They are the blood supply, the cerebrospinal fluid, the interstitial fluid, and the lymphatic fluid, which drains waste out of the brain.

Blood

Although the brain represents only 2% of the body weight, it receives 15% of the cardiac output, 20% of total body oxygen consumption, and 25% of total body glucose utilization.[4]

The blood supply carries oxygen, glucose, fats, proteins, ions, and other things to hungry brain cells. Its veins carry waste products like carbon dioxide, in deoxygenated blood, back to the heart and lungs. The brain is hugely demanding of bodily resources, and it needs to be. Brain tissue deprived of its blood supply loses a key fuel, ATP, in minutes. Without constant nourishment it rapidly dies.[5] So the brain's vascular system is critically important.

In healthy people, more nutrients are poured into the brain than it can use. In the cortex, for instance, blood flow can drop by up to four-fifths before serious acute harm is done. Chronic reductions in blood flow, however, may not need to be so severe to do damage. Low brain blood flow (hypoperfusion, measured by fMRI) and reduced glucose uptake by brain tissue (hypometabolism, measured by PET) are found in people at high risk of dementia, such as ApoE4 carriers, long before clinical signs of the disease are noticeable.[6] Association areas of the cortex are particularly affected, forming a characteristic pattern in patients with Alzheimer's.[7] Research on patients in the early stages of the disease found reductions of around forty-five per cent for glucose use and twenty per cent for blood flow.[8]

Interestingly, a recent small MRI study found similar, albeit temporary patterns of lowered glucose uptake in the brains of young, healthy people who had just consumed 50g of glucose, pushing up their blood glucose and insulin levels.[9] The decreases were much less—around five per cent—but statistically significant, and they hint at one of the more intriguing potential causes of dementia: blood sugar problems. Of this more later.

Hypoperfusion and hypometabolism are thought to occur when blood vessels stiffen (sclerosis) and become narrower (stenosis). Hardening of the arteries, arteriosclerosis, can occur throughout the body, and smaller blood vessels are thought to be similarly affected.[10] Sclerosis is probably best known as a contributor to heart disease, but it also raises the risk of dementia. The on-going fuel deficit places a prolonged metabolic stress on brain cells, with their high demand for glucose. Neuronal activity takes a lot of energy.

One cause of stiffening arteries is atherosclerosis, in which fatty, calcium-enriched material builds up into plaques on vessel walls. It has plagued humans for centuries, as mummified corpses from ancient cultures confirm under autopsy. Atherosclerotic plaques are partly made of cholesterol. This is why doctors encourage people to get their cholesterol checked, and if necessary make lifestyle changes, or take statins, to reduce it.

Blood is generously supplied to the brain, so that if one source is blocked it can still be fed. This is achieved by two pairs of arteries: the carotids at the front of the neck and the vertebrals at the back. These are the vessels blocked if someone is fool enough, or vicious enough, to grab someone else's throat and squeeze; the sprayers of gore when a throat is cut or a body decapitated. The carotids supply the front, top, and middle of the brain. The vertebrals fuse into the basilar artery, which supplies the back end and underside.

Two further pairs of arteries at the base of the brain connect the circulations of the left and right brain, and its front and back on either side. The result, clearly visible if a brain is removed from its bony vault and turned upside-down, is a ring of blood vessels known as the circle of Willis, after Thomas Willis, the great seventeenth-century doctor, anatomist, and founding member of the Royal Society. (Alas, the basilar artery is not named after a famous anatomist called Basil. It comes from the Latin word for basis: apt, given its location at the base of the brain and its critical role in keeping that brain alive.)

The circle of Willis allows the anterior (front) and posterior (back) circulations to back up each other's supplies. Up to a point: sclerosis in the circle is a common finding in post-mortem analyses of dementia. Carotid stenosis is another frequent problem in age-related brain disorders, thought to be involved in up to a fifth of ischaemic strokes (one of my relatives who had an operation for stenosis also had a minor stroke). Strokes themselves, as well as clogging arteries, increase the risk of dementia by up to tenfold.

Blood leaves the brain by way of cerebral veins, which flow into larger spaces, the venous sinuses.[11] These in turn exit mainly into the internal jugular veins but also via the vertebral veins which run down the back of the neck.[12] The jugulars lie near the carotids—the location can vary—and also near the vagus nerve, which regulates multiple organs and carries visceral information to the brain. Vulnerable things, necks.

Cerebrospinal Fluid

Cerebrospinal fluid (CSF) is a colourless liquid with similarities to blood plasma—what remains of blood when the cells are removed. It is produced in the centre of the brain by a specialized tissue called the choroid plexus, which pumps about half a litre, roughly a pint, of fluid into the ventricles each day.[13] From the ventricles the CSF flows into spaces between the brain's membranous outer wrappings, the meninges. There are three of these: the dura mater, arachnoid mater, and pia mater (and yes, the terms do translate as tough mother, spidery mother, and tender mother). Sloshing around the brain, CSF helps keep it chemically balanced and physically protected.[14]

CSF does not contain red blood cells unless something is seriously wrong. It does contain water, sugar in the form of glucose, and salt, and apparently tastes salty or metallic, like blood. We know this because of a condition called CSF leak, in which CSF can get into the mouth. Its most famous sufferer is probably the actor George Clooney.[15]

CSF also contains many proteins produced by brain cells. This makes it a desirable target for researchers, since measuring proteins in CSF provides much more useful information about brain function than measures from blood. Unfortunately, CSF is sampled by a procedure called lumbar puncture, which takes much longer than a blood sample, carries greater risks, and is one of the less pleasant experiences that modern medics see fit to inflict on patients. This is one reason why biochemical studies of dementia and other brain disorders are so expensive and difficult to do.

Windows on the Brain

When Paul Ehrlich injected his animals with dyes and observed that the brain was spared, he saw, as so often in science, the truth but not the whole truth. Later studies found that the blood–brain barrier has gaps or weak points: small areas around the edges of the ventricles where larger molecules could cross from blood to brain. These are the mysterious 'circumventricular organs' (CVOs). Typically more packed with blood vessels than other brain tissue, and less packed with defensive microglia, they have capillaries which often loop back on themselves, aren't sealed by tight junctions, and don't take up much glucose. So why have all those capillaries, if not for fuel?

The answer seems to be that CVOs are sampling stations, or border controls. They are open for trade between blood, brain, and CSF, but they check it as it crosses. Blood vessels are broad and circulation slow, giving CVO neurons time to sample the wares and detect warning signals. As befits a thriving marketplace, CVOs are full of commodities: chemicals and receptors for chemicals including neurotransmitters— acetylcholine, noradrenaline, dopamine, serotonin, GABA, and glutamate—and hormones like insulin (which lowers blood sugar), ACTH (which controls the body's stress responses), GnRH (which regulates oestrogen levels), and angiotensin (which raises blood pressure). All of these can affect the health of neurons, as we shall see; all have been implicated in dementia; and all can gain access to the brain via CVOs.

We know a lot about what CVOs contain, but we still aren't sure what they do, or even how many of them there are. They have been linked to everything from vomiting to attention (the quality of the evidence tends to decrease from basic to higher-level functions). Some, like the area postrema, seem to be chemical sensors reporting to a heavily interconnected network of areas in the brainstem called the visceral neuraxis. This receives information from both CVOs and nerves from the viscera, and it can send imperatives back to your squamous innards. If you get food poisoning, thank your area postrema for those nasty moments when the barf reflex takes over.

The visceral neuraxis includes the hypothalamus, source of numerous hormones, and also the locus coeruleus and the raphe nucleus, brainstem sources of noradrenaline and serotonin. These three areas regulate awareness, alertness, and mood— hence the proposed link between CVOs and attention—and they are among the first parts of the brain to fail in dementia. Via them, neural signals from CVOs have rapid access to the rest of the brain.

Any chemical hazards that CVOs let pass can also have a big impact. They can, for example, affect the hypothalamus, which in turn affects other CVOs like the posterior pituitary. This small gland pumps hormones into the bloodstream to regulate everything from stress to sexual development, appetite to growth. (One well-known example of this circuitry's importance is its role in the stress response, prompting the release of adrenaline and cortisol.)

CVOs are points where the environment, via the bloodstream, can have a major impact on the brain. CVO damage can cause a bewildering array of symptoms. Damage to the area postrema, for example, has been associated with severe developmental delay caused by hypoxia (lack of oxygen) at birth, with the effects of rattlesnake bites, and with anorexia linked to neuromyelitis optica. Even more subtle damage, however, may have a disproportionate impact. The brain areas affected earliest in dementia, such as brainstem nuclei and the hippocampus, are located close to CVOs, and Aβ protein is known to accumulate in them; they are also vulnerable to pathogens. That there is little research on their role in dementia is not because they are unimportant. It is due to the extensive technical difficulties of studying these small, inaccessible areas.

Interstitial Fluid

You may have come across statements that we humans are mainly water. All our organs sit in a chemical bath, and this interstitial fluid also soaks the brain. Cells need liquid to function, not least because the molecules that are their units of transaction need something to move about in. The closest human analogy may be those conveyor belt sushi bars in which customers choose their food as it travels past. For the cell's 3D perspective on interstitial fluid, you could imagine yourself submerged in a swimming pool where tasty snacks are floating all around you. Bear in mind, however, that interstitial fluid transports both nutrients and waste products, so your pool will also contain raw sewage.

Interstitial fluid is packed with long, interlocking strands of sugar-coated proteins.[16] This 'extracellular matrix' shapes and structures the environment in which cells live and move and have their being. Interstitial fluid and the molecules within it flow through narrow channels, not freely in all directions. Less like a swimming pool; more like a dense underwater jungle.

Interstitial fluid is supplied from blood, and also interacts with CSF via arachnoid villi. Villi in your gut are tiny protrusions of the gut wall that greatly increase the surface area available for processing food. Villi in your brain are tiny protrusions of the sub-arachnoid space—the gap between the inner two of the brain's three meninges—down into the brain, greatly increasing the surface area across which fluid exchange can take place. The villi form alongside blood vessels entering the brain, creating minuscule CSF-filled funnels known as Virchow-Robin spaces. Here CSF, interstitial fluid, and blood can meet and swap materials.

The Virchow-Robin spaces are sealed off at the base, where the blood vessel wall fuses with the brain tissue. Like the ventricles, they widen with age, and both are significantly enlarged in dementia. On neuroimaging scans the brain appears full of tiny holes called lacunae. In severe cases the phenomenon is known as '*état criblé*' and is a symptom of small vessel disease, which is classed as an early stage of vascular dementia.

Like amyloid deposition, however, brain lacunae are also found in some clinically healthy participants.[17] This is characteristic of age-related brain conditions: symptoms can also be found in people who don't have clinical problems. It is as if brains can tolerate a certain amount of damage before the effects on minds begin to show. This idea is the basis of theories about brain reserve (of which more later).

The term '*état criblé*', incidentally, was coined in 1842 by the French scientist and traveller Charles Louis Maxime Durand-Fardel, who also wrote on topics including mineral water, diabetes, and arthritis, as well as translating Dante's *Divine Comedy* into French.[18] Wide-ranging Max had an eye for metaphor: *état criblé* means 'like a fine-meshed sieve'.

Lymph

What goes in must come out, in the sense that the brain needs to maintain its fluid balance just as the body does.[19] If it fails, the results can be severe, like hydrocephalus—in which excess fluid crushes brain tissue and/or restricts its growth—and perhaps also brain lacunae and *état criblé*; some researchers think these could be due to drainage channels becoming blocked by excess protein, causing the Virchow-Robin spaces to swell.[20] The brain's drainage system is essential for its healthy function—not least because excess fluid in the brain exerts pressure on delicate brain tissues, and that can do damage in an organ so tightly boxed in by bone.

Fluid that drains out of organs is called lymph, and the body has a network of lymphatic channels—its other vascular system—that takes lymph back to the bloodstream. It was long thought that brains lacked specialized lymphatic networks. However, as I was writing this book news came through that just such a system had been discovered (or rediscovered) in mice: channels in the meninges capable of draining CSF from the brain.[21]

CSF enters the brain by flowing along the outside of blood vessels. It leaves in the same way, draining along the outside of veins back into the subarachnoid space (and hence into the blood) or into the meningeal channels (and hence perhaps to lymph nodes). Fluid can also flow through the spaces around cranial nerves, which carry information between the brain and the head and neck: areas above the spinal cord. These spaces, and the 'perivascular' spaces around blood vessels, form a 'glymphatic' network—the original brain drain.[22] Full of patrolling immune cells which monitor brain health, this system can clear amyloid from the brain.[23]

Glymphatic is short for 'glial lymphatic'. The term reflects the fact that the spaces around nerves and blood vessels are edged with astrocytes, a type of glial cell which, among many other things, regulates fluid flows within the brain.[24] Astrocytes— astroglia, 'starry glue'—are fascinating and underrated brain cells, once relegated to slave status or less: glue is stuff that holds other, more interesting stuff (i.e. neurons) together. But if astrocytes are neurons' servants, they are more like powerful butlers than lowly serfs—and neurons are more like needy, dependent children. Astrocytes supply them with fuel, alter production of neurotransmitters, and soak up excess glutamate from synapses. They also talk with microglia, influencing the brain's immune response as well as synapse development and function. They are remarkably varied in shape, size, and in the protein markers on their surfaces, and we do not yet know nearly enough about them.[25]

Astrocytes talk to each other by way of gap junctions—areas peppered with channels through which ions like calcium can pass from cell to cell, altering the electrical balance of their membranes. As in neurons, a change in this potential across the membrane serves as a signal—the astrocyte's equivalent of the action potential. However, I recall being told as a trainee neuroscientist that neurons can synapse with up to a thousand partners (a figure since updated to around seven thousand).[26] According to a recent review, astrocytes easily trump that. 'Each astrocyte envelopes several neurons, interacts with hundreds of neuronal dendrites, and contacts up to two million synapses in the human cortex.'[27]

The human brain's phenomenal ability to integrate, process and respond to continually changing and immensely complicated stimuli—a mass of data far beyond what we can currently handle—is not down to its networks of neurons alone. Astrocytes, the most plentiful cells in human cortex, also play a role. Not only do they coddle (and cuddle) neurons, they have also been found to be essential for memory.[28] And when they go wrong, the results can be deadly. Astrocytomas, the most common forms of brain cancer, 'remain fatal with no effective treatment'.[29]

For our current purposes, astrocytes are important because they can regulate the entry and exit of liquids from the brain. They do this using endfeet, which sound like something from a novel by Tolkien; but these are the 'feet' of brain cells, not mythical creatures. Astrocytes and microglia both extend these T-shaped protrusions, which form a layer wrapped around brain blood vessels. Endfeet, unlike human feet, are superbly sensitive organs, rich in receptors. They give microglia and astrocytes real-time information about what is coming through the brain's borders, and they also allow the control of those borders by the brain. For example, astrocytic endfeet contain aquaporin receptors, which allow them to transport water across the brain's borders, both internal (through Virchow-Robin spaces) and external (across the blood–brain barrier). Astrocytes can also control brain blood flow by affecting the diameter of capillaries.

On its way out, liquid waste borne by brain drains flows into specialized organs in the neck called cervical lymph nodes, and hence into the body's lymphatic system and ultimately the bloodstream. A person's waste can reveal much about their state of health, and so too for the brain, since fluid entering the cervical lymph nodes contains cellular waste products. It also contains antigen: material of interest to the immune system (technically, an antigen is anything, from pollen to pathogens, which can trigger the immune system to produce antibodies). Antigen includes molecules from bacterial cell walls, viruses, or dead cells—all signals of a potential problem.

Antigen is picked up by immune cells called antigen-presenting cells, which are constantly circulating in the blood and CSF. They cart the antigen off to lymph nodes: immune checkpoints where it is inspected and assessed for its threat potential. When a doctor feels your neck, and under your armpits, for tender lumps, she is checking whether your lymph nodes are swollen. The swelling is a result of immune cells in the nodes detecting a problem and calling for large-scale reinforcements.[30]

Flushing out Amyloid

Brainwashing is apparently best done while the person is asleep. A recent study suggests that the brain drains may flush out amyloid and other unwanted proteins more efficiently when the conscious self isn't getting in the way, with its imperious demands for blood and its aggravating habit of stirring up neurons.[31] Besides, people tend to lie down to sleep, and prone positions favour outflow via the larger jugular veins, whereas upright positions send more blood out through the vertebrals.[32]

It also seems that brain drains may work less well with age, especially if the person has cerebrovascular disease. Sclerosis of the arteries can reduce blood flow into, and therefore through, the brain. Stiffer arteries are less able to drive blood through them by contracting and then relaxing, and this pulsation is also thought to be what drives the glymphatic flow. When the brain's arteries become less energetic at flushing material through, so do its sewers. That makes harmful deposits—for example, of cholesterol or amyloid—more likely to build up.[33] Moreover, as Aβ accumulates around blood vessels—a condition called cerebral amyloid angiopathy, which is common in dementia—it also blocks its own exit routes from the brain.[34] Damage to blood vessels correlates well with cognitive problems.

The idea of blocked brain drains as a cause of Alzheimer's is appealing—so extra scrutiny is called for!—not least because it fits with research associating disturbed sleep with increased risk of dementia. People in whose brains amyloid is building up report sleep disturbance before they report cognitive problems, sometimes years before; it is also a common feature of diabetes. Shift work, late-night screen-watching, even over-lit bedrooms have all been targeted as potential contributors to poor-quality sleep; and quality matters more than quantity for your daily bout of sweet unconsciousness. High levels of the hormone orexin, which regulates sleep, have been implicated.[35] Animal studies applying orexin, or depriving the animal of sleep, found raised brain amyloid levels. Moreover, a small study of Alzheimer's patients and controls found higher brain orexin (and poorer sleep) in the patients.[36] So perhaps sleep problems lead to less efficient drainage, and hence to Aβ build-up and, eventually, damage to blood vessels and white matter, reducing the supply of fuel to neurons and damaging their axons and synapses. That's the theory. We await the required experiments on human volunteers.

Deportation

Apart from flushing out protein undesirables at night, brains have also evolved ways of deporting them. Specialized escort molecules such as ApoE and ABC transporter proteins bind Aβ and eject it into the bloodstream, where it is swept back to the liver and there destroyed.[37] It is thought that much Aβ may be cleared this way.

Destruction

Molecules that are not deported face execution by enzyme inside and outside cells. Most tau protein, for example, is taken back into cells for dismemberment into its constituent amino acids, which are then recycled. Aβ can likewise be chewed up this way, but it is also destroyed by extracellular proteins. Neurons are not the only cells to get rid of Aβ; astrocytes can also ingest and digest it. Microglia, the brain's immune cells, can take up and destroy Aβ when immune receptors on their surface are stimulated, and they can engulf and consume cells damaged by protein aggregates.[38] Problems with both internal and external waste disposal have been genetically linked to Alzheimer's, and if clearance of abnormal proteins is the central problem in dementia, as many researchers think, it is essential to understand how waste disposal works in the brain, and where it fails.

Internal Waste Disposal

Cells have three waste disposal systems. The first is autophagy. The term is Greek for 'self-eating': not common even in the ancient world, but in Ovid's *Metamorphoses* a king who offends the goddess of the harvest is punished by being made so hungry that he eventually eats himself, 'little by little'.[39] Autophagy is especially good at disposing of proteins like Aβ. The unwanted material is packaged into specialized vesicles called autophagosomes, which are then converted to lysosomes. These lipid bubbles enclose an acidic interior which contains protein-cleaving enzymes—proteases—such as cathepsins, whose levels are known to be altered in Alzheimer's brains.[40] Like internet trolls, proteases are activated by acid.[41] Lysosomes, like the (even more acidic) human stomach, break matter into pieces.

A second, linked system is used to get rid of unwanted proteins without employing autophagosomes. It involves specialist 'chaperone' proteins, which bind to the target and then transfer it directly to a lysosome. Among these chaperones are a family of proteins called 'heat shock' proteins (HSPs)—so called because they are produced by cells which get too hot.[42] HSPs have many roles, protecting the cell against 'hypoxia, ischemia, inflammation, and exposure to such cellular toxins as heavy metals, endotoxins, and reactive oxygen species' as well as high temperatures.[43] These versatile proteins also have another function. They help to sort out protein tangles—such as amyloid and tau aggregates—disentangling them to keep cells tidy.[44] HSPs have been implicated in neurodegeneration: research suggests that their levels may be lower, and drugs which boost their production appear able to dissolve abnormal protein aggregates in animal models. Such drugs are currently being explored for human use.

The third system, which targets mainly used, short-lived or misfolded proteins in the cell, is called the ubiquitin-proteasome system (UPS). A protein is doomed by being tagged for destruction: this is done by attaching a chain of ubiquitin molecules. These small proteins, named for their 'ubiquitous' presence in different cell types, then interact with the cell's protein-crunching mechanics, the proteasome, delivering the protein to its fate.

That the UPS is essential for brain health is clear from the rare genetic syndrome Machado-Joseph disease, a form of spinocerebellar ataxia. (Having any kind of SCA makes speech, balance, and movement increasingly wearisome and difficult, eventually confining the sufferer to a wheelchair; basic capacities like eating and drinking are also affected.) Machado-Joseph disease is caused by a faulty gene for a protein called Josephin, which regulates the UPS.[45]

Abnormal Josephin is also of interest in neurodegeneration for another reason. Like Aβ, it is an amyloid protein, and its aggregates are what trigger the SCA process. Neurodegeneration, therefore, need not be caused by Aβ: other proteins can also be a problem. Of this more later.

Autophagy, chaperones, and the UPS may be among the biochemical systems that weaken with age, and especially with dementia.[46] Attempts to boost their function in animal models have shown some promise in reducing neurodegeneration, though this is research in its early stages. Of course, cellular waste disposal doesn't happen in a vacuum. It is influenced by many other systems, from intracellular signalling to activation of surface receptors to changes in gene expression. It is this interconnectedness and multiplicity that makes the science of Alzheimer's so hard.

Outside the Cell

There are also extracellular enzymes, which can directly break down Aβ proteins. Among them are neprilysin, angiotensin-converting enzyme (ACE), and insulin-degrading enzyme. All three have been genetically linked to Alzheimer's, and the last two are also important in the metabolism of two major hormones, angiotensin and insulin. Any attempt to improve or stall dementia by targeting amyloid degradation must therefore be done with great care, for fear of side effects. As with Aβ's birth, its death illustrates the complex network of interactions in which it is embedded.

That vast complexity offers both danger and hope to researchers, clinicians, and their patients. The danger is that the difficulty of understanding, coupled with the desperate need to help patients, may lead to possible treatments being tested without their implications being understood. If the treatment succeeds, great. With Alzheimer's, however, potential treatments so far have had only modest effects; and some have done serious harm.

Even small benefits may help; and for dementia, small benefits are all we currently have. However, these must be weighed against the costs, both financial and personal. Dementia treatments can have nasty side effects. The popular drug Aricept, for instance, can cause diarrhoea, vomiting, and fainting: not as bad as dementia, of course, but then again, dementia patients have plenty to deal with already.

The same complexity that makes treatments so unpredictable, however, also means that neurodegenerative disorders are influenced by very many factors. This offers hope that we may be able to identify ways of reducing their prevalence that do not require invasive, potentially dangerous drugs: lifestyle, environmental, perhaps even social changes. Preventative medicine is part of this great endeavour, but it may also be possible to find ways of making life better for current patients as well as future ones.

To do this, we need to understand which risk factors make getting dementia more likely, and which protective factors lower its probability. Epidemiology—the science of who gets what illnesses and which factors are associated with which diseases—provides the suspects. This fascinating, difficult, and expensive science is our next topic.

PART 2

Risk Factors

...to preserve a man alive in the midst of so many chances and hostilities, is as great a miracle as to create him.

Jeremy Taylor, *Holy Living and Holy Dying*[1]

10

Interpreting Risk Factors

 News headlines often report on health risks. Here's an example from the *Washington Post*:

Study: Having just one drink doubles your risk of getting injured.[1]

Before we delve into the risk factors for Alzheimer's disease we need to look more closely at statements of this kind. They seem obvious, but their simplicity is deceptive.

For one thing, although it says 'your risk', it's extremely unlikely that you took part in the research. The scientists studied a group of people and derived the claim that when those people drank more alcohol they were more likely to get injured. (Who knew?) The implication is that this applies more generally, which is why the newspaper is applying the claim to all its readers. But readers—like drinks—vary greatly. Confirmed alcoholics drinking alone in the countryside run different risks from teenage novices out with their friends in a crowded city centre.

Note too that risks are often relative, as in the *Post*'s example. Your risk is doubled, it says. Compared to what? That is the crucial question, often left unanswered in health reporting.[2] In the original study the authors note that 'injured patients' alcohol consumption within 6 hours prior to injury is compared to their own alcohol consumption during the same time-period the previous week'. (In case you're wondering, the researchers also note as a limitation of their study the chance that participants might not have been able to recall their drinking accurately.)

The study does not give data about the baseline risk of getting injured, only about how much more likely injuries are after too much alcohol. Yet baseline risks matter. Clearly, a doubling of risk for something which normally affects one in ten people—to one in five—and the same change for a one-in-ten-million occurrence have very different implications, both for public health and for your individual chance of being affected.

To know how risk factors for dementia change your absolute risk of getting the disease, therefore, you would have to know your baseline risk. As we shall see, research can offer educated guesses about both baseline and additional risks. They are only guesses because of the complexity of the science, and because it deals in claims about studied groups, not unexamined individuals. That is, such claims apply to you insofar as you match the people in the groups in all relevant respects. Unfortunately, we don't yet know what all the relevant respects are. Having ApoE4 boosts the risk of dementia, for example, but drawing that gene card does not ensure your doom. You have many other risk and protective factors that can interact with ApoE and alter its effects on your body and brain.[3]

Too Much to Study

Epidemiology makes great headlines, but it is one of the murkier branches of medical research. Looking for connections, it is prone to seeing ones that aren't really there: statistical links which, on further examination, turn out not to be real.

Part of the problem is that there are so many potentially relevant covariates, and studies vary greatly in whether and how they take account of them.[4] For example, in Chapter 17 we'll encounter a meta-analysis of research on smoking and dementia (Cataldo et al., 2010).[5] A meta-analysis is a 'study of studies' that pulls together data from earlier articles; and as part of their work Cataldo and her colleagues list the covariates (variables other than smoking data and dementia status) recorded by each of the studies they assess. These range from age only—a poor effort!—to age, year of birth, ApoE status, BMI, blood pressure, cholesterol, vitamin E, alcohol intake, physical activity, total energy intake, history of cardiovascular disease, vitamin supplement intake, and education.

Needless to say, measuring all of these thirteen covariates is a good deal more time-consuming and expensive than simply asking people how old they are. This could be why Cataldo and colleagues found that only one of their forty-three studies took so many covariates into account; the other forty-two had seven covariates or fewer.

Defining what is being studied. As well as the problem of too many variables, studies are beset by differences in measurement and diagnosis. I have already mentioned that dementia is assessed in more than one way. The same is true of physical activity, diet, obesity, and medical history, to name a few important covariates.

Getting enough people to study. Problems with sample size are also common: understandably, since larger studies cost more. If the sample is too small, however, the study will simply not have the statistical power to detect significant relationships between variables properly. As a result, it may see relationships where none exist. It may also fail to represent the population it is sampling accurately enough to justify extending its conclusions to everyone in that population. For example, religiosity, lack of ambition, and not having a good relationship with one's mother have all been linked to dementia—in studies done on men. Even without such restrictions, many studies rely on volunteers: often people who are university students, have health concerns, or have time on their hands. Like readers of the *Washington Post*, these participants are not typical of the general populace.

Getting the result more than once. Replication of research—a scientific ideal more honoured in the breach than in the observance—is also a problem. Small, underpowered studies hinting at startling connections may suit sensationalist media outlets, but the promised link often fails to materialize in later research. (Then people complain that health science is contradictory.) So why do scientists bother doing small studies? Because they're cheaper and easier, and because funding agencies being asked to cough up for a large and well-controlled study like to see pre-existing evidence that the hypothesis being tested is worth pursuing.

Reverse causality. With complex conditions like dementia there is another complication: co-morbidity—that is, co-occurring medical conditions. For instance, cerebrovascular disease could be a risk factor for dementia; but it could also have been caused by the same underlying process (e.g. the build-up of Aβ). Indeed, conceivably both could be the case. This is especially problematic in dementia because changes are thought to take hold decades before the disease becomes clinically obvious. This long subclinical prelude can confuse cause and effect, a problem known as 'reverse causality'.

Here's an example. Studies have found that retirees who left work later and who developed dementia tended to be diagnosed after longer periods than those who retired more promptly. Should we conclude that working for longer maintains a healthily active brain? Perhaps—if we have ruled out other explanations. One is selection bias: people who choose to work for longer tend to be healthier. Another is reverse causality. Instead of later retirement delaying dementia onset, perhaps the beginnings of dementia caused some people to retire early.

Despite their disadvantages, epidemiological studies are needed because—thankfully—scientists are limited in what they can do to human beings. Many experiments that might establish causality would be unethical, as they would involve deliberately giving people Alzheimer's disease. Epidemiological studies can establish correlations between variables. In doing so, they point to factors worthy of further investigation by other means, such as animal models, stem cells, or bigger, better, and longer studies on people. Causal links are more difficult to establish, and the gold standard for them would be a randomized controlled trial, which is extremely costly.

From Quality to Quantity

The caveats that apply to the statistical detection of relationships between variables only intensify when scientists turn from the question of whether the relationship exists at all to the question of working out how strong it is. For example, if you go online you will find various sources offering risk calculators for various illnesses. I tested one for a medical condition that I happen to have and it assured me that my risk was low. This made me somewhat sceptical of the genre; it may be worth keeping a doubtful eyebrow poised to lift. All risk estimates should be taken with a large, albeit entirely metaphorical, pinch of salt.

That includes estimates from published scientific papers. For example, a study of home or workplace exposure to cigarette smoke found that it raised the risk of dementia by seventy-eight per cent.[6] Yet the equivalent increase in risk from actually dragging on the cancer sticks themselves has been estimated at twenty-seven per cent by a meta-analysis.[7] This seems unlikely. In general, risks are likely to be exaggerated, as noted by a commentary in the British Medical Journal which is well worth reading.[8] Even meta-analyses should not be taken as gospel. Repeated meta-analyses...well, maybe then our eyebrows can relax.

Dissecting the Numbers

So how do researchers measure risk?

Look at the article reported by the Washington Post, and the abstract mentions 'injury risk doubling at one drink [odds ratio (OR) = 2.3–2.7]'.[9] This introduces a common way of measuring risk: the odds ratio. An odds ratio of two or thereabouts is interpreted as meaning 'double the risk'. An odds ratio of one represents no more risk, an odds ratio of 0.5 represents half the risk, and so on.[10]

To see how to calculate an odds ratio, here is a made-up case. Suppose you want to know whether eating broccoli in childhood is a risk factor for getting Alzheimer's later. Luckily, you have a sample of people who, sixty years ago, filled in a form at school about their eating habits, and you have followed them up to see how many have developed dementia. You have identified 1,000 broccoli lovers and 2,000 who never touched the stuff. They do not differ significantly on any of the other variables you have chosen to measure (this is an imaginary study, remember). Of the veg fans,

100 have been diagnosed with Alzheimer's and 900 are well. Of those who missed out on the joys of broccoli, 500 are ill and 1,500 are well.

What is the odds ratio of getting Alzheimer's if you didn't, or did, eat broccoli? As the name suggests, it is the ratio of the odds that the 600 Alzheimer sufferers didn't eat broccoli to the odds that the 2,400 healthy people didn't. The odds of a patient not eating broccoli versus eating it are 500:100, (or 5 to 1). The equivalent odds for healthy people are 1,500:900 (1.67 to 1). So the odds ratio is 5/1.67, or 3, telling you that anti-broccolarians are three times (300%) more likely to get Alzheimer's than their veg-munching peers. Equivalently, eating broccoli—in this example—reduces the risk of Alzheimer's to a third (i.e. by 67%) of the risk for people who don't eat broccoli.[11]

Now that we have had a look at the statistics used to quantify and compare risks, let's look at some of the risk factors for dementia.

11

The Inescapables—Age,
Gender, and Genes

B rains are vulnerable to many forms of damage, internal and external. Some of
these, as we shall see, can be avoided or their risks reduced. Such modifiable
risk factors offer many options for lowering the likelihood of getting dementia.
There are some factors, however, which cannot be so easily adjusted. Ageing, gender, and genetic make-up all have a big influence on dementia risk.[1] Let's look at
these in turn.

Getting Old

...people are living longer—by about 30 years—than they did in Alzheimer's day

Claudia Kawas and Maria Corrada,
'Alzheimer's and dementia in the oldest-old'[2]

This is the big one (see Figure 7). At ages sixty-five to sixty-nine, the prevalence of
dementia is estimated by the Alzheimer's Society at somewhat under two in every
hundred.[3] Ten years later, at seventy-five to seventy-nine, it has tripled to six per hundred (6%). By ages eighty-five to eighty-nine it has tripled again to about eighteen per
cent, nearly one-fifth; and from there to age ninety-five and older it more than doubles, to forty-one per cent.

Put another way, nearly three-fifths of people aged ninety-five or over will not
have dementia, but that leaves an awful lot of people who will.

Hope You Die Before You Get Old?

Since the biggest risk factor for dementia is growing older, the first step in trying to
assess your risk is to ask how likely you are to reach old age. The answer is: very,

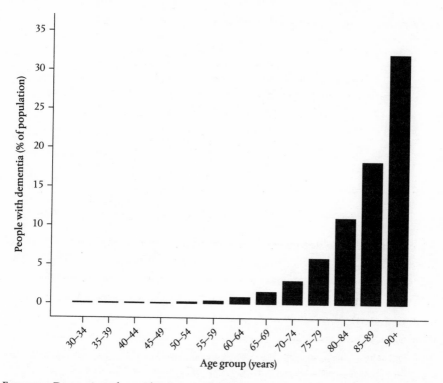

FIGURE 7: Dementia and age. The estimated percentage of people with dementia, relative to the total UK population, for each 5-year age group from 30 to 90 and older. Data on dementia prevalence are taken from a 2014 Alzheimer's Society report; population data are from the Office for National Statistics for 2013. From the seventh decade onwards dementia becomes much more common.

and the younger you are, the better your chances. Death rates rise considerably past age eighty-five, yet in Britain, around half of 2014's babies are expected to make it to age ninety-five. According to the latest available UK government data, ninety-five of every hundred baby girls born in the year 2014 will reach age sixty-five. Beyond that, eighty will see their eighty-fifth birthdays and fifty-six their ninety-fifth. For baby boys the numbers are ninety-three, seventy-two, and forty-seven, respectively (see Table 2). Put another way, life expectancy for girls born in 2014 was almost eighty-three years, and for boys just over seventy-nine years.[4] For comparison, US life expectancy in 2014 was eighty-one years for girls and seventy-seven years for boys; while life expectancy in Malawi, ranked by the World Bank as the poorest country in the world, was sixty-four years for girls and sixty-two years for boys.[5]

Table 2: Percentage of people expected to reach ages 65+ in the UK

		% of men surviving to age			
Age in 2014	Birth year	65	75	85	95
0	2014	92.6	85.7	71.7	47.2
20	1994	90.4	81.9	65.3	38.3
40	1974	86.7	76.4	57.2	29.0
60	1954	82.3	69.9	48.3	20.3
		% of women surviving to age			
Age in 2014	Birth year	65	75	85	95
0	2014	95.3	90.6	79.8	56.3
20	1994	93.9	88.0	74.9	48.1
40	1974	91.4	84.2	68.6	38.9
60	1954	88.1	79.1	60.9	29.6

Table 2 shows life expectancy data for the United Kingdom, separately for males and females. Data are shown for four ages: nought, twenty, forty, and sixty, and are as of 2014. The first two columns give the age and equivalent birth year; the other four columns give the percentages of individuals of that age/birth year who are expected to survive to the ages of sixty-five, seventy-five, eighty-five, and ninety-five.

For those of us born somewhat before 2014, the chances of reaching old age are lower, as shown in Table 2 for UK twenty-, forty-, and sixty-year-olds. Just over one-fifth of men, and nearly one-third of women born in 1954 can expect to reach age ninety-five.

No wonder experts are worried about the implications of people living longer. Paradoxically, older people are generally at *less* risk of getting dementia than the young, unless they are already approaching their seventh decade, because they are more likely to die before they reach the age when dementia risk rises fastest. We can get a feel for the data by taking current figures for dementia prevalence and combining these with the likelihood of survival. (This assumes that nothing changes over the next century: no cures, no reduction in risk factors, no apocalypse wiping out chunks of the population.)

The resulting estimates of the chance of getting dementia, for different age groups, are shown in Table 3, and they show how the risk generally decreases for currently older people. A sixty-year-old man in 2014 has a little less than half the risk of having dementia at age ninety-five, compared with his newborn grandson; but then he has less than half the baby's chance of reaching that age. The picture for the other half of the population is similar: a sixty-year-old woman will have a little over half the risk of her newborn granddaughter.

Table 3 also illustrates the logic behind attempts to delay the onset of dementia. With even a year or two's delay, the grim reaper will remove more people from the pool of potential patients before they fall ill.

Why does age have so profound an impact on the brain and body? The glib answer is that life's wear and tear is responsible; but what does the wearing and tearing? Why does the body's capacity to maintain itself weaken as we grow older, its systems becoming ever less efficient until they fail catastrophically?

Table 3: Percentage of people expected to get dementia in the UK

		% of men with dementia at age			
Age in 2014	Birth year	65–69	75–79	85–89	95+
0	2014	1.39	4.54	10.83	13.59
20	1994	1.36	4.34	9.86	11.04
40	1974	1.30	4.05	8.64	8.36
60	1954	1.23	3.71	7.29	5.86
		% of women with dementia at age			
Age in 2014	Birth year	65–69	75–79	85–89	95+
0	2014	1.71	5.98	16.12	24.90
20	1994	1.69	5.81	15.14	21.24
40	1974	1.65	5.56	13.85	17.21
60	1954	1.59	5.22	12.29	13.08

Table 3 shows calculated estimates of the percentage of individuals in the United Kingdom who are expected to develop dementia. As in Table 2, data are shown separately for males and females, and apply to people who were nought, twenty, forty, or sixty years of age in 2014 (age and birth year are shown in the two left-hand columns). Estimates are given for the likelihood of having dementia between the ages of sixty-five and sixty-nine, seventy-five and seventy-nine, eighty-five and eighty-nine, and ninety-five or older (shown in the four columns on the right). They were calculated by combining the life expectancy data in Table 2 with 2014 data on dementia prevalence in the United Kingdom from the Alzheimer's Society (see the main text for details).

DNA Damage and Repair

One major reason is that gene expression alters as we age. This is not least because DNA suffers damage from many sources, including ultraviolet light (hence skin cancer) and other ionizing radiation (hence the rise in thyroid cancer after the Chernobyl nuclear accident). Like epigenetic changes made by the cell's normal mechanisms, damage can change the DNA's chemistry, and hence its function. As a review in the journal *Neuron* puts it, 'All biological macromolecules are susceptible to corruption'; but corrupted proteins, membranes, and organelles can be replaced, to some extent. DNA must be repaired.[6]

And there is a lot of damage to repair. Estimates suggest that on any given day the number of wounds inflicted on a cell's DNA purely by internal events—by the business of metabolism—may be between 100,000 and 120,000.[7] Add the effects of ionizing radiation, drugs and food, air pollution, and other environmental damage, and the need for specialized DNA repair systems is clear.

Cells have a variety of such systems, involving thousands of proteins. They need to be fast, accurate, and capable of identifying and accessing damaged areas. This is no simple task, since the roughly three billion base pairs of human DNA which make up our twenty-three pairs of chromosomes share with computer cables the irrepressible urge to tangle and curl. Some areas of the genome, however, appear to be particularly vulnerable to DNA damage.

On the ends of chromosomes sit telomeres, sections of genetic material which shorten with age, so much so that their length can serve as a measure of cellular ageing. A study in mice was able to show that artificially inflicted DNA damage caused cells to show features of ageing, and that telomeres were especially likely to be the focus of such damage.[8] Such features included damaged mitochondria and also 'senescence markers'—the cellular equivalent of liver spots, slowed gait, and turning up the volume on the television.

Shorter telomeres and DNA damage have both been linked to diseases which cause accelerated ageing in humans, and to diseases of normal ageing. They have also been linked to severe stress and to some mental disorders, notably depression. Remarks about trauma adding years to people may now have scientific support.[9]

Scientists distinguish between biological ageing, which seems to occur at different speeds in different people, and chronological ageing. (The number on the birthday card may not match the telomeres' records.) Biological ageing is the risk factor for dementia. A 2015 study in young people noted that 'Already, before midlife, individuals who were aging more rapidly were less physically able, showed cognitive decline and brain aging, self-reported worse health, and looked older.'[10] The role of DNA damage and telomere shortening, and how to reduce these, is thus of great interest to dementia researchers.

Another study showed that artificially extending cells' telomeres caused them to proliferate—to make more of themselves, indicating youthful vigour.[11] Before you conclude that scientists have found the key to immortality, the work was done on cultured cells, not on people (cultured or otherwise). Besides, immortality isn't always a good thing; cancer cells are immortal. Furthermore, the cells did eventually stop dividing and display senescence markers. Ageing cannot be so easily escaped.

Neurons are among the more vulnerable parts of the body when it comes to DNA damage. They are highly active—activity which produces many molecules capable of damaging DNA. Animal studies have suggested that certain kinds of DNA damage are found very early in neurodegeneration. This implies that gene trouble may be among its first events.[12]

Mutations in DNA repair genes have also been linked to neurodegenerative conditions, as well as to accelerated ageing syndromes—some of which also involve severe neurodevelopmental and cognitive problems. The importance of having effective DNA repair systems is cruelly demonstrated by these conditions. An example is early-onset Cockayne syndrome, which leads to problems including deafness, small brain and body size, delayed development, extreme sensitivity to light, muscle and movement problems, and greatly reduced life expectancy. Such mutations are horrible tragedies for those affected. Children with the most severe form of Cockayne syndrome generally don't survive for more than five years.

Growth and Ageing

One source of errors in DNA is the process of cell division and replication. This is a particular problem as organisms age, because cell division is always risky, and life's wear and tear increases the error rate.

When I first learned about cells (ah, the joys of meiosis and mitosis in school biology!) they were presented in a very child-centric way, in that the exciting events took place during development. Adult cells settled down and got on with their boringly adult jobs. (Except for neurons, the body's privileged media outlets, which from cradle to deathbed were thrillingly full of chatter and activity.)

It is now clear, however, that adulthood need not mean stasis. Immature cells 'differentiate' into their mature forms by passing through a set of stages—which varies by cell type—but adult cells can also enter a variety of states. Immune cells such as microglia, for example, can become activated in response to immune signals, entering a state of defensive readiness. Some cells can even re-enter mitosis, which is part of the cell cycle by which cells divide and proliferate. The cell cycle underlies our transformation from minuscule blobs to multi-trillion-cell organisms, by way of individual cells repeatedly splitting into pairs.[13]

Human cells can divide around fifty times—unless they have become cancerous, in which case they can proliferate indefinitely.[14] Blood, skin, and immune cells are prolific dividers, as they need to be. Neurons, by contrast, are generally thought of as post-mitotic: no longer dividing, they must last a lifetime. However, recent evidence suggests that under extreme stress they can be prompted to re-enter the cell cycle. Stressors include a reduction in blood supply or damage to blood vessels, chronically high levels of neural activity (e.g. in epilepsy or early Alzheimer's), UV radiation or chemical poisoning, high levels of pro-inflammatory cytokines, and oxidative stress (of which more shortly).[15] Unsurprisingly, the number of neurons re-entering the cell cycle rises with age. Equally unsurprisingly, cell cycle problems have been found in Alzheimer's—and they occur before the accumulation of amyloid plaques.

When a stressed or ageing neuron re-enters the cell cycle, something goes wrong; exactly what is not yet fully understood. The cell gets stuck in an intermediate state, unable either to exit the cycle or complete it by dividing into daughters. In experiments, the addition of growth factors which would normally prompt a cell to complete its division has no effect. Such cells are senescent. They can be distinguished from other cells because they have different proteins—senescence markers—on their surfaces.

Senescent cells can still function, for a while. Indeed, they may swell in size; a study comparing neurons from Alzheimer and control brains found that the former were roughly ten per cent larger.[16] They may also secrete more proteins than usual into the extracellular environment. (If they are immune cells, like brain microglia, those proteins will include pro-inflammatory cytokines, stressing nearby cells and potentially pushing them towards senescence; cell hands on misery to cell.) Over time, the swollen cells start to deteriorate, with failing mitochondria, damage to the cell membrane and cytoskeleton, and rising levels of cellular waste. Neurons lose their connections: synapses and dendrites die off and axons fail. Eventually the cell disintegrates.

With every division a healthy cell's telomeres shorten, and eventually it too enters a senescent state. But the fact that certain stressors can induce premature senescence independently of telomere shortening has made senescence of great interest to researchers studying neurodegeneration. Senescence can affect many cell types; but neurons are long-lived, whereas many other cells can die and be replaced. One might therefore expect cellular ageing to have a particular impact in the brain. And indeed, studies have found signs of increased senescence, in both neurons and glia, early on in neurodegenerative diseases like Alzheimer's. This may mean that premature senescence is contributing to neurodegeneration, and that finding ways to stop it might lead to new treatments for dementia.

Failing Power Supplies

Another source of cell damage and death in ageing is problems with energy. A continuous energy supply is critical for the brain, and newer theories of Alzheimer's implicate failures in that supply, arguing that neurons effectively die of starvation. To understand dementia, therefore, we need to know how brain cells get their energy.

Carbohydrates, fats, and proteins can all be used for energy. The body tends to use carbohydrate when available, then fat, then protein if necessary, metabolizing them to glucose, used by all cells to generate energy. Glucose is then transported across the blood–brain barrier to brain cells.

We pay for the energy which powers our many gadgets, but waving a ten-pound note at a kettle won't make it boil. Instead we give money to companies which provide us with electricity. Likewise, our blood delivers glucose to intracellular processes which provide the cell with energy stored in a molecule called adenosine trisphosphate (ATP). ATP's structure includes a chain of three linked phosphate groups, and the bonds between these release significant amounts of energy when they are broken.[17] When an enzyme chops off the third phosphate group, the bond is broken and its energy released to drive many processes.

When ATP loses its third phosphate it becomes ADP (adenosine diphosphate). To keep the cell going, its ADP must be converted back into ATP, which itself requires energy. The job is done by three interlocking processes: glycolysis, which happens in the cell's cytoplasm, and two mitochondrial processes: the Krebs cycle and the electron transport chain.

Glycolysis, 'sugar-splitting', takes place in the cytoplasm, and it converts glucose into a versatile molecule called pyruvate, which can provide fuel for neurons.[18] (I think of pyruvate as neural brandy, since the word comes from the Greek for 'fiery' and the Latin for 'grape'; but that's by the by.) Pyruvate is also used to make two other key molecules, both suspects in dementia: cholesterol and acetyl-CoA.[19] Cholesterol is needed for cell membranes, so if at-risk brains are taking up less glucose for years before the signs of dementia appear, as researchers think may be the case, this could affect not only cells' energy budgets but their essential maintenance and repairs. Acetyl-CoA is required for many biochemical processes, including the production of the neurotransmitter acetylcholine, so cells using acetylcholine might be particularly impaired by lack of glucose; and as we have seen, such cells are early casualties in Alzheimer's.

Acetyl-CoA is taken up by mitochondria, where it is used in the second stage of cellular energy production, the Krebs cycle.[20] This produces carbon dioxide, water, intermediate molecules such as NADH (needed for the third stage of production), and ATP.[21]

The final stage of energy production, the electron transport chain, is yet another demonstration of the primal importance to biology of being able to relocate electrical charges. It takes electrons from NADH and passes them along a chain of complicated proteins embedded in the inner of the two mitochondrial membranes. The effect is to build up positive electric charge between the two membranes, and at the end of the chain that stored energy is used to power the conversion of ADP back to ATP.[22] Oxygen is needed for this process.

Mitochondria are organelles with an unusual double membrane. They also have their own DNA. Scientists speculate that, long ago, a single-celled organism engulfed a smaller colleague and found that doing so was good for both of them: one offered protection, the other some useful new biochemistry. Now mitochondrial DNA is passed from mother to child. Cells make as many mitochondria as they need to service their energy demands, and transport them to where they are required; but mitochondria seem to become less efficient as we get older. Some researchers think that mitochondrial dysfunction is a major cause, perhaps even *the* cause, of Alzheimer's.

Consistent with this, it seems that the risk of getting dementia is higher if your mother has it than if your father does. Furthermore, genetic variants in mitochondrial proteins have been linked to stroke and to changes in the rate at which people progress from normal cognitive function, through mild cognitive impairment, to Alzheimer's (they are also linked to the rare, devastating disorders which researchers hope to treat with so-called 'three-parent' embryo techniques).[23] Mitochondria contain the γ-secretase enzyme which releases Aβ from APP, and Aβ, tau, and excitotoxicity all seem to impair mitochondrial function.

As well as using glucose and oxygen to produce ATP, mitochondria make other things, among them reactive oxygen species (ROS). The production of ROS increases with age and also when mitochondria—or people—are unwell. This is of great interest to researchers working on ageing and the brain, for two reasons. First, neurons need a lot of energy. They can't survive long without glucose and oxygen; this is why speed is crucial in treating stroke patients. Secondly, one of the most relentless triggers of cell cycle re-entry and DNA damage—and a major suspect in ageing and dementia—is oxidative stress. And that involves ROS.

Oxidative Stress

Many cellular reactions, including those of mitochondria, make ROS. Oxygen is a key fuel, but it is a dangerous friend to cells because it is a highly reactive atom, hungry for the two electrons it needs to attain stability.[24] It readily engages with other molecules to form ROS, so its use in cells must be tightly regulated to prevent excessive ROS production.[25] These lively molecules include free radicals, the bodily scourges you are encouraged to suppress by taking anti-oxidants like vitamin C, eating fruit, and drinking red wine rather than strong spirits (though that last exhortation may also have other rationales).[26] The best-known ROS is probably hydrogen peroxide, H_2O_2, used the world over for everything from bleaching hair to disinfection to teeth whitening.

Apparently hydrogen peroxide is also good for removing earwax. Given the importance of oxidative stress in dementia, Alois Alzheimer would surely have been intrigued at this link between his two interests.

Anything that can bleach hair or dissolve earwax is clearly a force to be reckoned with, but ROS have other roles than as agents of biochemical apocalypse. They are important signals of cellular health. For example, hydrogen peroxide released from damaged neurons appears to act as an 'alarmin', triggering healing responses in nearby cells. When mitochondria begin to fail, their ROS production rises, and so does cell damage.

ROS, as the name suggests, are prolific sources of oxidative stress.[27] Stripping electrons from other molecules, they alter their electrical forces, their shape, and their behaviour. The resulting damage accumulates with age and seems to play a major part in both depression and diseases of ageing, including dementia, Parkinson's disease, and stroke. Oxidative stress has been shown to shorten telomeres and to be triggered by environmental pollutants like car emissions and cigarette smoke. ROS are also increased by infection and by other stresses such as UV radiation, low oxygen levels (hypoxia), and certain drugs. If your tan has left you wrinkled, blame oxidative stress.

ROS greedily bind to fatty acids, proteins, and nucleotides. Of the 100,000 or more daily assaults on DNA, at least four-fifths are thought to be oxidative events. Oxidative stress can thus affect gene expression and numerous biochemical pathways, as well as damaging structures like mitochondria and cell membranes.

When ROS levels rise too high for too long, overwhelming a cell's anti-oxidant capacities, they can trigger cell death. This capacity to kill is used by immune cells to attack pathogens as part of the inflammatory response to infection. (Inflammation and oxidative stress are closely related.) Activated immune cells can produce a pulse of ROS called a respiratory burst: chemical warfare which sprays the enemy with the cellular equivalent of strong bleach. As in war, collateral damage is inevitable, so more inflammation is likely to create more oxidative stress.

Cells have evolved a range of methods for mopping up ROS and repairing the damage they do, including damage to DNA. Enzymes like superoxide dismutase and anti-oxidants like glutathione and vitamins C and E bind to ROS and neutralize their impact. Oxidative wear and tear, however, builds up with age, while cellular systems for controlling ROS grow weaker—not least because they are themselves damaged by oxidative stress.

This is why moisturizers promising 'younger-looking skin' contain anti-oxidants, and why health food shops sell glutathione. Large industries have formed on the assumption that artificially supplying these molecules will help repair oxidative damage. So far, the evidence of effectiveness is weak, especially when it comes to staving off Alzheimer's. Fruit and vegetables, however, are also good sources of anti-oxidants, and the evidence for their benefits is stronger, as we shall see.

Damage repair is hard work and makes considerable energy demands on cells. This may make neurons particularly vulnerable to problems with energy supply. They have weaker anti-oxidant capacities than many other cells, putting them at greater risk of oxidative damage; and they are avid consumers of brain fuel to run their communications.[28] Furthermore, a study of cultured neurons and glia derived from human stem cells found that adding Aβ oligomers to the culture reduced their energy metabolism and glucose usage.[29] Thus amyloid may starve brain cells of the energy they need.

Being Female

Given how many reasons there still are for not wanting to be a woman in this world, you might think that an increased risk of dementia is the least of ladies' worries. The gender gap is, however, noticeable: by age eighty, according to the Alzheimer's Society's 2014 report, for every two men there will be three women with dementia. Figure 8 shows how the prevalence of dementia changes beyond the age of sixty-five for men and women.

(For any women readers demoralized by this information, it could be worse, and it has been. Historians think that some of the victims of the Western mediaeval witch hunts may have been suffering from dementia. At least European states no longer sanction the burning of unwanted elderly women.)

There has been much discussion of sex-related factors which might enhance female susceptibility to dementia. These include biological differences between the sexes (e.g. in immune function, susceptibility to stress, and levels of sex hormones) which might be modifiable with treatment. They also include gender-related cultural differences (e.g. in the readiness to go to a doctor, to assume cognitive incompetence in a female patient, or to put the blame on hormones), which can be rather difficult to adjust.

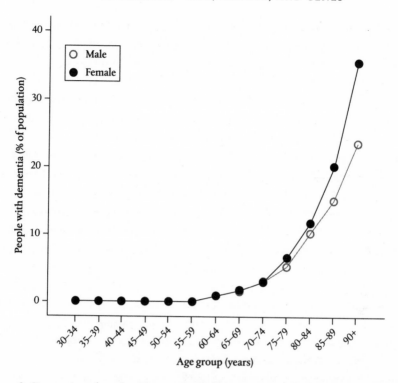

FIGURE 8: Dementia and gender. The estimated percentage with dementia is for each 5-year age group from 30 to 90 and older. Data are for the United Kingdom. The grey circles/line show the data for men; the black circles/line show the data for women. In older age groups dementia becomes noticeably more common in women than in men.

There is, however, another way of looking at this. Instead of asking what makes 'the weaker sex' succumb to dementia, we might challenge the notion of weakness. As Table 2 clearly shows, more women survive to extreme old age.[30] That advantage starts early: the risk of stillbirth in males is estimated at ten per cent higher than in females.[31]

In addition, more men die earlier from diseases which boost the risk for dementia, such as heart disease. Men who survive to old age are therefore likely to be the healthiest; this is less the case for women.

Cognitive problems are common, if not universal, in normal ageing. They seem to affect men and women similarly, at least between sixty and eighty years of age (more research is needed into the brain function of the healthy oldest old). A 2014 systematic review of the literature found that most studies detected no significant differences between the rate of cognitive decline in healthy men and women in their sixties and seventies.[32] Studies of new cases of dementia found that any sex differences were small.[33] Dementia may affect the two sexes differently, but findings vary considerably from study to study, so there is no consensus at the moment, any more than there is about sex differences in healthy brains.

This is not something you're likely to hear Alzheimer's researchers saying—especially not male ones—but there is a feeling that dementia ought to hammer women more severely, because it would make such good physiological sense. Not only do men generally have larger brains and hence more cells to start with, but men do not experience that well-known change in sex hormones known as the menopause. Testosterone does diminish with age, but not as dramatically. Oestrogen has many effects in both brain and body: two of the most significant are that it is neuroprotective and it influences glucose metabolism. Falling oestrogen levels during menopause have been linked to a rising risk of diabetes as well as of cognitive decline. This could be one reason why women get dementia more than men do.

However, if plummeting oestrogen is a major contributor to dementia, hormone replacement therapy should help prevent the disorder; and it doesn't seem to offer much benefit. At the least, this suggests that the relationship between levels of sex hormones and cognitive function is complicated, and that sex hormones may not make an enormous contribution to the risk of Alzheimer's.[34] Reality can sometimes be stubbornly gendered when we would prefer it not to be; for dementia, however, it may be that reality is less gendered than expected. The evidence is currently lacking to say definitively one way or the other.

Having Certain Gene Variants

If you worry about your memory, one question you have almost certainly pondered is whether there is any history of dementia in your family. In some cases of dementia there is a clear pattern of inheritance. Having certain rare genetic variants, for example in the genes for APP or presenilin, makes the disease inevitable—though environmental factors can still affect when it strikes. Such genetic bad luck is uncommon: a few per cent of all dementia cases. That is still a lot of suffering, especially as the disease tends to strike in midlife. In the United Kingdom more than 40,000 people are thought to have early-onset dementia.[35]

Most dementia is late-onset, striking in the seventh decade or after. Many risk factors contribute to its onset and trajectory, including multiple genes. However, this kind of dementia is termed 'sporadic' precisely because there is no clear pattern, no obvious cause. (Scientists contrast sporadic diseases with epidemic ones, which usually arise quite suddenly, spread fast, and have relatively simple causes such as pathogens. Dementia meets none of these criteria, which is why media talk of an 'epidemic of dementia' is ill judged.) The genes in which rare varieties cause familial Alzheimer's also have more common variants, but these do not seem to be linked to sporadic dementia.[36]

If you have family members with dementia, but it is not early-onset, you are still at higher risk of getting it yourself; but risk isn't certainty, even if the person who has it is your twin. Unless they were diagnosed early, your anxiety is probably better directed towards risk factors you can change instead of the genes you can't. (Until, that is, we learn how to turn those genes on and off safely and precisely; and despite all the excitement over gene editing techniques like CRISPR, that may take a while.[37])

There is one risk gene, however, that is definitely cause for concern: ApoE4. Not only does it raise the risk of Alzheimer's significantly, it also interacts with numerous lifestyle factors to increase their dangerousness. ApoE4 carriers will have to work harder at virtuous living than their luckier peers. To see why, let's take a closer look at that useful molecule, apolipoprotein E.

APOE AND CHOLESTEROL

Apolipoproteins are fat truckers.[38] Made in the liver, they transport lipids—cholesterol, triglycerides, and phospholipids, sourced mainly from dietary meat products—around the body, and, if unused, back to the liver for excretion or recycling.[39] They bind to receptors on cell surfaces, enabling the lipid molecules to be ingested. Cells use lipids for fuel if glucose is low, or for maintenance and repairs on cellular membranes.

The two most important membrane lipids are cholesterol, high levels of which are suspects in dementia and cardiovascular disease, and phospholipids, which are needed for supple cell membranes.[40] Suppleness matters because cell membranes are not static. They are constantly changing the proteins embedded in them, forming vesicles to suck material inside the cell, or fusing with vesicles to secrete material. More flexible membranes make such changes easier and cells more rapidly responsive.

The suppleness of a lipid bilayer depends on which fatty acids are in its phospholipids. If they are saturated, the phospholipid molecules are quite straight and can pack closely together, resulting in a tight but less flexible membrane. Polyunsaturated fatty acids like EPA and DHA, kinked by their plentiful double bonds, do not pack so closely, making the membrane more fluid. Thus a diet high in unsaturated fatty acids may assist your brain in other ways than by their beneficial effects on inflammation.

Cholesterol comes from your diet or is made in the liver.[41] Statins, widely prescribed for high cholesterol, inhibit its production.[42] The body uses cholesterol to make other steroid hormones, such as the glucocorticoid stress hormones and the sex hormones oestrogen and testosterone.[43] If you are a man, you also need cholesterol to make sperm, and both sexes use it to make bile. About one-quarter of your body's cholesterol, however, is not assisting your sex life or digestion, or clogging up your arteries; it is making itself extremely useful in your brain. There it is essential for signalling, repair, making myelin to keep cells insulated, and building synapses.

When apolipoproteins latch on to lipids like cholesterol they form globules of different sizes and compositions. (Your blood is full of fatballs.) The largest, chylomicrons, are mostly triglycerides. As the size shrinks the density increases, from low- to high-density lipoprotein (LDL and HDL, respectively). HDL particles, the smallest, are roughly half and half cholesterol and phospholipids, but have much less triglyceride.[44]

Larger LDL particles tend to do outward supply—transferring fat to cells— whereas HDL tends to do the recovery phase—collecting 'spare' cholesterol from the blood and returning it to the liver.

HDL is sometimes called good and LDL bad cholesterol. This is because high LDL is thought to be a risk factor for vascular and other chronic inflammatory diseases. LDL's larger lumps are more likely to stick to, and clog up, blood vessels, contributing to atherosclerosis. LDL can link up with molecules on vessel walls, and in doing so it converts to a more reactive and dangerous form, oxidized LDL (oxLDL).[45] This in turn triggers an inflammatory reaction, releasing cytokines which attract white blood cells called macrophages.[46] These hungrily suck up excess oxLDL. Macrophages bulging with fat give atherosclerosis its characteristic blubbery, foamy appearance; hence their other name, foam cells. Ingesting oxLDL stimulates them to boost their own inflammatory response.[47] The result is a spreading inflammatory sore.

ApoE, which shifts fat around the bloodstream, is the main apolipoprotein made in the brain. Neurons need a lot of fat, especially during early development when the brain is growing fast: long axons and sprouting dendrites require extensive cell membranes. Animal and cell culture studies implicate ApoE in on-going brain function and repair as well as in growth, making it relevant throughout the lifespan. It transports fat needed for neurogenesis, synaptic plasticity, membrane repair, and intracellular management (e.g. building vesicles), as well as for manufacturing useful substances like oestrogen, which is made in the brain as well as in the gonads.

(Neurogenesis, incidentally is the production of new neurons, a phenomenon once thought not to happen in human beings and now of great interest to researchers studying brain repair. Of this more later.)

After damage, ApoE is released mainly from glia, along with cholesterol. This stimulates neurons to grow new synapses and fix damaged membranes.[48] Such post-injury remodelling is vital for nerve repair. In the brain, it allows the formation of new connections which can, to some extent, compensate for permanently damaged tissue. (This is why physiotherapy is a common treatment for stroke patients. If brain cells could not form new connections, patients would be unable to recover any function; in fact they often do.)

APOE AND DISEASE

The human gene for ApoE exists in three common flavours, or alleles. Called epsilon (ε) 2, 3, and 4, they are commonly abbreviated to ApoE2, ApoE3, and ApoE4. ApoE3 is the most frequent and ApoE2 the least, though the exact proportions vary greatly across the globe.[49] The differences between them affect only two of their 299 amino acids, but the effects of those changes are considerable.[50]

ApoE4 prefers to bind with LDL; the other two prefer HDL. ApoE4 is also a less efficient cholesterol carrier, which is particularly significant for the brain. Animal research suggests that ApoE4 may damage the blood–brain barrier, unlike ApoE3. As noted earlier, ApoE4 seems to enhance the transport of Aβ into the brain while reducing its removal from brain to bloodstream. Furthermore, ApoE4's 3D structure makes it more vulnerable to having bits of itself chopped off by passing enzymes, and the resulting fragments seem to be harmful to neurons.[51]

In some populations two in three Alzheimer patients carry at least one copy of the ε4 allele, compared with perhaps one in seven of the population in general.[52] Having one copy is thought to at least double, perhaps quadruple, your risk of Alzheimer's. Having two may increase it by eightfold or more.[53] ApoE4 is by far the best-established gene for late-onset Alzheimer's, and has also been linked to early-onset forms. Having the ε4/ε4 genotype, however, does not guarantee a future with dementia.

Note that most of the research into ApoE—and indeed Alzheimer's—has been done on Western, mainly white people. Much more work is needed to understand dementia in other ethnic groups. Existing data hint that geography and race both make a difference. For example, ApoE4 prevalence seems to vary with location, being higher in very hot or cold climates. Hispanic/Latino and African/African-American samples do not show the links between ApoE4 and Alzheimer's (positive) and ApoE2 and Alzheimer's (negative) as clearly as do studies on Asians and Caucasians; and the different ethnic groups also seem to have different chances of getting dementia, even when they have equal access to health care. A recent sizeable Californian study (*n* = 274,283 people aged sixty-four or older) calculated 'the percent of individuals expected to develop dementia before death over a hypothetical follow-up period' of twenty-five years, for six ethnic groups. The figures were: '38%

African-Americans, 35% AIANs [American Indian/Alaska Native], 32% Latino, 25% Pacific Islanders, 30% white, and 28% Asian-Americans'. The reasons for this considerable variation are not yet clear.[54]

Like gender, ApoE4 does not appear to alter the speed with which Alzheimer's develops once it has been diagnosed. Being ApoE4-positive, however—and especially having copies of this allele from both parents—does seem to increase the chances both of getting it in the first place and getting it earlier. Even in elderly people without dementia, having ApoE4 is linked to higher levels of amyloid and tau in the brain. There is also some suggestion of sex differences in ApoE4's impact (in men's favour).

ApoE2, the most unusual variant, is thought to protect against Alzheimer's, nearly halving the risk of getting it.[55] Carrying two copies of ApoE2, however, can cause a rare condition called hyperlipoproteinemia type 3, in which patients have high blood levels of triglycerides, LDL, and cholesterol, often with atherosclerosis. Atherosclerosis raises the risk, among other things, of heart disease and vascular dementia. ApoE2, therefore, is not ideal.

ApoE3 is considered a neutral variant. If you have two copies of this allele, lucky you, as far as we know.

Research suggests that ApoE4's prevalence may slowly be diminishing. This may have something to do with the risk it brings of an earlier demise: a large 2014 study found that average life expectancy was about four years shorter in ε4 carriers.[56] Having ApoE4 doesn't just increase the risk for Alzheimer's. It is also linked to high cholesterol, atherosclerosis, and cerebral amyloid angiopathy; and to worse recovery from brain injury and bleeding, carbon monoxide poisoning, and perhaps chemotherapy.

People with ApoE4 may show faster shrinkage of their cortex and hippocampus. They also seem to have less efficient brains, as measured by the amount of glucose used, long before their senior years. This pattern has also been found in individuals with midlife high cholesterol or insulin resistance. As we shall see, insulin resistance is a risk factor for dementia, and some researchers think the same is true of midlife high cholesterol, although the evidence is not yet clear.

On the other hand, having ApoE4 has also been associated with better survival of some infections, like childhood dysentery, although it may increase the risk for others, like malaria. It has moreover been linked, tentatively, to higher blood levels of vitamin D and to protection against lead poisoning. These beneficial effects could help to explain ApoE4's persistence, given the impact of infections, vitamin D deficiency, and lead pollution on children—particularly poor children at high risk of malnutrition. Global estimates reckon that about 4.88 million children under five years old were killed by infectious diseases in 2010.[57] Vitamin D deficiency, which causes rickets and other bone disease, is a common problem worldwide, though more so in some countries (e.g. China, India) than others (e.g. Thailand, Japan).[58] Lead exposure, meanwhile, is linked to about 143,000 deaths per year—and many children survive with intellectual impairment.[59]

To date, the relationship between mortality and illness, ApoE, and cognition remains unclear. A study of ApoE genotypes in children from high-income families found no effects of having ApoE4 on general cognitive ability. However, other research has found that underfed survivors of childhood infections can suffer long-lasting cognitive deficits. A small study of extremely poor children in Brazil found that those with ε4 genotypes were less likely to be thus impaired.[60] Thus it may be that ApoE's effects will vary depending on how well fed the child is.

Unfortunately, there are still areas of the world where further research would be able to confirm or disprove this link.

Alleles with multiple effects are called pleiotropic, and genes which have opposing effects at different stages of life—for example, beneficial in childhood and damaging in old age—are said to show antagonistic pleiotropy. Some researchers think ApoE4 may be such a one. Historically, it offered the benefits of lower child mortality to the very poor; but as child poverty diminishes that useful role becomes less crucial. Meanwhile ApoE4's harmful impact grows as more people live longer.

Antagonistic pleiotropy has also been proposed as an explanation for Alzheimer's. One idea is that genes with mutations linked to dementia—many of which seem to have to do with cellular communication or with synapses—have brought humans extra powers of synaptic flexibility; but the price for such cognitive prowess is paid in late-life failure.[61]

Immense amounts of work have gone into studying the ApoE gene, not just because of its associations with diseases, but because its three alleles are unique to humans. Other primates have only one, similar to ApoE4, from which it seems ApoE2 and ApoE3 evolved around 200,000 years ago. This is puzzling: if ApoE4 is so dangerous, why do our closest primate relatives not succumb to atherosclerosis—or dementia? Heart disease is common among long-lived captive chimpanzees, but cardiovascular disease is rare. It is also rare among hunter-gatherer populations who eat a high-fat, mainly meat diet.[62]

The answers may lie with other factors which contribute to the harmful effects of ApoE4. There are three in particular which began affecting most of us only recently, in evolutionary terms, and their impact on human society, especially in the West, has been transformative. Hunter-gatherers and apes don't have them—although some formerly isolated tribes are now acquiring them—and only the richest few of our ancestors achieved the kinds of lifestyles they promote. Where humans do obtain them, the effects of ApoE begin to make their damaging mark.

They are the car, the personal computer, and the modern food industry, and they lead inevitably to those favourite mantras of modern health care, diet and exercise. Before we leap joyously into that quagmire, however, let us take a look at some other factors linked to dementia.

12

Injury and Surgery

Modern science teaches that the brain is part of the body and that it and other organs are interdependent. One of the aims of this book is to show how greatly affected brains—and minds—are by happenings elsewhere in the organism, and beyond.

Many people do not believe this, and even those who believe it intellectually may not feel it to be true. We experience the mind as located in the head, not the liver; on a higher plane than the wet gurglings of our viscera. Some regard their essence as nonphysical, and the body as a temporary cage. Some accept that brains give rise to selves, but seem to imagine their cerebrum as a lord in a bony castle, profiting from the slaving organs beneath but detached from them and indifferent to their privations.

But brains are neither bridges to the spirit world nor pampered parasites. They are more like hard-working managers who use others' labour but also respond to their demands. Your brain needs a healthy body: *mens sana in corpore sano*. When the *corpus* is no longer *sanus*, the *cerebrum* and the *mens* will suffer.

Damage can come from outside or from within. External attacks on our fragile brains can result from accident, malice, or sport; brute force can crack a skull, burst blood vessels, or inflict tissue-crushing pressure. Chemical assault can also do damage. Pathogens may penetrate and infect brain tissue, even occasionally taking up residence. And infections in the body may affect the brain.

Internal sources of damage are also numerous. Ageing, stress, and exposure to toxins lead to oxidative stress and inflammation, which damage both cells and their DNA—and its repair mechanisms, impairing cells' efficiency. Some mutations can lead to tumours, which in turn can crush nearby tissue as they grow.

As well as these cellular programming failures, wiring faults may arise due to white matter damage, whether from clogged-up waste or failing blood vessels. There may also be supply problems, ranging from malnutrition or lack of specific nutrients to poor blood oxygenation or delivery.

This chapter considers two kinds of external stressor that are thought to raise the risk of later dementia. We begin with the more obvious one, brain injury, and then look at one less often mentioned: medical treatment, in particular surgery.

Traumatic Brain Injury

Traumatic brain injury (TBI) is a major concern for people of all ages, and it is a growing problem. In the United States, 'Each year, an estimated 1.7 million Americans sustain TBI of which ~52,000 people die, ~275,000 people are hospitalized and 1,365,000 people are treated as emergency outpatients' (the ~ reminds us that approximation is a feature of epidemiology).[1] About one per cent of people in the West experience TBI sufficient to cause clinical symptoms, such as loss of memory, anxiety, and depression.[2] Head injury, as a recent study notes, looks set to be the third most common cause of death worldwide by 2020.[3]

TBI is one of the better-known risk factors for dementia. Thanks to the bizarre human habit of trading blows to the head as a form of sport there have been many cases of what used to be called *dementia pugilistica* and has since been labelled chronic traumatic encephalopathy (the clinical validity of this term is much debated). A study which used MRI to predict healthy brain ageing patterns found that moderate or severe, but not minor TBI appeared to accelerate brain ageing and atrophy.[4] A 2014 review estimated that suffering TBI may quadruple the risk of later dementia.[5] Boxing, heading footballs, contact sports like rugby and American football, and other sporting efforts are, however, a small contributor to the head injury statistics. Common causes include fights and assaults, car crashes, falls, and other accidents.

Another source of injuries to brain tissue is the pressure waves from explosions. TBI is a big concern for the military, especially since recent conflicts have seen extensive use of improvised explosive devices, which cause blast injuries with effects akin to those of shellshock. (So a century of progress in warfare has brought us back to the First World War.) Other risks of soldiery for dementia include chemical exposure, combat exposure, and post-traumatic stress disorder.

Brains are soft in their natural, unpickled state, and can easily be damaged if sudden acceleration slams them against the skull. Evolution didn't equip us for dealing with car crashes, falls from high places, and other perilous interactions with natural forces: physics can be very unforgiving. Yet for all their fragility brains can survive remarkable pressures, as divers and boxers bear witness. Their most obvious protection is that they are surrounded by a hard, bony skull and the three layers of membrane, the meninges.[6] To see a neurosurgeon in action is to realize that the outermost meninx, the dura mater, is well named: this is one tough mother. Cutting through it without then plunging into the brain beneath requires excellent motor skills and considerable force.[7]

Between the two inner membranes, the arachnoid and pia, is the sub-arachnoid space. This is where CSF from the ventricles flows, providing an extra cushion against the forces experienced by a brain attached to a walking, running, fighting, or falling body. CSF is mostly water, and water is buoyant: that is, it exerts an upward force proportional to the weight of the thing sitting in it. (Remember Archimedes, slumping into his bath and feeling lighter?) Thus a brain in a bath of CSF is lighter than a brain lacking such protection. Much lighter: a 1,250 g brain supported by CSF would effectively weigh around 40 g. Thus when it is moved by some force its momentum—mass × velocity—is much lower, reducing the stresses which rupture brain tissue.[8] As Newton's Second Law reminds us, force = mass × acceleration, so the forces which act on human heads have to be much greater to send a CSF-soaked brain smashing against its skull—though a fall or a car crash can still do it.

Together, membranes and fluid offer a lot of protection from physical injuries. Anything that overwhelms the brain's inbuilt protections, however, crushing its delicate tissue against its confines, can do damage. And it seems that the risk increases with age; in elders, even a mild injury can increase the chance of developing dementia. Other risk factors for dementia, such as poor nutrition and lack of exercise, can also affect how well someone recovers from brain injury.[9]

Research in rodents suggests that besides directly harming neural tissue, TBI briefly lowers heart rate and blood oxygen levels. It also sets in motion many secondary events with the potential to cause long-term damage.[10] TBI increases markers of brain inflammation and cellular stress, and it damages the 'glymphatic' pathways for toxin clearance, thus affecting the brain's ability to cleanse and repair itself.

An imaging study of mild TBI (concussion) found a pattern of white matter damage 'strikingly similar to the distribution of pathologic abnormalities in patients with early Alzheimer dementia'. The authors say that this finding 'may help direct research strategies'. It may also frighten anyone who has ever suffered a bang on the head, so please bear in mind that not all head injuries cause TBI.[11]

Please note too that although concussion is well known to cause short-term problems, including both cognitive failings and emotional disruption, there is intense controversy over its long-term effects—particularly for single events. Not all researchers use the same definitions for TBI, and it can be hard to control for covariates—for example, to disentangle emotional reactions like anxiety after a car crash from emotional disturbances due to the injury itself.[12] Research on more severe TBI suggests that it may increase the risk for dementia to a lesser extent in individuals who are living 'pro-brain' lifestyles: that is, people with plenty of protective and few risk factors.

Surgery and General Anaesthesia

'He was never quite the same after the operation.' Patients, friends, and families have long commented on the presence of cognitive problems after heart surgery and other major operations, but the deficits are often subtle, more noticeable to a family member than to a busy clinician. Recently research has confirmed that there may indeed be problems, especially among elderly patients and those whose cognitive status before the operation was less than ideal.

A big study of the Taiwanese population's medical records suggests that the type of surgery may be relevant. Surgery under heavy sedation was not associated with greater dementia risk, whereas anaesthetic use increased it by between one-quarter and one-third (odds ratios ranged from 1.25 to 1.34). The pre-operative health of the patient and—as with TBI—the number of events also seemed to influence the risk.[13]

Other studies and reviews, however, have found inconsistent evidence, so the question of whether general anaesthetics are a risk for dementia—and whether that risk differs at different stages of life—remains to be settled.

If there are effects, inflammatory processes may be key contributors, as studies of cardiac surgery have observed that it triggers cytokine production and inflammatory cascades. Unfortunately, having a working hypothesis as to the mechanisms is only the beginning. At present, as a 2014 article notes, 'Clinical data are emerging from longer-term studies to support this concern, but evidence for effective preventive or therapeutic strategies is limited.'[14] To recognize the problem, in other words, is not to solve it. Surgery may harm cognitive capacities, but surgery is not performed just because surgeons feel like a challenge. These are patients with urgent medical needs.

Nonetheless, the hope is that there may be ways to modify the body's responses to injury and surgery so as to reduce the risk of damage to brain tissue. To understand how that damage occurs, we need to look at one of the most important processes in the body (and, many people think, the ageing brain): inflammation. It has been much mentioned; now is the time to dig a little deeper. Inflammation is central to how our bodies react to another major risk factor for dementia: infection. That lifelong hazard is our next topic.

13

Infection and Inflammation

We know that there is virtually no disorder of the CNS in which the immune system—or parts thereof—is not involved.

Frank L. Heppner, Richard M. Ransohoff, and Burkhard Becher, 'Immune attack: the role of inflammation in Alzheimer disease'[1]

The Fragile Brain is not an immunology textbook, although it could have been. It must, however, sketch out some of that difficult science, because the immune system is a suspect—some say the prime suspect—in neurodegeneration. Inflammation triggered in response to pathogens helps our bodies to fight them off, but inflammation can spiral out of control, or become a chronic problem. Both of those situations can damage the brain.

That damage can be severe. Infectious and inflammatory diseases, even early in life, have been found to increase the risk of dementia, or worsen already-present cognitive deficits.[2] With respect to infections, it is known that some viruses, like HIV, can affect thinking skills; patients with AIDS are at increased risk of dementia. Yet people caring for patients with dementia often remark on the fact that they get worse when they catch even minor infections. In animal studies, prenatal infections such as HIV and herpes can produce signs of neurodegeneration in later life. And inflammation may explain the otherwise puzzling observation that poor dental hygiene and tooth and gum disease are risk factors for both dementia and cardiovascular disease.

But what is inflammation, and what triggers it? For that, we need to look at the immune system in a little more detail.

Three Functions of the Immune System

Scrape away the jargon, and the language of immunology is the language of war, of a fight for survival.[3] This reflects its best-known function: warding off invading micro-organisms. However other humans may perceive you, to pathogens you are intensely desirable. Your cells and fluids offer a paradise of plenty where they could feast and grow and reproduce—if only they could get past your defences.

Some already have. We human beings prize autonomy, but in one sense we are not independent organisms but walking cities, gigantic tenement blocks for colonies of microbes that move in shortly after we are born, on a life tenancy. Even the cleaner, publicly visible parts of your body are populated by these invisible guests. Their collective DNA, and by extension the creatures themselves, are known as the human microbiome.[4]

Most of the microbiome is in our colon, a previously unfashionable research area which microbiome science is doing its best to gentrify. Many of the micro-organisms seem to be essential for our healthy development and our capacity to extract nutrients. They calibrate and regulate immune function, both in the body and in the brain, and the chemicals they produce form part of the 'gut–brain' axis, which links the neural networks in our stomachs (the enteric nervous system) with their more famous cousins in our heads. We know how a stomach upset can affect our mood, energy levels, and ability to focus, or how stress can do unpleasant things to the gut as well as the brain. Research on the gut–brain axis is now identifying the hormonal, neural, and immune signals involved.

The bacterial gardens of the microbiome are affected by many environmental factors, providing an important interface between the world and the brain. Diet and antibiotic use are obvious influences, as is stress. One less obvious factor that has recently emerged as a microbiome modifier is access to the natural environment, especially in early life. Nature provides a wide variety of stimulants to calibrate children's immune function, teaching their bodies what to attack and what to leave in peace.[5]

Growing up with your microbiome, you tolerate its presence. With respect to other invaders, however, your riches are well guarded; and your bodyguards are primed to kill. Like the garden of death created by James Bond's enemy Ernst Stavro Blofeld, you are full of lethal dangers.[6] But whereas Blofeld had poisonous plants and carnivorous fish, you have hungry white blood cells and blood full of alarm signals: chemicals poised to trigger inflammatory responses as soon as an intruder is detected.[7]

I have written of war and defence, but there is another language of immunology: the language of peacekeeping, repair, and healing. This is the second function of the immune system. Its cells may destroy pathogens, but they also bring a Marshall Plan for affected areas, prompting the rebuilding of tissues and the regrowth of blood vessels. The defenders that rush to sites of pathogen invasion bring orders for building materials as well as weaponry. Immune cells express receptors whose activation leads to anti-inflammatory gene expression, such as the glucocorticoid and vitamin D receptors. Cholesterol and fatty acids are shipped in to rebuild membranes. Omega-3 fatty acids like EPA are also used to produce 'resolvins', chemicals that damp down the inflammatory response.

We associate inflammation with injury and sickness, but well-managed inflammation is needed for us to heal. In a healthy body, the inflammatory response is a chemical symphony, from the initial problem detection to the recruitment of supplies for rebuilding, the repair of damaged tissues, and the final damping down of inflammatory stimuli. Researchers are still a long way from fully understanding the intricate techniques by which the body fixes damage, and the reasons why those techniques seem to fail as we grow older—and may fail more severely in dementia.

The third function of the immune system, as of government, is surveillance: information gathering about its own citizens as well as immigrants. We have already come across one example: the antigen-presenting cells which report brain cell problems to the cervical lymph nodes. There are plenty of ways in which a cell can malfunction, and when it does it can become a hazard to its neighbours. As cells malfunction, however, they change the expression of certain 'marker' proteins on their surface. If patrolling immune cells detect the change, this can stimulate their activation, an inflammatory reaction, and the cell's disposal.

What is now clear is that inflammatory processes occur in the brain as well as elsewhere, and that the brain's capacity to fight off infections, repair itself, and monitor its milieu for dangers is considerable. It is far more sophisticated than neuroscientists used to believe in the days—not so long ago—when we were told that brain function peaked at age eighteen and no new neurons were created after birth. In late life, however, immune capacities appear gradually to crumble under the pressures of existence, as cells become senescent and DNA errors accumulate. Scientists hope that, as their technical mastery of cellular processes improves, artificially adjusting the brain's defence, repair, and surveillance systems may become feasible options for ageing brains. This will not be easy, however. To see why, we need to know a little more about the forces massed against them.

The Enemies

It is a testament to the rich complexity of the human body that we can be attacked by a phenomenal range of other creatures. Among the smallest (though their numbers are uncountable) are pathogens: micro-organisms which can affect the brain directly or—by provoking reactions in the body—indirectly. Immune responses have evolved for each of the four major classes of pathogen: bacteria, viruses, fungi, and parasites.

Only rarely do any pathogens affect the brain. Its defences—the blood–brain barrier and the immune cells beyond—are so effective that most find the challenge insuperable. Brain infections are not as rare as we might think, however. In England, where my teenage relative had encephalitis in 2012, estimates for its incidence have recently been revised upwards from 1.5 to 4.3 per 100,000 annually, making her one of as many as 4600 sufferers that year.[8]

When they do occur, brain infections can have appalling consequences. One of the best-known and most dangerous is bacterial meningitis, which is thought to affect two to three thousand people in the UK every year.[9] Its pathogens, which have evolved to hijack blood–brain barrier transport mechanisms, kill about ten per cent of meningitis victims.[10] Others are left with cognitive deficits as well as a raised risk of later cognitive impairment. Compare this with the most common source of food poisoning, *Campylobacter*, which as anyone who has had it will know all too well, attacks the gut rather than the brain. It averages 50,000–280,000 infections per year, but the annual death toll is around 100.[11] At the most generous estimate that is about 0.2 per cent of victims.

Bacteria are a common source of brain damage.[12] *Streptococcus pneumoniae* and *Neisseria meningitidis* cause meningitis. Like other bacterial infections, they are also suspected of contributing to neurodegeneration. *Treponema pallidum*, a spirochaete bacterium, is the agent of syphilis, which in its later stages can have a well-known impact on personality and cognition (even that master of racing thrillers Dick Francis has a syphilitic villain, in *Bonecrack*).[13] Spirochaetes have likewise been proposed as contributors to Alzheimer's. A post-mortem brain analysis found them to be present in over ninety per cent of cases, significantly more than in controls.[14]

Cerebral threats also include viruses like HIV, which can lead to dementia, and rabies, which is so adept at following nerve pathways into the brain that neuroscientists use it to track brain circuits.[15] Herpes simplex, producer of coldsores, genital blisters, and sometimes encephalitis, can also exploit this access, and some researchers think it may have a major role in neurodegeneration. Research suggests that being infected raises the risk for later Alzheimer's, especially in people already at higher risk for the disease because they have ApoE4.[16] Herpes infection may show no symptoms at all, and can lie dormant for years, but it is reactivated—triggering renewed immune activity—under certain conditions, like severe stress.

Then there are fungi, like the yeast species *Candida*. These may live peacefully on the skin, or cause the mild symptoms of vaginal thrush, but if they enter the blood they can cause sepsis, an inflammatory overload that can be lethal or cause lasting cognitive impairment. Figures from an awareness-and-advocacy website give an annual death toll of well over a million people, with many more made ill.[17] If a hospital patient dies of 'an infection', you might assume it was bacterial or viral, but in the United States the fourth most common blood infection is due to *Candida*.[18]

The fourth class of pathogens is the parasites: organisms such as *Plasmodium falciparum*, *Toxoplasma gondii*, and *Taenia solium*.[19] *P. falciparum* is carried by mosquitoes and linked to malaria, which in its cerebral form can cause brain swelling, an increase in brain blood pressure, and coma. *T. gondii*, famous in scientific circles for brainwashing rats, causes toxoplasmosis in humans.[20] Normally a mild flu-like infection, toxo can, like malaria, herpes, and syphilis, cause encephalitis—or, in pregnant women, foetal damage or abortion. As for the tapeworm *Taenia*, which like *T. gondii* deposits cysts in the brain, it produces a seven-syllable nasty called neurocysticercosis, which can cause hydrocephalus. *Taenia* is also a major cause of epilepsy.[21]

As we shall see, pathogens can also act indirectly on the brain by way of their effects in the body. An extreme example is pneumonia due to *Streptococcus* infection, called 'the old man's friend' because it ends so many long lives. Even infections that cannot normally pass the blood–brain barrier—like the *Salmonella* species and *Escherichia coli*, notorious for food poisoning—can be dangerous to the very old and very young, the immune-impaired and the already-sick.

So much for the attackers. Now for the defenders.

The Detectives

Evolution developed two immune systems. The earlier, more 'primitive' set of responses is known as innate immunity. Innate immune processes react rapidly to hazards, and healthy humans are born with them, but they are less tailored to individual threats. Later came the processes of adaptive immunity, such as the activation of B and T cells. Adaptive immunity takes longer to react to new threats, but it allows the body to recognize threats it has encountered before and deal with them faster and more efficiently. This capacity for immune memory is one reason why a child's parents may catch the virus brought home from school while the grandparents escape, having met the bug before. Adaptive immune systems are fine-tuned over a lifetime.[22]

In responding to an immune threat, bodies tend to deploy both innate and adaptive mechanisms, with the former becoming active first and guiding the latter's reactions. Initially, threats are detected by the innate immune system, which then stimulates activation of adaptive immune processes. Imagine a peaceful, law-abiding city street, crowded with shoppers, in which a fire breaks out. The first people to react are likely to be nearby members of the public (innate immune cells), and it is their emergency calls that bring the specialist responders (adaptive immune cells) to help. Those calls, and the response, will vary depending on the type of fire. Passers-by may be able to quench the flames, if the fire is small. Police and fire fighters have the necessary equipment to kill larger conflagrations.

In this brief overview I will focus on the innate immune system. Many scientists think that neurodegenerative disorders like Alzheimer's have something to do with immune dysfunction; but most would point the finger at innate more than adaptive immunity. That is not to say that adaptive immunity has no role in the brain. Adaptive immune cells (such as T cells) may struggle to pass a healthy blood–brain barrier, but illness can weaken the barrier and let both native and pathogenic invaders through, as well as harmful chemicals. Such invasions characterize many brain disorders, including MS and stroke as well as infections; but they occur at later stages, whereas our concern is with earlier events, potential causes of neurodegeneration.[23]

Signs of Danger

Pathogens, like cells, are coated with surface molecules. Some of these are so characteristic that immune systems long ago evolved to recognize them and react accordingly. For example, bacterial infections like *E. coli* have surface molecules called lipopolysaccharides (LPS). Injection of LPS triggers a strong, potentially fatal immune response, whether or not the bacterium itself is present. (This is why LPS is also called endotoxin.)

LPS is a PAMP: a pathogen-associated molecular pattern. Like the clues of voice and dress by which people instantly judge each other's status, PAMPs involuntarily announce that their bearers are 'not one of us'.[24] For the immune system, they are the equivalent of a paedophile's image collection or the traces of explosive in a terrorist's car. While a terrorist can survive without bombs, however, microbes need PAMPs. This is a weakness of which our immune systems take full advantage. The invaders have, of course, developed many tricks in response.

There are also DAMPS: damage- or danger-associated molecular patterns. These are signals given off by unhealthy cells, and they too can prompt immune reactions. PAMPs and DAMPs are both types of antigen.

Cells and Chemicals

How are PAMPs and DAMPs detected? Like any other chemical signal: by receptors, in this case located on innate immune cells such as the brain's microglia. There are many kinds of these pattern recognition receptors, specialized for PAMPs from different sources.[25] (Evolution used Adam Smith's division of labour long before Smith named it.) Together they offer wide-ranging immune coverage.[26]

Our innate defences, however, rely on both cell-mediated forms of immunity, such as receptors, and a more liquid kind. This so-called humoral immunity involves chemicals in the blood—and in other body fluids.[27] Skin, our most familiar immune organ, releases lipid-filled sebum from sebaceous glands (which impedes pathogens by acting rather like the wax on a waterproof coat), while the sweat and tears which wash over it are laden with chemical defences against invaders.[28] Tears contain lysozyme, a product damaging to bacterial walls and membranes, while sweat, like many household cleaning products, contains ammonia.[29] Saliva, nasal mucus, and sticky secretions from the cells lining other orifices are laden with trapped and damaged bacteria. We evolved to find these substances disgusting because disgust prompts avoidance, and thus reduces the chances of infection.

The Naming of Names

One of the most interesting players in the humoral, wet arena, for neuroscientists, is complement, a set of around thirty proteins. This group of evolutionarily ancient molecules is named by the letter C and successive numbers: C_1, C_2, C_3, and so on. Lower-case letters are stuck on when researchers find that a molecule exists in more than one variety (e.g. C_{3a} and C_{3b}, or C_{1q}). R, with a number if needed, is added to name a receptor for the protein; thus $C_{1q}R_1$ is one of the receptors for C_{1q}.

Complement is on a growing list of immune proteins now known to multitask elsewhere.[30] Evolution has no qualms about repurposing, and complement is required for normal brain development. Without it neurons do not form connections properly. More particularly, they cannot get rid of excess synapses. We think of young brains as growing strongly, and so they do, but after birth much of their development depends not on adding neurons, but on adding glia and reducing synapses. This helps the brain learn by removing unused neural connections. Any stimulus can potentially trigger many pathways from sensory input to motor reaction. Reducing the cloud of possible routes—by pruning those least-travelled—speeds up reactions and reduces the energy needed to process the response.

Complement proteins can attach to unused synapses. This tagging attracts nearby microglia, which carry complement receptors. The microglia then eat the synapse.[31] When complement is highly active, therefore, as it is in inflammatory brain disorders and in Alzheimer's, more synapses may be tagged for elimination. Loss of synapses is thought to be among the earliest events in neurodegeneration. Overenthusiastic microglia, stimulated by overactive complement, are on the suspects' list.

There is another biochemical naming system beginning with C: the CD cell surface marker proteins, of which there are over 300. These proteins, which stud and speckle cell membranes, serve a vast array of functions, from signalling the cell's identity (like PAMPs) or health (like DAMPs) to helping it move or attach itself to its neighbours (like cytokines and chemokines). Some CD proteins have been identified as unique to certain cell types, such as microglia—this useful fact allows scientists to label or manipulate specific cells without targeting others. For many, their roles and relationships are yet to be discovered.

Some CD proteins are part of the immune system. We have already met the 'Don't eat me' signal CD47, for instance, while CD33 regulates both inflammatory responses and oxidative stress; it is one of the genes associated with late-onset Alzheimer's, albeit not as strongly as ApoE.[32] Some CD proteins are even part of the complement system. CD11b, for example, is linked to the autoimmune disease lupus, but it also leads a double life as integrin αM. Integrin αM is part of the complement receptor CR3 and of a cell surface receptor known as Mac-1, these being the same entity.[33]

Having just one name for every molecule would be so much less fun.

Immunology reminds me of trying, in my teens, to read Tolstoy's *War and Peace* (someone told me not to, otherwise I would have left it until my brain was old enough to cope). Most of the characters, being Russian, had at least three names, and sometimes French equivalents and titles as well. Trying to remember who was who, let alone who was related or married to whom, was excellent preparation for a scientific literature in which so many molecules have been identified in multiple contexts, or given different names at different times. So if you want your child to be an immunologist...

As research fields mature, one name for each scientific object tends to predominate, so perhaps the confusion here is a sign of the discipline's youthful vigour. Certainly neuroimmunology is one of the most exciting and fast-changing areas of brain research.

Go Forth and Multiply

Complement proteins are crucial players in immune function, as shown by the fact that variations in complement genes can cause severe immune disorders.[34] CR3 binds bacterial LPS. Mac-1 helps immune cells stick to pathogens, an essential step in their destruction.[35] And complement genes are associated with Alzheimer's. Complement activation has even been proposed as a 'biomarker', to be used by clinicians diagnosing dementia.

Complement proteins can be activated by binding to bits of pathogens or damaged areas of body tissue, or by adaptive immune proteins such as antibodies. They can also be switched on by molecules like C-reactive protein. CRP is used as a marker of inflammation, often included in blood tests on people with diagnosed or suspected autoimmune disease. It is a remarkably ancient molecule. I have not come across many studies whose animal model is the horseshoe crab, but apparently this evolutionary relic can survive doses of LPS that would kill a mouse, and it uses CRP to activate its potent innate immune response. The protein binds to LPS and then to C1, setting off the complement cascade.[36]

Complement proteins are amplifiers, magnifying innate immune responses using feedforward loops. In these, an earlier stage in the process (e.g. the activation of C1) affects later ones (e.g. C1 activates C2 and C4, which in turn trigger other proteins in the cascade). This results in exponentially fast reactions.[37] Feedforward loops are a great way to get a quick result, but they must be handled with care. The complement system is under tight regulation to prevent your bloodstream seething with proteins the first time you catch a cold.[38] Mutations in one of the regulatory proteins, CR1, raise the risk of Alzheimer's, supporting the idea that over-active complement may be a suspect in dementia.[39]

The Counter-attack

As in scanning for danger, when responding to it our immune systems use both cellular and humoral processes.

Cell-mediated immunity, as the name suggests, involves both innate immune cells (like monocytes, neutrophils, and natural killer cells) and adaptive immune cells (such as B and T cells).[40] Both types, like all blood cells, originate from stem cells in the bone marrow and thymus.[41] The latter is a small organ near the heart; it may be one of the body's least-known viscera, but it is immensely important.[42] In these two nurseries new blood cells are created at a rate of about a trillion a day, mostly red blood cells (erythrocytes), but also platelets and the white blood cells (leucocytes) of the immune system.[43] This astonishing fecundity is the reason why some ancient human bones, and some not so ancient, have been found with signs of butchery and cannibalism: the long leg bones cracked open to extract the nutritious marrow.

Innate Immune Cells

Bone marrow and thymus, however, have much more to offer than food value. The neutrophils and natural killer cells to which immune stem cells give rise have an important role in innate immunity, and may also be called into the degenerating brain by cellular distress signals.[44] Are they helping, or making things worse? We don't yet know; so I will focus on the third type of innate immune cell, monocytes. These are of interest in dementia because they are very similar to microglia. Indeed, researchers are not sure how much of the immune activity seen in Alzheimer's is due to microglia, and how much to peripheral (blood-borne) monocytes that have slipped across the blood–brain barrier to lend assistance to their cerebral cousins.

Monocytes demonstrate two of the immune system's core functions: destruction of the enemy, and analysis of its identity. They circulate in blood until summoned to a particular tissue where damage or infection has occurred. There they differentiate to become activated macrophages, ready to eat and destroy. This pattern—of cells circulating in immature form and only taking on their final characteristics when they reach the tissues where they are required—is a way of protecting healthy tissue, in this case from over-enthusiastic immune cells. It is akin to soldiers not drawing their weapons until they directly engage the enemy, in order to spare civilians in the area. In both cases the control systems sometimes fail.

Macrophages, like T cells, are phagocytes (the term means eater-cells).[45] Phagocytes detect microbes, cell debris, or cells with problems, and destroy them for the greater good. Your body is a police state where suspected criminals, the sick, and illegal immigrants are executed as soon as they are detected. Phagocytes can also react to abnormal proteins. Microglia, for instance, consume amyloid.

Macrophages and other phagocytes are analysts as well as killers.[46] They are antigen-presenting cells (APCs), and having eaten a pathogen, or an antigenic protein, they chop it into fragments to display on their surfaces. (One thinks of soldiers' sometimes gruesome trophies.) They then move to the lymph glands, where T cells are plentiful. Like a child saying, 'Look what I found!' as it holds out some appalling object to its mother, APCs warn T cells that there is a problem and give them enough information to take appropriate action. They thus link the early responses of the innate immune system to the more specific responses of adaptive immunity: the antibody-producing B cells, and the hunter-killer T cells.

Adaptive Immune Cells

One of the most talked-about developments in dementia is the possibility of immunotherapy: using the immune system against the disease. Much of the research has focused on antibodies. One such drug, solanezumab, made headlines in July 2015 by showing some signs of slowing the disease in early-stage patients, though the results need to be confirmed—a trial is due to report at the end of 2016.[47] To understand how such drugs work, we need to know a bit about antibodies.

B cells, like other immune cells, continuously patrol the body's waterways. Once activated by the innate immune system they turn into plasma cells and produce antibodies—molecules specialized to detect and lock on to particular antigens. Antibodies can mop up extracellular threats, such as viral particles in the bloodstream. (T cells, meanwhile, kill infected cells, whose virus-filled innards antibodies cannot reach.)

The adaptive immune system tackles so vast a range of antigens that it is thought to need about 100 million different antibodies, known as antibody specificities.[48] This is roughly 5,000 times the number of human genes, so antibodies cannot be produced by having a gene for each protein. Moreover, we can react to evolutionarily novel antigens; many people are allergic to plastics, for instance. We can also produce new antibodies in response to a vaccine—as is currently being tried for Alzheimer's.

How is all this possible? By the same power that gives us the riches of our native tongue: recombination. Human languages have relatively few basic grammatical elements—nouns, verbs, etc.—and a vocabulary perhaps one-thousandth the size of our lifetime antigen repertoire; yet we can easily create an original sentence.[49] We do it by combining words in new ways according to grammatical rules implicitly acquired as we learn language.

The immune system does likewise, only with genes, splicing together unusually variable segments of DNA in different ways.[50] Lots of different ways: the number of possible combinations—i.e. antibody specificities—has been estimated at more than ten trillion. (Unravelling the details won Susumu Tonegawa—a man who endearingly reports failing his university entrance exam on the first attempt—the physiology Nobel Prize, outright, in 1987.[51]) In practice the number of B cells is thought to be a mere 100–200 billion. That's still a hefty arsenal for life's immune threats.

When a threat is first encountered it takes time to make an antibody to match it. That this can be done at all is due to the fuzzy nature of chemical identity. The interaction between any receptor (including an antibody) and its ligand (or antigen) is not like a computer's data-matching systems. When you type your password into an online site you must get it exactly right to gain entry, but receptors are more tolerant. The matching process is a matter of which atoms are attracted to which others, so the match can be partial. Saying that 'chemical X binds to receptor Y' means that X and Y are physically attracted and move closer to each other. It does not imply that either X or Y would stay faithful, given a better electromagnetic offer. Insulin binds to the insulin receptor and to insulin-degrading enzyme, but so does Aβ. (This may mean that insulin changes could affect how much amyloid is degraded in the brain, and is one reason why diabetes is of interest to dementia researchers.)

When an antibody achieves even a partial match, the B cell producing it replicates, and better matches lead to more replications, so over time there will come to be more high-affinity B cells, honed to detect specific antigen. This process of speeded-up evolution is called affinity maturation.[52] Once matured, some B cells turn into a long-lived type called a memory B cell, which float around the bloodstream looking for their particular kind of antigen trouble. These weapons with memory provide us with fast defences against familiar pathogens: the remembrance of bugs past.[53]

The effects of infection, or autoimmune disease, can last a lifetime, not only when they directly damage brains, but because of immune memory. Pathogens like T. *gondii* or herpes viruses can lie dormant for years; but when they do reactivate, the immune system's response is swifter and stronger thanks to memory B cells. That may help you fight off infections, but repeated inflammatory surges can stress and eventually damage your native cells.

Immune memory has another consequence. Each immune reaction you experience changes your reaction to the next one. Apart from making you the victim of your own history, this makes experimental immunology extremely difficult to do well. Researchers do experiments by comparing two groups, which should, ideally, only differ on the one variable of interest. Thus dementia patients and controls should be the same in every respect, except that one group is ill and the other isn't.

Not a chance. The immune system, like the brain, behaves differently depending on its history, making each of us unique in even more ways than we usually assume. This helps protect us, and no doubt makes us fascinating individuals, but it's a thorough nuisance for the people trying to study us.

The fuzziness of affinity is also a problem, since it means that drugs to treat neurodegeneration must be developed with extreme care (viz. the abandoned trial of the Alzheimer's treatment semagacestat).[54] The same imprecision applies to immunotherapy. Typically, antibodies react to one small part of their target ligand, the epitope. This is why vaccines work: the epitope of a pathogen is not the same as the bit that does the damage. Carefully inactivated samples in a vaccine can therefore trigger an immune response without causing full-blown illness.

However, antibodies may also react to other molecules with a similar structure. If one of those happens to be a native protein, the antibody may bind to it as well—and trigger immune responses against the cells expressing it.

This cross-reaction is thought to be a key mechanism of autoimmune diseases. Autoimmune reactions to the body's own proteins can have horrible effects, such as lupus or arthritis. When the target is the brain (as in MS) they can be lethal. Because the brain's environment is so specialized, many molecules found there are not found elsewhere, and if these rare species get into the blood, the peripheral immune system (i.e. outside the brain) may react as if to an alien, forming antibodies which may then get into the brain and cause massive damage. Antibodies to a type of brain glutamate receptor called NMDARs, for instance, can cause a terrifying illness called anti-NMDAR encephalitis. It brings severe psychiatric symptoms like depression, memory loss, odd behaviour, and psychosis, as well as movement problems and seizures, and it can lead to coma and death.[55]

The hope for Alzheimer's is that Aβ-targeting antibodies like solanezumab, or vaccines which stimulate antibodies to proteins like Aβ and tau, will prompt their removal and thus, in theory, cure—or at least delay—the disease.[56] This will work if the proteins are causing the disease and if the antibodies don't target other proteins. So far, initial attempts have not been successful. In January 2002 a clinical trial of an Alzheimer's vaccine was halted, and the vaccine permanently withdrawn, after what the company described as 'some setbacks'. Four patients had developed serious brain inflammation and more would follow.[57] Work on vaccines is, however, on-going, and the data on solanezumab are exciting, if tentative.

Free-floating antibodies lock onto their specific antigen. This tagging makes antigen more noticeable, labelling it as a tasty snack for passing phagocytes. The technical term is 'opsonization', from the Greek word for prepared meat. Opsonins, like Lewis Carroll's Walrus with his oysters, get antigen ready for dinner.[58] Unlike the Walrus, however, antibodies are not lethal by themselves. Once they have caught their prey, other agents, like T cells or microglia, must destroy it.[59]

Fluid Defences

Complement proteins are also opsonins, and they interact extensively with other immune system components like T cells. They can alter blood vessels' permeability—how readily they let material through—and, in severe situations, they help to put the body into anaphylactic shock. C5a production, for example, is thought to drive the onset of fever.[60]

The complement system can distinguish home grown, 'normal' cell damage from abnormal injury. In both cases, if it is working properly, it marks damaged cells for consumption, but it triggers inflammation only for damage caused by invasive threats. Of course, in neurodegeneration it may not be working properly.

Some complement proteins—C5b, C6, C7, C8, and C9—have another strategy for killing foreign cells: stabbing. They join together, creating a tube-like structure called the membrane attack complex. The membranes in question are those of pathogens, and the effect is not unlike that of pricking a water-filled balloon. The membrane attack complex binds to the surface and punctures the cell membrane, a process called 'lysis', from a Greek verb meaning 'destroy'. (The people who gave us the *Iliad*, the world's best-known war poem, had many such verbs.[61]). Cytoplasm leaks out; *finis* invader.

Amyloid proteins can employ a similar strategy against native cells. Research suggests that Aβ oligomers can form ion channels that insert themselves into cell membranes, allowing calcium ions to flow into the cell. Calcium, as we have seen, is dangerous in excess, and these extra pores can damage neurons' communication capacities by lowering the number of synapses—or can even kill the cell.[62]

As we noted earlier, microglia and other phagocytes devour their prey, but they have other weapons. One is the respiratory burst: squirting ROS to damage pathogens. Oxidative stress and inflammation are frequent companions, and the same molecules that can wreck a neuron's membrane can also damage or kill bacteria. Microglia also release a variety of chemical signals that activate many immune processes. These include immune proteins called cytokines which, like complement, are of great interest to neuroscientists because of their newly discovered roles in the brain. They are important because their levels rise with age and in early Alzheimer's, and because some of them have the capacity to kill brain cells.[63]

Cytokines

Cytokines are produced by immune cells like microglia and macrophages to drive the body's inflammatory responses.[64] Raised cytokine levels have been linked to very many medical conditions, including heart disease, atherosclerosis, insulin resistance and diabetes, infections, and, more recently, dementia.

And not just dementia. Multiple lines of research now link increased levels of cytokines with Alzheimer's, Huntington's, stroke, depression, chronic fatigue, schizophrenia, TBI, encephalitis, and other brain dysfunctions. Symptoms such as fatigue and reduced activity have been attributed to cytokine overproduction. Life circumstances and personal choices—including childhood abuse, poverty and deprivation, smoking, poor diet, and obesity—have an impact too, and some medical treatments such as chemotherapy can also affect the body's inflammatory status, altering cytokine levels in the blood. That in turn affects the brain. For example, people treated with certain cytokines (e.g. for cancer) sometimes develop severe depression.

Furthermore, cytokine levels tend to rise with age. So does the severity of the immune system's responses to stimulation—so much so that some researchers use the term 'inflammaging' for the wear and tear inflicted by life on the body via the immune system.

Cytokines are small proteins, sometimes with sugars attached (glycoproteins). The name comes from Greek words for 'cell' and 'movement', as some cytokines can affect how cells move about. Brain microglia, for instance, may change shape and migrate in response to cytokines. (Brains are usually thought of as static, but that soft solid stuff in your skull doesn't all stay put. Quite apart from the shrinkage that comes with age, and the brain's overall movement within the skull, brain cells are remarkably dynamic. Microglia migrate even in adulthood; neurons grow new branches; cells are pushed aside by tumours or excess fluid; blood vessels are rebuilt in response to damage; and so on.)

Cytokines carry influence from one cell to another. They can engage with their receptors locally, like neurotransmitters, altering the behaviour of neighbour cells or sometimes the cell that produced them; or they can act at a distance, as hormones do. Cytokines are involved in normal cell signalling. But they are also critical to the immune response and especially to inflammation.[65]

The Signs of Inflammation

Traditionally—that is, at least since doctors in ancient Rome took the word '*inflammatio*' from the verb for 'to set on fire'—inflammation was recognized by four cardinal signs: '*rubor et tumor cum calore et dolore*' (redness, swelling, heat, and pain).[66] Even the smallest skin punctures show this pattern. Cytokines mediate all four signs. Released by innate immune cells in response to injury and infection, they stimulate production of many other molecules, including pro-inflammatory lipids like platelet-activating factor as well as chemokines and adhesion molecules. These activate platelets and phagocytes and stimulate them to move towards the site of damage (chemokines) and then park themselves there (adhesion molecules).

As well as calling the emergency services and giving them directions, cytokines also dilate blood vessels, providing easy access to the wound or infection source. This leads to swelling, redness, and warmth around the area. With *tumor*, *rubor*, and *calor* comes *dolor*: both pain processing and depression have been linked to cytokine levels.

Cytokine teamwork, aided by chemokines, adhesion molecules, and other factors, is also central to the processes of blood vessel regrowth and tissue repair, *aka* remodelling.[67] The phagocytes they attract will clear pathogens and cell debris. Cytokines also recruit other cells involved in wound healing, such as platelets, keratinocytes (skin cells), endothelial cells to build blood vessels (when repairs require new supply lines), and fibroblasts, which produce new extracellular matrix and also collagen for connective tissue, knitting both cells and organs into place. The net result of all this chemical action is a shifting balance: first inflammation to destroy the problem's source, then repair of the damage caused.

Inflammation involves pro-inflammatory cytokines, including interleukins 1 and 6 (IL-1, IL-6) and tumour necrosis factor-α (TNFα).[68] Raised blood levels of pro-inflammatory cytokines have been found in patients with mild cognitive impairment—often considered pre-clinical dementia. This suggests, as does work in

PART 2: RISK FACTORS

animals, that the effects of inflammation on neurodegeneration, like those of amyloid, may be at their most damaging early on in the disease.

Anti-inflammatory cytokines, such as the interleukins IL-4, IL-10, IL-13, and IL-37, damp down responses (as do certain chemokines, vitamin D, and also resolvins made from omega-3 fatty acids).[69] In addition, anti-inflammatory cytokines alter production of pro-inflammatory cytokines: IL-4, for example, inhibits IL-1, IL-6, and TNFα. Anti-inflammatory cytokines may also be anti-neurodegenerative. Tests on blood macrophages taken from Alzheimer's patients found that applying both vitamin D and resolvins encouraged the cells to eat more Aβ and protected them from Aβ fibrils which could otherwise kill them.[70] Needless to say, such findings have prompted great interest in methods of boosting levels of these cytokines.

The balance between attack and repair alters as we age, as repeated infections, illnesses, and stresses—and the inflammation they cause—exert an increasing toll on the body's resilience. The immune system learns from experience, and tends to react more quickly and strongly to repeated stimuli. Alongside this, accumulating oxidative stress, low levels of dietary micronutrients, ageing mitochondria, and DNA errors all tend to weaken the body's ability to damp down inflammation and make rapid, efficient repairs.

Reaching the Brain

The brain is not impervious to these changes. Cytokines are sizeable molecules, and for a long time it was thought that they could not pass the blood–brain barrier; but we now know that they are important signalling molecules in the brain. Neurons and glia produce them, have receptors for them, and use them to communicate. Some cytokines, notably TNFα, IL-1, and IL-6, have roles in learning and memory processes such as long-term potentiation, one of the key ways of changing synaptic strength. Microglia also produce cytokines, especially when they are activated. Microglial release of TNFα, for example, can affect neurons' synaptic strength and their numbers of glutamate receptors, altering their activity and connectivity. Conversely, microglia are affected by neural activity. Thus immune status can influence cognition.

The implication is that brain cells might be affected by high levels of systemic cytokines (i.e. cytokines in the blood) as well as by those produced locally; and indeed, this seems to be the case.[71] Inflammation in the body can affect the brain.

This is thought to be why some chemotherapy drugs, such as doxorubicin, can impair cognitive function in cancer survivors ('chemo brain' or 'chemo fog'). The drugs cannot themselves pass the blood–brain barrier, but they push up levels of peripheral (blood) cytokines, which then affect brain tissue. It is also why repeated infections increase the risk for neurodegeneration; the inflammation they cause boosts not only peripheral but brain cytokines to damaging levels.

How could peripheral cytokines affect brain tissue? One answer is that the brain is kept informed about the body's immune status by the vagus nerve, which sends visceral information to the brainstem, midbrain, and insular cortex. This mighty nerve lets your heart and guts talk to your brain, and it has numerous cytokine receptors. Another potential access route is via the brain's circumventricular organs, the border crossings where peripheral cytokines may stimulate neurons to produce their own inflammatory molecules. As well as being made by brain tissue, cytokines are also produced by the endothelial cells of the blood–brain barrier, which could affect neurons and glia. Finally, some cytokines may also be actively transported across the blood–brain barrier. Whatever the routes, it is clear that the brain is susceptible to repeated inflammatory stress.

That vulnerability may be most noticeable late in life, but it begins early. Cytokines are important during brain development, helping to guide newborn neurons to their correct positions. In excess, however, they can cause problems: raised cytokine levels—including levels in the mother's bloodstream—seem to damage the foetal brain. A study of immune developmental programming in mice suggests that raised levels of cytokines during pregnancy can leave the baby mice with higher cytokine levels of their own throughout their lives, and more likely to develop Alzheimer-like signs (such as abnormal Aβ and tau) later in life. If the unfortunate rodents are then given a second immune challenge their brain pathology becomes much worse.[72] Thus a stressor in the womb can make the offspring more vulnerable to later stressors.

Cytokine effects on areas of the brain such as the hypothalamus are also thought to control sickness behaviour. This is the suite of behaviours seen in illness or injury: lethargy, drowsiness, low mood, fever, nausea, and vomiting.[73] When you have flu or a gastric infection cytokines make you feel pale, sweaty, bloated, and reluctant to work. It is even thought that the anticipation of an aversive—or pleasant—event can alter cytokines, and that this may be why placebos work. (Psychoneuroimmunology, the wild frontier of neuroimmune science, studies how beliefs and expectations can influence the immune system.[74])

Clinically, if inflammation is causing neurodegeneration you would expect treatment with anti-inflammatory drugs to cure it, or at least stall it. Some studies have found statistical links between the long-term use of non-steroidal anti-inflammatory drugs like aspirin and lower risk of dementia; but trials using NSAIDs to treat or prevent dementia have so far failed.[75] Worse, the drugs can have nasty side effects like cognitive problems and stomach bleeding—and, trials in dementia patients suggest, brain bleeding too—so there are significant costs associated with taking them. If inflammation is doing its worst in the early stages of the disease, however, perhaps future trials with high-risk younger people may find some preventative effects. Such trials may also be required for drugs that specifically target amyloid.

Alternatively, NSAIDs may not be the right kind of anti-inflammatory drug for the inflammatory processes involved in neurodegeneration. This is hinted at by a study of the brains of people who had used glucocorticoids, but not non-steroidal drugs, to treat inflammation: it found fewer signs of dementia in the glucocorticoid users.[76]

Context is Everything

The sources and drivers of an immune process, in body or brain, are not simple matters. Cells and humoral factors can both contribute—and interact in many ways— with each other and also with neural signals. Injury type, location, and duration make a difference.

In addition, immune chemicals do not act in an empty theatre. The chemistry of the fluids already percolating through the injured tissue, together with its cells and their secretions, will affect how severe the reactions are. Other events such as exercise or hypoxia can also affect immune responses, triggering changes that facilitate or suppress inflammatory processes.

And, of course, aged tissues react differently from young ones. This is the rationale behind attempts to stall or reverse ageing in mice using parabiosis, in which an old mouse's blood supply is linked to a younger one's. Results so far have been intriguing enough to garner excited headlines about vampiric seniors; but it's very early days. Excitement has greeted many anti-ageing findings which later prove problematic— and mice have died in parabiosis experiments for reasons that are not yet understood—so more research is needed before we accept young blood transfusions as a useful strategy.

As well as the cell/humoral and innate/adaptive divisions, a third dimension on which immune processes can be classified is time. How long an immune response lasts affects how, or indeed whether, the tissue recovers. Many of the chemicals involved are like the stress hormone cortisol in that they appear to do good in the short term, adapting the body to deal with threatening situations. If they linger, or if too much is released, then they may make things worse. In lethal infections, the shock of the inflammatory reaction is usually what kills.

In a healthy body immune processes are tightly controlled, with multiple layers of regulation so that if one fails the others can still prevent inflammation from going on too long. This is the kind of control we see in nuclear power stations, and the logic is the same: dangerous material needs careful handling. And for much of our lives it works. The redness fades as the damage heals, the pain subsides, the cells return to normal, healthy function. Sometimes, however, the resolving mechanisms fail, and inflammation becomes a chronic problem. The triggers of this shift from temporary to permanent are not well understood, but they are the subject of intensive research, because chronic inflammation is increasingly being linked to all sorts of problems, including the slow decay of ageing brains.

Our tour of the immune system has brought us back to where we started: the fragile brain. To close the circle we need to bring immunology and neuroscience together, and look at the brain's immune cells, microglia.

Microglia

Microglia, guardians of the brain, make up between ten and twenty per cent of its cells.[77] They were distinguished from other brain cells in 1927 by the Spanish neuroanatomist Pio del Rio Hortega, but it took decades before they were recognized as being immune cells.[78] Now we know that, like peripheral macrophages, they can participate in inflammatory responses. They are activated in brain infections, and express pro-inflammatory cytokines like IL-1 and TNFα. They can also act as phagocytes, engulfing not only abnormal proteins, synapses, cell debris, and pathogens but other phagocytes like neutrophils—which in severe infections and other disasters like stroke are allowed through the blood–brain barrier.

As well as eating things, microglia that are activated by, for example, Aβ can change their shape and move through the brain towards areas of damage. They do so in many neurodegenerative diseases, including dementia. When activated by pro-inflammatory molecules such as IL-1, Aβ, or LPS, they trigger the transcription factor NFκB. As we saw earlier, this controls the expression of many inflammatory genes, ramping up production of pro-inflammatory cytokines and other innate immune molecules, like complement, as well as receptors for the anti-inflammatory vitamin D and glucocorticoids. Microglia then secrete pro-inflammatory cytokines and also produce respiratory bursts of ROS.

When activated by anti-inflammatory cytokines like IL-4, however, microglia follow a different pathway. They increase the expression of anti-inflammatory and repair molecules like chemokines and the neurotrophin BDNF. Thus microglia can switch their production line from promoting inflammation to resolving it, depending on the signals they receive. It is thought that ageing pushes the balance of those signals towards a more inflammatory pattern, in the body and perhaps in the brain as well.

Even 'resting' microglia are far from quiet. They arrange themselves in a grid throughout brain tissue, extending many short filaments to probe their environment, continually on the alert for warning signs. When they detect something amiss they are thought to retract their branches, taking on a more rotund and compact, macrophage-like shape, ready for action. They are continually in contact with neurons, by way of surface proteins that bind to proteins on neuronal membranes; it is thought that, like fretful toddlers with their mothers, the contact keeps the microglia quiet. And they are receptive to many chemical signals emitted from healthy neurons, such as neurotransmitters, as well as heeding signals of distress.

Neuroinflammation

So microglia are the brain's macrophages and they drive 'neuroinflammation' in the brain, just as their peripheral cousins drive inflammation in the rest of the body. Correct?

Numerous scientists think so.[79] Since the term 'neuroinflammation' entered the literature in 1996 it has become widespread. After all, why would brain cells produce RNA and receptors for inflammatory molecules unless they are using them? As often happens, however, the concept of neuroinflammation has undergone considerable mission creep, expanding from clearly inflammatory conditions like spinal injury to a range of other disorders, including neurodegeneration.[80]

Meanwhile, new technologies—from microscopes to antibody markers—have given researchers improved ways of identifying, extracting and analysing activated microglia in post-mortem tissue.[81] Methods of tracking them in living brains, using PET neuroimaging, are also being developed. Then there is the genetic evidence, reinforcing the idea that neurodegeneration involves the increased transcription of inflammatory genes.

Yet there are problems with assuming that neuroinflammation is a contributor—perhaps even a major cause—of neurodegenerative damage. For example, inflammation in the spinal cord is often used as an experimental model; but this may not be the same as neuroinflammation in the brain. Studies testing the assumption that they are the same—of which there are rather few—note significant differences.[82] There are also species differences.

Another difficulty is due to conceptual vagueness. As we have seen, inflammation started out being defined as a set of symptoms: *rubor*, *tumor*, etc. Yet these are problematic even in the body, let alone in the brain. People with congenital insensitivity to pain due to a genetic mutation, who cannot feel pain from injury, may nonetheless show signs of inflammation such as redness and swelling; brain tissue is also insensible to pain.[83] Inflammation is now recognized as a much more complex process which includes:

- vascular changes (blood vessels must become more porous, allowing cells to exit through their walls);
- cellular activities such as infiltration (white blood cells must enter the target area);
- chemical changes (e.g. rises in pro-inflammatory cytokines).

A brain infection, or an inflammatory disease like MS, satisfies these criteria. The blood–brain barrier is penetrated; neutrophils, macrophages, and T cells enter the brain; cytokine levels rise. It is not clear, however, that the same is true in neurodegeneration.

Microglial activation, which is accompanied by their proliferation, does increase in ageing and in neurodegeneration. There is also more expression of genes for immune proteins such as complement. A 2012 study found that 'essentially all pathways of the innate immune system were more active in aging'.[84]

Interestingly, the same study found that the changes mostly took place during ageing, and much less so when aged brains became Alzheimer brains. The authors interpret this as a hint that the immune changes may be an early factor in Alzheimer's. One could also infer that the immune system has much to do with ageing, but that something else is pushing brains towards dementia.

A 2014 study compared the genes expressed in an accepted inflammatory brain disease, MS, and the degenerative disorders Alzheimer's and Parkinson's. The authors found distinctly different genetic signatures, 'demonstrating that very different sets of genes are involved'.[85] They argue, therefore, that inflammation and microglial activation are not the same. Activation may lead to a full inflammatory reaction, but it need not always do so.

The brain is a very different environment from the rest of the body. It has long-lived cells which mostly no longer divide, and which are part of life-long, highly complex networks. This puts cell preservation at a premium, since the brain cannot afford extensive collateral damage. When a horde of eager neutrophils or T cells invades tissue, like soldiers called in to protect a territory, collateral damage can be extensive. So it makes evolutionary sense for the brain to exert tight control over inflammatory reactions—which are indeed rare—and to manage its environment without calling for reinforcements, if possible.

What brains do need is micromanagement of their networks: removal of old or weak synapses, growth of new ones, remodelling of dendrites, and protection of neurons' far-reaching axons. We have already noted how microglia interact with complement to prune synapses, for example. As a 2011 review observes, 'These normal synapse and spine modulating functions of microglia are likely to be much more important than their functions as part of an inflammatory response which are utilized only under exceptional circumstances.'[86]

In short, perhaps microglial activation is less about full-blown inflammation, about destroying pathogens, and instead more like cerebral gardening. As any gardener knows, keeping the place tidy takes continual effort: monitoring, pruning, sometimes removing dead plants. Like brain maintenance, it gets harder with age; and it involves active renewal and reshaping as well as just sweeping up leaves. Likewise, a review of how microglia clear away cell debris after injury remarks that it 'is more than simply tidying up, but instead plays a fundamental role in facilitating the reorganization of neuronal circuits and triggering repair'.[87] Interestingly, one of the key receptors involved in microglial clearance of dying neurons is a protein called TREM2. Mutations in the gene for TREM2 have been repeatedly linked to Alzheimer's disease, suggesting that a weakness in microglia's ability to tidy their brain gardens might contribute to neurodegeneration.[88]

Weakened Before You Were Born?

Animal studies also imply that healthy microglia are needed for the development of neuronal networks during childhood, as well as in adults, and that problems with microglia could contribute to brain disorders. For example, work on young mice has found that a diet deficient in anti-inflammatory fatty acids like EPA and DHA can lead to microglial changes, higher levels of pro-inflammatory cytokines, and alterations in genes involved with synapse maturation. Prenatal infection or early exposure to toxins can also alter the immune systems of the offspring, tilting them towards a more pro-inflammatory profile and affecting many other aspects of physiology, such as hormone production, via effects on the developing brain. In addition, gut microbiota, the tiny billions in our bowels, are crucial for microglial development and function; mice without them have defects in microglia and innate immunity.

It is thought that their effects on microglia may be a reason why infections in pregnancy, such as flu or toxoplasmosis, can be bad news for baby as well as for mum, linked to a greater chance of children growing up with psychiatric and neurodevelopmental disorders like bipolar depression, autism, and schizophrenia. (A sizeable recent study confirms, however, that getting flu vaccine during pregnancy does not seem to do any harm.[89]) Epigenetic mechanisms offer a plausible means of achieving this intergenerational messaging, but the details are only beginning to be worked out.

As well as affecting childhood and young adulthood, early changes may have neural consequences much later in life. For instance, a study that exposed newborn rats to lead found that brain levels of Aβ rose briefly and then fell. Thereafter the exposed rats showed no differences from control animals—until their old age. Then their amyloid levels increased, despite no further lead being added to their water.[90] Again, we see the pattern of an early stressor setting the stage for later vulnerability.

As well as being triggered by infections and toxins, inflammation can result from autoimmune diseases and allergic reactions. Both are more prevalent in highly developed countries with good hygiene and public health systems, and, within these, in kids who grow up less exposed to the outdoors or to household pets. The hygiene hypothesis of immune dysfunction proposes that too much cleanliness, whatever it may do for godliness, may not be good for health, because humans need dirt to develop properly.[91] More specifically, the immature immune system needs dirt—i.e. exposure to pathogens—to tune its reactions and avoid excessive inflammation, just as eyes and brains need exposure to light to develop normally.[92]

Dementia shows the same pattern of higher prevalence in countries with lower microbial burdens. It has therefore been suggested that over-cleanliness may be bad for the ageing brain as well as for the immune system. Just as animals deprived of visual experience during the brain's 'critical period' for vision fail to develop normal sight even if their eyes are later opened, so it seems the immune system may need stimulation early on for optimal effect. Suboptimal immunity may lead to excessive inflammatory reactions—particularly with age, which brings more exposure to pathogens. Ageing also increases the chance of the immune system over-reacting to signals from sick cells. More work, however, is required to confirm this idea, especially given all the other differences between countries with high and low levels of infectious disease.

Stressors in the womb may alter the baseline settings of the immune system, and lack of childhood stimulation may leave it ill prepared and overly aggressive. Later stressors can also tip the balance towards accelerated neurodegeneration, however, and those stressors include much more than the bad luck of catching an infection. In Chapter 14, therefore, we turn to some other illnesses that stress our ageing brains.

14

Big Killers

I take pills every day, and I am not alone. In England about fifteen million people—roughly a quarter of the population—have at least one chronic medical condition. Many have more than one: diabetes and heart disease, or cancer and depression.[1] Often, like dementia, they involve inflammation, and often they must be managed rather than cured. They are also among the most common causes of death.[2]

Some people are also now taking pills for conditions they don't actually have but have been told they may get, or for conditions like high cholesterol which are considered risk factors for serious diseases. Preventative treatment is another fast-growing trend in medicine, especially for diseases like MS and Alzheimer's, where potentially modifiable factors have a big role. Some researchers think that prevention is our best hope for the common scourges of Western health care. Some fear Western health care can't afford anything else.

The Heart and the Blood

The tale is not one of unrelieved despair, however. Cardiovascular diseases are the world's number one cause of death, accounting for about thirty per cent of deaths according to the World Health Organization: yet there is evidence that making lifestyle changes can effectively reduce their impact. In the United Kingdom, rates of coronary heart disease have been falling for years (as indeed have overall mortality rates). A study by the British Heart Foundation noted a drop from around 166,000 in 1961 (when heart disease caused more than half of all deaths) to around 80,000 in 2009.[3] This remarkable decline is attributed to better treatments, better diet, and less smoking.

Despite the changes, cardiovascular diseases remain enormous health problems, ranking among the top five killers for both men and women in the United Kingdom in 2013.[4] Also on that list are cerebrovascular disease (by number of deaths, it ranks fifth for men and third for women) and dementia itself (second for men and first for women).

It is thought that downward trends in heart and vascular disease may in part explain why, as we saw in Chapter 3, the prevalence of dementia may be stabilizing, or even starting to fall, in Western Europe. These conditions are major risk factors for dementia. The idea that lifestyle and treatment changes beneficial to the heart and circulation may have already begun to lower the risk for dementia is immensely encouraging, for individuals and governments.

Why are these illnesses such big risk factors for dementia? Because they starve brain cells. Doctors often remark that what is good for the heart is good for the brain, and that statement works in many ways. Hungry brain cells need a healthy heart and arteries. The amount of blood pumped out by the heart per minute (cardiac output) falls with age, and reduced cardiac output—even without obvious heart disease—is thought to raise the risk of age-related brain conditions like Alzheimer's. Blood vessel blockage, stiffening, and narrowing—thrombosis, sclerosis, and stenosis—reduce blood flow and disrupt the distribution of nutrients to and through the brain. Heart failure reduces cardiac output. Atrial fibrillation, in which the heart beats fast and irregularly even at rest, also disrupts blood flow. All become more common as we age.

In addition, many of the same factors that cause cardiovascular problems, such as diabetes, obesity, and smoking, also particularly affect the brain. Organs like the skin and liver can repair themselves after damage, but the brain's capacity for regeneration is more limited, making it vulnerable.

Failures in blood supply are one of the most common causes of lethal age-related brain conditions. Strokes alone kill over six million people a year.[5] Haemorrhagic strokes—brain bleeds—occur when a blood vessel ruptures, but they are relatively rare: about five in every six strokes are ischaemic.[6] Before they reach breaking point, blood vessels can swell, forming aneurysms—the term is from the Greek word for 'widening'—which may remain unnoticed until they burst. If the vessel is a large one, the resulting haemorrhage is often fatal. My family includes two aneurysm survivors. One event was cerebral, the other aortic: an emergency operation on a rupturing 12-centimetre bulge. The aorta, the body's largest artery, is particularly aneurysm-prone. The largest aneurysms I can find reported are 13 and 15 cm, so my relative, who was in his eighties at the time, is a lucky man to have survived his. Brain aneurysms can do damage before they burst as well as after, since pressure from the swelling vessel can crush surrounding cells.

The Vulnerable Border

Both kinds of stroke, like aneurysms, can be lethal. All three are extreme manifestations of a problem with how the blood vessels are working—a problem which also contributes to dementia. Blood vessels are most vulnerable where they are thinnest, so it is no wonder that blood–brain barrier damage, common in ageing and illness, is closely linked to brain ill health.

Some researchers think that the vascular system is so central, not only to dementia but to many of its risk factors, that Alzheimer's is better viewed as a vascular disorder with resulting neurodegeneration. Post-mortem studies suggest that most people diagnosed with Alzheimer's also have detectable problems with brain blood vessels, such as cerebral amyloid angiopathy due to Aβ build-up; the same is true of many elderly people. Research comparing patients diagnosed with Alzheimer's and with vascular dementia found significantly lower brain blood flow in both, compared with healthy people of the same age.[7] Lower brain blood flow has been detected years before the clinical signs of cognitive impairment. A study of flow rates through major vessels found that they varied depending on the individual's anatomy, but that they declined with age as the total blood flow to the brain diminished.[8]

Vascular dementia, in which damage to blood vessels predominates, tends to progress in fits and starts, as small strokes damage tissue. It is often diagnosed after an abrupt change in clinical symptoms, whereas more gradual cognitive impairment is presumed to be due to neurodegenerative processes. Yet slowly accumulating problems with the blood supply—potential causes of gradual cognitive decline—can quietly precede a more noticeable stroke or heart attack, as many people learn to their cost each year.

Hypertension (high blood pressure) in midlife or earlier has long been seen as a risk factor for dementia, particularly vascular dementia, although not every study agrees.[9] Once again the causes are intertwined. Blood pressure is affected by genotype and stress and tends to rise with age, inactivity, and poor diet—with high salt intake being the prime suspect.[10] Higher pressure also strains the heart and blood vessels. Think of an elastic tube being repeatedly stretched and relaxed. The more forceful and prolonged the stretching, the sooner the tube begins to lose its elasticity. Anger, which raises blood pressure, seems to increase the risk of a heart attack or stroke shortly afterwards.

Research suggests that treating high blood pressure might help to prevent dementia, although the data are far from conclusive. The time lag between blood pressure rising and cognitive impairment may be years, or decades, with many other factors meanwhile contributing to brain decline. Moreover, blood pressure has been observed to fall as Alzheimer's sets in. Nonetheless, when an international panel of eight experts (Deckers et al., 2014) reviewed research on dementia prevention they listed hypertension—in midlife—as the fifth most important risk factor for dementia prevention, 'associated with a 61% increased risk of developing dementia'.[11]

Blood pressure is controlled by the hormone angiotensin, which raises the pressure by narrowing—tensing—blood vessels. (Angiotensin can also contribute to neurodegeneration in other ways: it inhibits the release of acetylcholine in the brain and promotes both inflammation and oxidative stress.[12]) There is some evidence that taking angiotensin receptor blockers for high blood pressure may protect against dementia and stroke, improve brain blood flow, and reduce brain changes associated with Alzheimer's disease. Angiotensin is converted to its active form by angiotensin-converting enzyme, ACE, some genetic variants of which have been linked to late-onset Alzheimer's. However, as with most of the risk factors for Alzheimer's, we cannot yet be sure how big a role angiotensin plays in the onset of dementia.

Diabetes

Second in the Deckers *et al.* (2014) ranking, and high in other lists of dementia risk factors, is that scourge of civilized living, type two diabetes. The Deckers estimate is that diabetes may raise the risk of having dementia by almost one-half (47%). This effect is thought to be independent of the effects of high blood pressure; but diabetes also increases your chances of acquiring this and other risk factors, such as vascular disease and later-life depression.

Diabetes mellitus, type two, which makes up nine in ten cases of diabetes, was named from its effects on urine. The Greek verb *diabainein*, meaning 'to pass through', references the characteristic increased production, while the Latin adjective *mellitus*, meaning 'sweet' or 'like honey', notes the equally characteristic smell and—apparently—taste. What the Greek doctor who named it would not have known was how that sweetness did its damage.[13] Smelly urine is an embarrassment. High blood sugar can be fatal; and even when it is not doing obvious damage it is now recognized as a major risk factor for dementia.

The Glucose Trap

When you eat a meal your blood glucose levels rise.[14] In response, your pancreas produces one of the world's best-known proteins, insulin. Its release into the bloodstream is stimulated by the sight, smell, and taste of food, via the vagus nerve, and also by glucose, some hormones, fatty acids from dietary fat, and some amino acids from dietary protein.[15] Sugar is thus not the only type of food to trigger a rise in insulin, which is why cutting out sweets may not be enough to spare you diabetes.

Insulin stimulates cells to take up glucose for fuel. It also encourages liver cells and astrocytes in the brain to store glucose as glycogen, in case of need. Insulin can in addition affect those other energy depots, fat cells (adipose tissue). They turn blood fatty acids into stores of triglycerides, and they can likewise convert protein and sugar—amino acids and glucose—into fats. Insulin increases the liver's conversion of glucose into fatty acids, while suppressing fat cells' conversion of stored triglycerides back to fatty acids.

Insulin's overall effect, therefore, is to withdraw glucose from the blood into cells, which are using it, storing it, or both. It does other things too, like stimulating cell growth and division, and acting as a neurotrophin in the brain.

When blood glucose levels drop the pancreas releases another hormone, glucagon, which stimulates the liver to turn glycogen back into glucose, to boost supplies. The stress hormone adrenaline can also stimulate this form of glucose production, which makes sense, since stressful situations often demand high-energy responses. Insulin is inhibited by stress. Exercise, which imposes mild stress, also reduces insulin levels.

Cells detect insulin via receptors on their surfaces, of course, but cells are not passive recipients of chemical messages. They can tune their production of receptor proteins, and move them to or from the cell membrane, in response to how much those receptors are being used. When the amount of activating ligand is small, and thus the signal is weak, cells can increase their sensitivity by producing more receptor molecules and shipping them out to the cell membrane. When there is a lot of ligand around—a strong signal—cells can turn down the gain by producing fewer receptors and removing or inactivating existing ones.

If insulin is frequently released in large amounts, cells are liable to react by inactivating some of their insulin receptors (this is done by phosphorylation, the addition of a phosphate group to the receptor molecule). Over time, this will make insulin less effective at stimulating cells to take up glucose: the problem of insulin resistance. As a result, more glucose stays in the blood, prompting the pancreas to release more insulin, which increases receptor inactivation. The slide into the vicious spiral of insulin resistance has begun. Eventually the pancreatic cells become exhausted, producing less and less hormone.

Meanwhile, resistant cells have less glucose. In the midst of biochemical plenty they begin to starve, as insulin resistance pushes the body towards prediabetes.

The Dangers of High Blood Sugar

Estimates suggest that about one-tenth of people defined as prediabetic go on to become diabetic every year, and that over their lifetimes seven in ten will develop diabetes.[16] Prediabetes is widespread in Western populations. Between 2009 and 2012 the US government estimated that over one-third of US adults and one-half of senior citizens were affected. Nearly ten per cent had full diabetes, of which around one-quarter were undiagnosed.[17] In the United Kingdom the proportions are about one-third for prediabetes, nearly five per cent for diabetes.[18] And the trends, unlike those for heart disease, are upwards. A UK study of prediabetes found that between 2003 and 2011 its prevalence tripled from 11.6% to 35.3%. Older and overweight people are more likely to be affected.[19]

Insulin resistance and high blood sugar have other damaging effects. They promote chronic low-level inflammation, which itself makes insulin resistance more likely. They raise levels of pro-inflammatory cytokines and Aβ in the brain. And they worsen the wear and tear of oxidative stress.

While type two diabetes involves insulin resistance, in type one the pancreatic cells fail to produce enough insulin, often due to autoimmune damage. This rarer form of diabetes is also thought to raise the risk of later dementia, especially if it strikes at a young age (which is likewise the case for type two).

In what follows, for simplicity, 'diabetes' refers to type two diabetes.

Diabetes can be life threatening. Swings in blood sugar levels (hyper- or hypoglycaemia) stress the body and brain, and can in extreme cases lead to unconsciousness, or even coma. When the body cannot meet its energy demands—because the cells can no longer take up available sugar—it resorts to alternative methods of making glucose from fats and amino acids. In moderation, this can result in gradual weight loss. In diabetes, however, blood levels of acidic ketones (products of the reactions which turn fat into sugar) can rise to dangerous levels. This can cause hyperventilation, irregular heartbeats, confusion, coma, and organ damage. In the brain ketones can be used as fuel, protecting it to some extent from metabolic stress; but that protection is far from absolute.

Diabetes, and to some extent prediabetes, have been linked to heart and vascular disease as well as to high cholesterol, hypertension, and common cancers. Associated eye diseases like glaucoma and diabetic retinopathy can cause blindness. Diabetes can damage the kidneys—sometimes necessitating dialysis—and blood vessels elsewhere—sometimes necessitating amputation.[20] (Kidney problems have also been identified as a risk factor for dementia.) In the United States, diabetes is the seventh leading cause of death.[21] It also damages many other body systems—such as blood vessels—whose healthy function is needed for a healthy brain.

Epidemiological evidence supports a relationship between diabetes and dementia, finding that diabetics are more likely to suffer cognitive impairment and dementia patients more likely to have diabetes. For example, in a US study '81% of cases of Alzheimer disease had either type 2 diabetes or IFG' (impaired fasting glucose, a warning sign).[22] The Deckers et al. review noted nineteen studies of diabetes as a risk factor for dementia, of which seventeen found increased risk; the other two found no link.[23]

Your Energetic Brain

Insulin resistance affects cells' ability to produce energy, and neurons need a lot of energy. A 2007 review states that 'between 50% and 80% of the energy consumption of the brain appears to be devoted to signaling associated with the input and output activity of neurons'.[24] That energy comes mainly from glucose. In an awake and healthy brain it is consumed at a rate of, on average, 0.33 micromoles—or 59 millionths of a gram—per gram of brain tissue per minute. The rate is higher in cortex, lower in hippocampus and cerebellum.[25] For a brain weighing 1400g, that implies consumption of about 120g of glucose per day—equivalent to about 3.5 cans of Coca Cola.[26] There is, of course, no need to drink cola or eat sugary snacks, because sufficient glucose can be obtained from many common foods like fruit, bread, and dairy products. Brains can also use other molecules, such as glycogen, lactate, and ketones, for energy.

In early Alzheimer's, the rate of brain glucose uptake has been found to be almost half the normal rate. Old age is often portrayed as bringing a quieter and less active life, but the idea that the brain's need for sugar drops by fifty per cent upon retirement, or diagnosis (or in the years preceding these events), seems, shall we say, improbable. The brains of people with the first stages of dementia still need fuel, but they seem to be having trouble getting it. It's as if, in dementia, brain cells are starving to death.

Insulin and the Brain

By now you may be thinking, 'Wait a moment. If lack of fuel is a problem in dementia, shouldn't high blood sugar be a good thing, not a risk factor?' If only it were so simple, and we could all eat cake to our hearts' content, secure in the knowledge of cerebral benefits (until we got cardiovascular disease, kidney problems, and diabetes). Of course we can't. It's more complicated than that—not least because when dealing with insulin the brain is rather different from the body.

That brain tissues do have insulin receptors has been known since the 1970s, but brain levels of the hormone are generally low in healthy humans. How brains use it is more controversial, since neurons—unlike, for example, muscles—do not need insulin to take in glucose. Indeed, the brain was initially thought to be insulin-insensitive because its overall glucose uptake was not affected by blood insulin levels. (Note that no overall change could mask regional variations.[27]) Even if high blood sugar were to lead to insulin resistance in the body, therefore, neurons would presumably be spared.

So why, in the competitive field of dementia hypotheses, has research on brain insulin become so significant a player that some researchers call Alzheimer's 'type 3 diabetes'?[28] If neurodegenerative diseases like dementia do involve brain insulin resistance at an early stage, why might that be a problem?

Here are some reasons. First, insulin's role in regulating glucose may be lessened in the brain, but it has many other responsibilities. It is an important neurotrophin. In the hypothalamus, it regulates body metabolism, for example by altering body temperature, appetite, and how fat is processed and stored. In the hippocampus it seems to improve learning and memory through effects on synaptic plasticity and glutamate receptors. And as well as promoting the survival of neurons and the growth of new synapses, it affects their conversations, modulating neurotransmitters like acetylcholine and noradrenaline. Insulin resistance, therefore, could have a considerable impact on brain function irrespective of any effects on brain glucose uptake.

Research on Alzheimer patients has shown changes in the expression of brain genes involved in insulin processing, and this is borne out by research on human brain cells. A study of neurons from the hippocampus and cerebellum of people without (diagnosed) diabetes found evidence of brain insulin resistance.[29] The insulin signal seemed normal but cells' detection of it wasn't, because many of the insulin receptors had been inactivated, as happens in the insulin-resistant body.[30] There were more inactivated receptors in the hippocampus of people who had had Alzheimer's than of people who had died with milder cognitive impairment, and more in the hippocampus (which is typically severely affected in Alzheimer's) than in the cerebellum (which is generally less damaged). Neurons were still able to suck up glucose, but those from Alzheimer patients took up only about one-third as much as those from healthier people. As new research techniques have become available, the initial finding of insulin insensitivity, like so many initial findings, has given way to a more nuanced picture.

The exciting implication of the insulin hypothesis is that pre-existing treatments for diabetes might help people with dementia. A study comparing diabetics who had or had not used metformin found that long-term use of this common diabetes drug halved the risk of cognitive decline.[31] Research administering insulin, or its longer-lasting analogue insulin detemir, via nasal spray is also showing promise for staving off cognitive and memory decline, and work examining its effects in early Alzheimer's is on-going.[32] Nasal sprays can affect the brain without exerting unwanted metabolic effects elsewhere in the body, making them potentially very useful.[33] Plus, the high costs of pharmaceutical development are big incentives to use existing drugs if possible.

That said, despite its appeal there is a lot of work to be done on the insulin hypothesis.[34] Although brain insulin resistance *may* starve neurons of their glucose fuel, it is not yet certain that it *does* so in living brains. The initial problem might lie not within the brain itself but elsewhere: with the endothelial cells of the blood–brain barrier. Glucose must be transported across the barrier before it can nourish brain cells; and in an animal model, reducing this transfer produced effects like those seen in dementia, including vascular and blood–brain barrier damage, and neurodegeneration.[35] So perhaps the problem is at the borders, more than within the brain's own territories.

Furthermore, not all Alzheimer sufferers have—or have had—diabetes or prediabetes, as far as we know. That could be a methods problem: many studies have not recorded their patients' blood sugar levels. At present, however, high blood sugar does not appear to mean that senility inexorably beckons. Dementia and diabetes share common risk factors, such as ageing and depression, but that does not make them the same disease. Diabetes might worsen the progression of dementia by other means than by affecting brain insulin—for example, by damaging blood vessels.[36] So perhaps 'type 3 diabetes' is too strong a claim. More research will be needed before researchers—and more importantly, patients—can give a final yea or nay to the insulin hypothesis.[37]

Needier Cells Die Younger?

Insulin is not the only possible cause of changes in brain energy metabolism; others include mitochondrial dysfunction and reduced blood flow. Whatever the cause, a drop in the brain's energy consumption does seem to occur in people at high risk for dementia, and long before the disease is diagnosed (as we saw in Chapter 9). Irrespective of where neurons get their energy from, it is clear that they need a high and continuous supply.

Some neurons require more energy than others, however, and this has interesting implications for the pattern of symptoms typical in dementia. Among cortical neurons, GABA-using inhibitory interneurons are especially demanding. As noted in Chapter 5, these cells are crucial to the process of making sense of experience. They keep the synchronized patterns of brain activity generated by successive stimuli from blurring into an incoherent mess. Other cells with high energy demands are the big-bodied cells of the deep subcortical nuclei, such as the acetylcholine cells of Meynert's nucleus basalis. Thus the neurons most vulnerable to lack of energy are not those dealing with primary processes like interpreting sensory information or commanding movements. Rather, starvation will first affect the cells by whose activity we 'hold it together'. They give us mood and meaning, stitching hordes of tiny electrical surges into coherent representations of, and responses to, our environment, external and internal. (How apt that the nucleus basalis of Meynert was named after a neuroanatomist who was also a poet.[38])

This is why syndromes which alter brain energy metabolism—syndromes like diabetes, chemo brain and probably chronic fatigue, cerebrovascular disease, and the reduced brain blood flow which seems to precede dementia—begin not with primary motor or sensory symptoms like falls or hallucinations, but with more subtle problems: slowed decision making, apathy, mental tiredness, mood disturbances, and 'brain fog'.

Cancer

In the UK, cancer charities have worked extremely hard to reduce the fear and stigma facing patients. Dementia charities are beginning the same long process. The two conditions have a certain amount in common. Both are mainly diseases of ageing; though they can strike at younger ages, dementia affects children and young adults only in exceptionally rare genetic tragedies. Both carry a heavy burden of terror, uncertainty, grief, and physical as well as emotional pain. And both inevitably change the sufferer, uproot settled lives, alter family dynamics, and impose all kinds of costs, not just financial ones. The main difference is that dementia always kills its prey, unless pre-empted by accident, infection, or suicide; whereas cancer is increasingly surviveable with modern treatments.

Intriguingly, some researchers have speculated that the two conditions might also share an underlying mechanism. This is because, remarkably, epidemiologists have found that some cancers, unlike many illnesses, do not raise the risk of later dementia. Instead, repeated studies have found that the chance of getting some neurodegenerative disorders—especially Alzheimer's—appears to be significantly *lower* in people who have had certain types of cancer.[39] The reverse also seems to hold true, suggesting that neurodegenerative disorders may somehow protect against certain cancers.[40]

Cancer involves uncontrolled cell division and replication—i.e. a failure to control the cell cycle—whereas dementia involves cell death and, as we saw in Chapter 11, senescent neurons which have re-entered the cell cycle and got stuck. Researchers have thus proposed that both cancer and dementia involve disruption to the proteins which control the cell cycle, but in opposite ways. There is genetic evidence to support this. Genes that are altered so as to produce less protein than normal in dementia tend to produce more protein than normal in cancers, and *vice versa*.

One leading candidate is the tumour suppressor protein p53, which is mutated or deleted in many cancers. When activated, p53 can either trigger cell death or bring the cell cycle to a stop, so overproduction of p53 might plausibly contribute to neurodegeneration.[41] A 2015 study of gene networks in Alzheimer's implicated p53 as an important regulator, and it has also been found to be important for synaptic function.[42] It seems to be vulnerable to oxidative stress, which can change its shape—and therefore its behaviour. And p53 not only interacts with amyloid (research suggests that $A\beta_{42}$ inside cells can activate p53 and thereby trigger cell death), but is also itself an amyloid protein, accumulating in Alzheimer brains alongside $A\beta$.

The p53 protein is well studied in cancer but has only recently begun to be considered as a potential therapeutic target in dementia. This means that researchers studying neurodegeneration can call upon the pre-existing knowledge of cancer scientists, which is a boon. However, it is also a warning that treating Alzheimer's will require careful work to avoid disturbing delicate physiological balances. No clinician wants to prevent, stall, or cure one illness only to inflict another, and with an illness as complex as dementia that risk is sizeable.

For an example of such risks we need look no further than cancer itself, and its life-saving treatment chemotherapy (which involves a varying collection of drugs, of which newer ones are generally safer than older ones). Research on long-term cancer survivors is beginning to find that chemotherapy, blessing though it be in granting them life, may not be so generous with the quality of life, especially as they grow older. I have already mentioned that certain drugs may impair cognitive function—the notorious 'chemo brain', which can last for decades after treatment—possibly via effects on inflammatory cytokines, oxidative stress, and brain glucose metabolism. Another hazard of some forms of chemotherapy is damage to reserves of neural stem cells, one of the tools with which brains make repairs.

Stem Cells

Stem cells were once thought to exist only in developing brains, their repeated divisions filling up foetal skulls with neurons and, later, glia such as astrocytes.[43] (Microglia, whose source is bone marrow, invade and settle in the growing brain.[44]) However, it is now known that adult brains continue to house puddles of stem cells, especially around the lateral ventricles. Consequently, and contrary to what was once believed, some neurons—in the hippocampus, for instance—can be replaced in adulthood. Other cells, such as the oligodendrocytes which form white matter, can also be replenished. The brain's supply of microglia can be supplemented with monocytes from bone marrow, if required.

The continued presence of neural stem cells in adults has to be one of the greatest discoveries of modern neuroscience, at least in terms of its potential for clinical medicine. This is because in theory stem cells are 'pluripotent': they can turn into any kind of body cell. As each stem cell divides, however, it undergoes fate restriction, a narrowing of its career options akin to that traditionally imposed on human teenagers. Some stem cells become neurons; others take alternative paths; and some remain immature.[45] Like bone marrow stem cells waiting to become blood cells, these junior brain cells can be held in reserve until needed, whereupon they differentiate into mature cells.

Scientists are beginning to untangle the complex processes that govern a cell's fate. Clever chemical tweaking can even change one kind of brain cell into another, or back into a neural stem cell. Such cells have recently been successfully extracted from adult human post-mortem brain tissue and differentiated into astrocytes, neurons, and oligodendrocytes. The hope is that implants of stem cells could be used to reverse neurodegeneration by regenerating brain tissue. (The potential for any implants to turn cancerous will, of course, be carefully assessed in clinical trials.)

Meanwhile, stem cell technology is generating intense excitement amongst Alzheimer researchers, not least because it makes studies of brain tissue very much easier.[46] This is because human skin or blood samples can be converted into stem cells and thence into functioning brain cells. These are otherwise rather difficult to get hold of unless the patient either dies (and has donated their brain to research) or has a brain disease that requires invasive surgery (and has consented to a brain biopsy).

Furthermore, studying stem cells facilitates research on the genetics of dementia, because taking samples from patients with a particular gene profile ensures that the resulting neurons or glia will have the same mutations. This eliminates the need to mess around with transgenic techniques, by which genes are artificially added to healthy cells—or animals—to make them malfunction (e.g. by producing more Aβ). Patients' samples can be stored for years before being converted into stem cells, and hence to brain tissue cultures; this preserves a great deal of information about the donor even after their death. Stem cells also speed up the testing of new drug candidates, reducing the need for animal research. They are thus immensely useful experimental models in themselves, quite apart from the tantalizing prospect of brain repair they offer.

That's the dream: a way of rebuilding lost brain matter, personalized to each individual because the source of the stem cells is their very own skin or blood. It's a vision that could revolutionize the treatment of neurodegenerative disorders like dementia. Every vision has its critics, however, and the stem cell dreamers will need to listen to their critics, as well as do a staggering amount of work, if the vision is ever to materialize.[47]

Troubled Bodies, Troubled Minds

In this discussion of risk factors we have seen how malfunctioning brains and bodily illnesses can also affect the mind. That makes sense: we know that when we feel sick we also feel mentally dull and unenthusiastic, and may struggle with tasks that previously seemed simple. It also makes sense that a mind that struggles to cope with life's stresses and trauma may be at increased risk of failing later on. Yet many people are unfamiliar with the idea that both trauma and mental illness may be risk factors for dementia.

Clinical depression and schizophrenia have both been associated with a greater chance of cognitive impairment. Severe stress—particularly in childhood—is considered a major risk factor for both of these disorders and may also raise the risk of dementia in its own right. Many researchers think that early life abuse or other trauma can disrupt the way the body reacts to stress, putting children at greater risk of later depression, chronic disease, and suicide. Studies of affected children have found 'a significant decrease in lifespan, and a doubling of the incidence of premature coronary artery disease. The incidences of premature diabetes and osteoporosis are also substantially increased.'[48]

If there were any justice in how fates are meted out, people facing such problems in earlier life would have filled their quota of suffering long before they reached retirement age. Of course it doesn't work like that; fairness is a human concept, not a law of nature. Many medical conditions are sociable: they tend to cluster. Depression, diabetes, heart or cerebrovascular disease, and later dementia is one pattern; depression, heart disease, and cancer another. Often the depression strikes first, sometimes years before the other illnesses occur.

Depression

If cancer and dementia still carry stigma, how much more so does depression. And stigma is a big medical problem. In the West, fewer people now openly espouse the ancient idea of sickness as divine punishment, but the idea is still around in secular disguise: if you don't do X (eat your greens, exercise, whatever) you'll fall ill (and you'll have only yourself to blame). The idea that sickness reflects some moral weakness—such as failure of will—is also still surprisingly potent. At this moment there are children dying of cancer, and terrorists planning an atrocity. If you catch yourself wondering why the terrorists couldn't have had cancer instead of the children, you will understand the continuing power of the link between illness and morality. (And yet being nice does not spare people from depression, or cancer, or dementia.)

These ancient beliefs are an extra burden for the sick, especially when their illness is low in that lingering hierarchy which grades broken legs as real and broken minds as less solid, less visible, and less true. (This is why dementia charities work so hard at reducing stigma, and do so in part by emphasizing brain research and biological mechanisms.) Being ill is nasty. Being ill, being blamed for it, or being thought a cheating malingerer is worse.

To be clear: when talking about risk factors, it's a big step from 'Doing X raises the risk of dementia' (or depression) to 'Doing X may cause dementia'. Even when this move is justified by the evidence, the further jump to 'If you do X, you are to blame for your illness' is not. Therefore, discussing the financial costs of dementia should not be seen as a licence to judge patients more harshly for 'taking' resources. And finally, both depression and dementia involve life-threatening disruption of numerous physiological systems, and both are among the world's most serious health concerns. Depression is estimated to affect over a third of a billion people, about one-twentieth of the global population, with huge costs in medical care, lost productivity, and suffering.[49] It is not something dreamed up by life's losers, any more than dementia is an invention of life's has-beens.

Depression may nearly double the risk of dementia, according to the expert consensus of Deckers *et al.* (2014). It considered depression *the* most important risk factor to be considered in attempting to prevent dementia.[50] Long-term/recurrent depression is associated with memory problems, and effects on hippocampal size and function have been observed. In later life, the risk appears to be especially strong for vascular dementia. Two meta-analyses found raised risks—up by over two-thirds for general dementia, more for vascular dementia—in people with depression.[51]

Once again, inflammation is thought to play an important role. Raised levels of pro-inflammatory cytokines such as IL-6 and TNFα, and of the complement-activating protein CRP, have been found in human patients with depression. They are also much studied in animal models (if you're wondering, depressed mice don't move much, hide away if they can, and go off their food).[52] People with autoimmune disorders are more likely to have depression—and not just because the illness gets them down. The role of inflammation may help to explain why taking traditional antidepressants—which target neurotransmitters, not cytokines—does not seem to lower the risk of getting dementia, and quite often doesn't help the depression either.

Schizophrenia

Schizophrenia has also been linked to dementia (it was after all originally called dementia praecox), as we saw in Chapter 5. It too is thought to be at least partially an inflammatory disorder, as well as one made worse by stress. Prenatal and later infections are thought to increase the risk of getting schizophrenia, as do autoimmune disorders. It is thought that their effects on immune function may in turn affect many other aspects of brain and body, predisposing an infant to later mental illness and mood disturbance. If the world is hostile—full of pathogens—then a pregnant mother who catches an infection may be 'warning' her unborn baby, by way of raised pro-inflammatory cytokines, to come prepared.

Stress

Abnormal stress responses have been implicated in both schizophrenia and depression. Since stress is also thought to contribute directly to dementia, as well as via its effects on mental health earlier in life, let us look more closely at how bodies react to danger.

The stress response is a physiological alarm signal. It is responsible for our reaction to threats, from the shakes you'll have had if you've ever narrowly escaped an accident to the ground-down tension caused by workplace overload or a disintegrating relationship. What counts as a threat has broadened considerably over the course of evolution, especially since we started talking and living in groups. Like an individual's risk of developing dementia, the palette of what he or she perceives as stressful is uniquely coloured by personal history, especially by the formative experiences of early life.

Some researchers have found that personality may also influence people's susceptibility to stress. Studies have found that more neurotic types are likely to suffer long-lasting psychological distress in midlife, and that this is associated with greater dementia risk, as well as with a higher chance of dying from something else, like heart disease. High conscientiousness and openness to experience, on the other hand, have been tentatively linked to lower dementia risk.[53]

Dementia itself, of course, also stresses both victim and carers, especially when it causes personality change or challenging behaviours like wandering and assault. Some varieties of dementia—such as frontotemporal disease—are more likely to cause these symptoms, which can be terribly distressing. I once saw a video of a patient with frontotemporal dementia which showed a previously pleasant grandmother acting like a rude, abusive racist; the clinician doing the interview must have been gritting her teeth. (Next time you encounter someone behaving appallingly, could they have damage to their frontal lobes?) The behaviours usually wane as the disease progresses, which may be little consolation to traumatized carers.

The body's stress response is triggered by the hypothalamus, one of the brain's prime executives. It activates the sympathetic nervous system (SNS), a network of nerves extending from the spinal cord to organs as diverse as the eye, the liver, and the adrenal glands, which produce the stress hormone adrenaline.[54] This prepares the body for 'fight or flight', pushing up heart rate and blood pressure and diverting resources from less urgent processes like digestion to immediate priorities like energy for muscles.

Even as the SNS jolts adrenaline into our bloodstreams, the hypothalamus is triggering a second, slower stress response: the release of adrenocorticotropic hormone (ACTH) into the blood. This prompts the adrenals to release another kind of stress hormone: glucocorticoids such as cortisol. The system is known as the hypothalamic-pituitary-adrenal (HPA) axis.[55]

Glucocorticoids have many effects on body and brain. Activating glucocorticoid receptors has been found to affect around 6,000 human genes, more than one-quarter of the total.[56] Among the targets is NFκB. Glucocorticoids inhibit this transcription factor, hence reducing the production of inflammatory molecules. This is why they are often, despite side effects such as osteoporosis, used to treat inflammatory diseases like rheumatoid arthritis.

'Anti-inflammatory' is not always 'good', however. Glucocorticoid hormones also seem able to prime innate immune cells such as microglia, making them more likely to react strongly—perhaps too strongly—to the next stimulus that comes their way, whether that be debris from a dying cell, a synapse tagged with complement, or a bundle of amyloid. (Inflammation management now; pay later.) Glucocorticoids also have a particular impact on the hippocampus, an area that is densely packed with their receptors.

The hippocampus is closely bound to the HPA axis and can, when working normally, inhibit its function. Needed for retaining new memories, it shows signs of damage and decay early in Alzheimer's—later than brainstem nuclei, but earlier than almost all of cortex. Chronic activation of the HPA axis, producing constant stimulation from glucocorticoids, is thought to damage the hippocampus and contribute to neurodegeneration. It lowers production of the neurotrophin BDNF, reducing neurogenesis and synaptic plasticity. Mutations in the gene for BDNF have been linked to depression, bipolar disorder, and schizophrenia, to abnormal hippocampal function, and to poorer episodic memory.[57] Changes in brain BDNF and glucocorticoids have been linked to severe depression, to childhood abuse, and to suicide.

The HPA axis illustrates an important principle of body function: hormesis, a word derived from the Greek for 'all things in moderation'.[58] Hormesis is the notion that human physiology is like elastic.[59] Stretch it a little and it can easily recover its original state. Stretch it too far for too long, however, and it warps into a new, dysfunctional shape. Thus a cell, organ, or body exposed to some kind of stress, like a toxin or a surge of cortisol, can adapt as long as the stimulus is not too great.

Hormesis has been observed in multiple body systems, and in the brain. As we have seen, for instance, low doses of Aβ seem to be beneficial for memory and neuron health, whereas high doses appear to be harmful. The concept of hormesis is closely related to that of homeostasis. This is the idea of a natural balance, or comfort zone: a normal range of body functions within which the organism can sustain itself without damage. Various physiological stressors disrupt the balance, and this activates mechanisms that evolved to restore it (which is why when you eat something salty you then get thirsty). The fast, adrenaline-producing stress response evolved to deal with immediate threats—at the cost of temporarily pushing cells out of their comfort zone. Slower HPA responses damp down the adrenaline rush and, via their effects on the hippocampus, help the brain to learn from experience.

Body systems become less efficient at restoring homeostasis as people get older, however, and eventually the stressors on cells accumulate to overwhelming levels. In the brain, neurons react much as we would: cutting down on expenses like mito-chondria, sacrificing non-essentials like synapses; then tipping over into unsustaina-bility as cell maintenance fails, axons are retracted, and waste builds up; followed by the final collapse, either expiring from starvation or committing suicide.

The principle of hormesis implies that mild, brief stress, now and again, can toughen us up, and therefore help prepare our bodies for future stresses—like age-ing—especially if we can control the source of the challenge. Chronic, inescapable stress, however, is highly damaging, especially to developing brains. (Inescapable stress is a standard way of inducing depression-like symptoms in animal models.) Short-term responses to acute stress helped to keep our ancestors alive. But long-term dysfunction in response to chronic stressors can make people sick or kill them.

And if traumatized individuals survive to reach old age they then face an increased risk of dementia. Age alters HPA axis function, pushing up cortisol levels, and more in women than in men. This is unsurprising given the effects of menopause, with its fall-ing oestrogen levels. Oestrogen and glucocorticoids tend to have opposite effects on body and brain—oestrogen is neuroprotective, whereas glucocorticoids have been linked to cell stress and damage—and oestrogen can damp down the impact of gluco-corticoids. So if with age oestrogen and other neuroprotective factors fall and cortisol rises, brain cells will find it harder to stay within their homeostatic comfort zone.

The behavioural effects of depression, such as social withdrawal, may initially help failing brains to deal with a world that has begun to overload them. In the long term, however, the defence itself does damage, because synapses need stimulation to stay alive.

So far, this exploration of risk factors has concentrated on bodily phenomena that seem to push up the chances of getting dementia. Unfortunately, even if your risk is known to be high you can't buy a new set of genes, or replace your ApoE4s with ApoE3s (not yet, anyway). Nor can you avoid all of the pathogens, environmental hazards, and other stresses that will interact with you and your genes to determine how you person-ally succumb to the grim necessities of fate. However, there are some aspects of your lifestyle that you can alter—and probably should, if you want to lower your chance of getting dementia (and depression, heart disease, stroke, diabetes, and other chronic diseases). It is to these more obviously modifiable risk factors that we now turn.

15

Consumerism, Literally

Chapter 15 plunges us into the bear pit of free will, choice, and personal responsibility. Its topic arrives dragging noisy chains of guilt, shame, anxiety, and moralizing smugness; I will do my best not to rattle them. The topic, of course, is 'lifestyle': specifically, what we eat and how active we are.

Today's society makes life easier in many ways. For moving about, the effortful horse, or even more effortful trudge, has given way to the far less demanding car. For food, we don't even need to move from our ubiquitous screens, thanks to online shopping. And yet, when it comes to other aspects of living, such as finance or technology, we are expected to deal with highly—and increasingly—complicated matters. Do you understand how your computer, smartphone, pension, or government works? If so you are in a small minority. Or perhaps individual citizens are not expected to understand, but to consume.

Consumerism generates desires and then supplies products that are marketed as satisfying those desires. It must do so rapidly and continually to keep the economy growing. The problems with this model are well known. Most relevant for us is that it is biased against products that actually satisfy desire unless they also foster more desire—and so is biased towards more pleasurable and addictive products.[1]

The consumer model works well in many ways. It has given us immensely efficient manufacture and transport systems. It allows a good many of the seven billion plus inhabitants of this planet to live a life far better than their ancestors did, and spend a much smaller proportion of their income on food.[2] Yet when it comes to our health, consumerist incentives intersect catastrophically with the brain's prioritizing of present over future. As far as we know, we are rare among animals in having any sense of the future at all. The capacity evolved late, however; and although we have made great use of it in other ways, we are only beginning to apply it to our own bodies.

An ageing world compels us. And to age better, we need to start early.

Diet and Obesity

Nowhere is the brain's betraying weakness for instant gratification clearer than in what we eat and drink. The mismatch between the drive to give us what we want, now, and the soaring costs of expanding and unhealthy citizens is one of the most urgent challenges besetting governments.

Alas, what we want has been engineered with an eye to our short-term desires, not our long-term benefit. As a review of the topic remarks: 'The industrialisation of food processing in the twentieth century has led to increases in palatability and digestibility with a parallel loss of quality leading to overconsumption.'[3] Modern food engineering makes meals and snacks more palatable and more easily digestible because we prefer them that way. We evolved to store fat, and gobble sugary foods whenever we found them, because those of our ancestors who did that survived long enough to become ancestors in a world where dinner was often hard to find.[4] Now, however, our species has taken control of its food supply. But our genes still make us store and gobble, just in case.

It is, however, not just our genes which make us eat too much and do too little. We face endless marketing demands—'Your food industry needs you. Buy cookies!'—as well as a surfeit of social expectations about food provision which associate plenty with wealth and generosity. I come from a culture where it was taken for granted that any visitors would be offered tea or coffee plus scones, cakes, biscuits, or all three. Moreover, wasting food was a sin and refusing it downright offensive. In times of scarcity, this made good social sense, but for industrialized nations scarcity is a problem now found only among the very poor.

In China, by contrast, people traditionally leave a little on their plates to show they've had an elegant sufficiency. Even China, however, is acquiring Western lifestyles and their associated health problems. Greater wealth brings rising longevity and less child mortality; the downside is that 'Modern populations are increasingly overfed, malnourished, sedentary, sunlight-deficient, sleep-deprived, and socially-isolated.'[5] And, it seems, unwell. Initially the poor health manifests as an increase in conditions like diabetes, heart disease, allergies, depression, and so on; later it shows up in more age-related disorders like dementia. A 2013 study estimated that the number of dementia cases in China rose from 3.68 million in 1990 to 9.19 million in 2010.[6]

One of the most visible consequences of the easy availability of modern food is obesity. It is usually assessed by BMI, with the range between 18.5 and 25 seen as healthy and anything above 30 considered obese.[7] In the United Kingdom in 2010, on average, adult males had a BMI of 27.0, females 26.9. For the United States, the numbers were 29.3 and 29.9, respectively. Not every country is so overweight.[8] For the Central African Republic, one of the world's poorest nations, the average BMIs were 21.0 and 22.0.[9]

Food Quality and Food Habits

Note that people can be overfed—taking in too many calories from macronutrients (carbohydrate, fat, or protein)—and at the same time malnourished. This is because the body also requires small amounts of essential micronutrients such as vitamins, minerals, and fatty acids. Junk food diets provide copious macronutrients, but they are often low in micronutrients and fibre. Those are more typically found in lean meat, fish, some oils, nuts, seeds, fruit, and vegetables, especially dark green leafy ones. And if you find that list depressing, allow me to make it worse. Lentils are nutritionally magnificent: high in fibre and protein, low in fat and salt, and full of useful minerals and vitamins.

Unfortunately for swelling waistlines the world over, it can be much more agreeable to eat high-fat, high-sugar food than to chew on something virtuous, especially if you aren't used to lentils and don't have the time, equipment, or knowledge to prepare them.

Habit and context have much to do with what we eat and drink. The last time I was in a fish-and-chip shop I remember watching, awed, as a customer chatted away while holding the saltcellar upside-down over his chips. His brain had adapted to a diet so highly flavoured that many people would find it unbearable. Neuroimaging studies confirm this flexibility. The brains of obese and lean people respond differently to food, notably in areas associated with visceral, reward, and emotion processing. (Eating is rarely if ever just about nutrition.) A recent preliminary study also found evidence that the brain's adaptation to an unhealthy diet may be reversible.[10] Even adult brains can learn to prefer an initially unappealing food, such as bitter dark chocolate. Or lentils. I can vouch for this, as long as they're well spiced.

However, our physiology's powers of adaptation are not unbounded, and its resilience lessens as we grow older. A study of the effects of weight loss on hormones governing appetite and metabolism—such as leptin, ghrelin, and insulin—found that a year after the weight came off, hormone levels and feelings of hunger had not readjusted.[11] This may be one reason why weight loss is so hard to maintain.

Eating poor-quality food is bad for our bodies, and what is bad for our bodies damages our brains as well. The Deckers consensus rated diet sixth in its list of risk factors for dementia.[12] One of the effects of poor diet is on our vascular systems. Thickening blood vessels may be less obvious than extra inches, but are none the less harmful for only being visible on scans.

Poor diet also contributes to the health problems which often accompany obesity.[13] Excess fat can raise blood sugar, disrupt insulin metabolism, raise blood fats, and lead to inflammation and high blood pressure—all linked to cognitive decline and neurodegeneration. Cardiovascular disease, cancer, and depression are also frequent outcomes, perhaps because of the inflammation associated with obesity.

Passing on the Problems

The nutritional status of parents is, moreover, thought to affect their children, in the womb and later. Earlier we noted that epigenetic changes to DNA can change the levels of proteins made by cells. One cause of such changes may be hormones and other chemicals from the mother's blood that cross into the foetal circulation.

This phenomenon, known as developmental programming, has been much studied by Dutch researchers because of the Dutch Hunger Winter during the Second World War. Towards the end of 1944 the occupying Nazis squeezed food supplies so tightly that the population's daily calorie intake fell to between 400 and 800 kcal. That is far below what it should have been; recommended intakes are 2,500 kcal for men, 2,000 for women.[14] The children of mothers who were pregnant during this and other famines have since been found to be at increased risk for psychiatric illness and for obesity, heart disease, and dementia.

Again the concept of hormesis is relevant, because it seems that parental over-nourishment can also predispose the child towards obesity, metabolic disorders like diabetes, and perhaps some brain disorders too.[15] All things in moderation.

(Parental nutrition is not the only stressor implicated in developmental programming. As we have seen, there is evidence for the harmful effects of severe psychological stress, and animal research suggests that air pollution may have a similar, albeit lesser effect.)

Having a lot of fat is not always a physical problem—as opposed to drawing down social stigma—but it often brings problems to those who are both fat and physically unfit. This is because adipose tissue, particularly abdominal fat, is not just a passive energy store but an active source of chemicals. It produces pro-inflammatory cytokines, leading to chronic, low-level inflammation. It also produces substances called adipokines, such as the hormone leptin, which regulates appetite and blood pressure by acting on the hypothalamus.

We would thus expect that obesity in earlier life should raise the risk of cognitive decline and dementia. Studies indeed suggest that a very high BMI pushes that risk around a third higher—but being underweight also increases it, as does yoyo-ing. A 2015 UK analysis of nearly two million middle-aged people followed for two decades found that the risk from being thin (defined by the researchers as a BMI of less than 20) was thirty-four per cent higher than for normal weight.[16]

However, that study also found, contradicting earlier findings, that excess weight *reduced* the risk of dementia: by twenty-nine per cent for very obese people (BMI greater than 40). This raised eyebrows among academics and beyond. Possible explanations for the difference include the fact that the 2015 study was larger and controlled for more potential confounds than earlier research, or that overweight people, unlike underweight people, die earlier for other reasons. How this fits with findings in animals that calorie restriction promotes longevity has yet to be determined, and further investigations will be needed to settle the debate about obesity and dementia.[17]

Foods versus Diets

Excess weight has much to do with excess consumption, but it also has to do with the quality of what is consumed. To keep our brains healthy, we need to eat a high-quality, healthy diet. However, there are so many diets on the market, and so much apparently conflicting advice, that it can be tempting to ignore the lot and reach for a nice unhealthy snack. So what should we eat for the best chance of staying cognitively healthy long into old age?

Studies of dietary risk factors for dementia have uncovered plenty of associations. Here are some of the better-supported findings.

Low Levels of Micronutrients

Micronutrients including vitamins A, C, D, E, and the B vitamins, minerals such as selenium and magnesium, and omega-3 fatty acids have all been fingered as potentially lacking in dementia, for example in blood tests comparing dementia patients and healthy seniors. Conversely, diets rich in micronutrients seem to protect against dementia from early in life. Being breastfed—which supplies plentiful fatty acids—has been associated with reduced risk of Alzheimer's.[18] Eating fish, which is rich in fatty acids, selenium, and other micronutrients, also seems to protect against cognitive decline, although it is not clear that taking fatty acid supplements has the same effect. Eating plenty of fruit and vegetables has been associated with better mental health and well-being, as well as with better heart health. High consumption of green tea, which is rich in polyphenols, is said to protect against obesity, and possibly against cognitive decline. (Polyphenols in green tea have been shown to inhibit the aggregation of both Aβ and tau into more toxic forms—*in vitro*.[19] So if you're a cell on a petri dish, drink up! If you're a human, to my knowledge no one has yet found significant evidence that drinking green tea in moderation is harmful.)

Some micronutrients, such as vitamin D and omega-3 fatty acids, damp down inflammation and help in the repair of damaged cells. Others, such as vitamins C and E, are known for their anti-oxidant properties. Another possible link between micronutrient deficiency and dementia is via homocysteine, an amino acid that may promote atherosclerosis. B vitamins help metabolize (i.e. get rid of) homocysteine, so B vitamin deficiency might be expected to result in high blood levels of homocysteine, which in turn have been linked to both heart disease and dementia. However, not all research has found this link, and studies using B vitamins to treat dementia are so far inconclusive.

Red Meat and Dairy

High consumption of red meat, which is rich in cholesterol, saturated fat, and iron, has been linked to dementia.[20] Vegetarians are thought to have a lower risk of dementia, and dietary guidelines for the prevention of dementia have recommended reducing meat intake. Some research suggests that as nations adopt a higher-meat diet their dementia rates increase (though as always, correlation does not entail causation). Dementia is, of course, only one of many reasons why eating less meat might be good for many of us (and for the planet). Consumption of dairy products, on the other hand, may be beneficial: a long-term Japanese study found that people who ate and drank more dairy products had a reduced risk of developing dementia, especially Alzheimer's.[21] Further research is needed, however, before this finding can be considered definitive.

Iron and the physiologically similar metals copper and zinc are suspects in dementia.[22] All three metals are highly reactive, and their enthusiasm for shifting electrons makes them potent stimulators of ROS production and oxidative stress. They are also important co-factors, needed to make many biological reactions work—including mitochondrial energy production, gene expression, and cell defence systems such as anti-oxidants. All three interact with Aβ and with ApoE, so are of great interest in Alzheimer's research.

Dietary iron can be obtained from plants, but much more readily from red meat.[23] Zinc and copper can also be obtained from meat—especially if you're a fan of fried liver or devilled kidneys—but are also found in foods which are good for you, like dark green leafy vegetables. If you dislike both organ meats and broccoli, you may be risking mild deficiency of these micronutrients. If you are too poor to be able to afford meat you may be risking iron deficiency, which according to the WHO is 'the most common and widespread nutritional disorder in the world', particularly affecting women and children.[24]

Zinc and copper have important roles in normal neural activity. They are released along with neurotransmitters like glutamate, regulate the activity of their receptors, and are required co-factors for many important enzymes, including those that regulate gene expression.

Iron, like copper, is required for mitochondria to function. It is also involved in the making of neurotransmitters and myelin. It is abundant in the brain, but its levels are—in healthy brains at least—tightly regulated. Anaemia is a common result of iron deficiency, but too much iron can also be a problem. Mutations which lead to iron accumulation in the brain lead to movement problems, developmental delays, and later to parkinsonian symptoms and dementia. Yet iron, zinc, and copper are crucial to early development. Deficiencies during pregnancy have been associated with numerous problems, including brain disorders like schizophrenia.

Iron is transported as part of organic compounds called hemes, the best known of which is the blood protein haemoglobin. Hemes readily bind to amyloid proteins, competing with copper for binding sites. Heme levels have been found to be increased in Alzheimer's brains; and iron also builds up in amyloid plaques and in blood vessels damaged by cerebral amyloid angiopathy. (A 2014 genetic study found evidence that iron metabolism may be faulty in Alzheimer's disease.[25])

Iron also regulates production of APP, and hence Aβ. Higher iron levels encourage more APP production, but also seem to favour the neuroprotective α-secretase pathway, which leads to sAPPα, not Aβ. Interestingly, the pro-inflammatory cytokine IL-1 exhibits similar behaviour, suggesting that inflammatory stimuli may also boost APP levels.[26] Cell studies suggest that APP tends to push iron out of the cell, thereby reducing oxidative stress. Meanwhile, outside the cell Aβ rapidly binds iron (and copper) into plaques, likewise potentially acting as an anti-oxidant.[27] Perhaps one reason the APP gene evolved as it did was because it was a useful mopper-up of these reactive metals. And perhaps amyloid plaques can act as reservoirs for excess metals as well as other potentially dangerous material, like Aβ oligomers.

Processed Foods

High consumption of refined carbohydrates has been suggested as a potential health problem (e.g. brown bread and rice are considered better than their white equivalents), as has high consumption of fried food, barbecued food, and preserved or processed food containing transfats and other artificial components like sweeteners and emulsifiers. These are rich in sugar-protein compounds which activate the cellular receptor RAGE, which as we saw earlier is well placed to contribute to neurodegeneration.[28] Such foods also lack micronutrients and fibre found in their less processed (e.g. wholegrain) sources. Fibre is material that is eaten but not digested, and its presence has numerous benefits, helping to keep blood levels of sugar, cholesterol, and other fats within normal ranges.[29] This is why some researchers advocate adding high-fibre foods like beans and lentils, suitably mashed, to sausages, hamburgers, and other meat products as a way of reining in ballooning waistlines.

Processed foods often also contain high levels of sugar and/or saturated fat, though this may not always be clear to consumers. Some studies have implicated fructose as the top sugar villain. Others argue that it is the total sugar intake that causes the problems. Similarly for saturated fat; some researchers think the problem is more to do with how much people eat, and the abundance of food cues, than with which type of fat is eaten. High levels of dietary saturated fat and cholesterol have been linked to increased dementia risk, but the evidence is by no means conclusive. As we have seen with respect to diabetes, however, too much sugar affects the brain as well as enlarging the belly.

Quick Fix or Slow Change?

For consumers interested in adjusting their diet to reduce their risk of dementia there are two ways of approaching this massive—and often maddeningly nebulous—body of research (apart, that is, from curling up in a ball and weeping). The first is to look for a quick fix: a supplement or superfood to serve up better nutrition. The second is harder: to change overall eating patterns.

The quick fix approach is problematic, especially in clinically healthy folk (if you have been diagnosed with a micronutrient deficiency, such as low vitamin D, that is another matter). For one thing, much of the research in this field uses animal models, most often rodents. However, rats and mice do not process fats and carbohydrates in quite the way humans do, and there are other metabolic differences too, so it is not always clear how well findings in animals apply to people.

Furthermore, seeking a quick fix assumes that there exists some single product that will solve the problem. Yet the brain, as we have seen, is hugely complex and therefore vulnerable in many ways. Dementia and other age-related disorders are multifaceted. Each of the risk factors discussed here may shift the balance of probabilities slightly towards making them more likely to happen, and to happen earlier; but only a few rare genes make early-onset disease a certainty.

It is therefore highly unlikely that a single dietary change could solve the problems of poor brain ageing. Studies which have applied such changes—for example, with vitamin supplements—have not to date produced convincing evidence that their chosen factor brings the hoped-for benefits.

The list of dietary associations highlights another issue: our old acquaintance correlation. Many people who eat high-fat diets also consume large quantities of sugar and processed food. Red meat is often fried or barbecued, or served in a soft white bun. Fruit and vegetables may not feature highly, reducing the intake of micronutrients and fibre. Calorie-rich soft or alcoholic drinks may be favoured over green tea and water. And portions may be unnecessarily large.

In other words, it may be the eating pattern and amount of food that matters, not consumption of any particular food or supplement. This is what the science suggests. Strip away the media noise generated by promotion of particular foods or diets, and the underlying research looks a lot more consistent. Poor nutrition raises the risk for several conditions that, while serious in themselves, are also risk factors for dementia (like diabetes). Very poor nutrition in early life slows physical growth, resulting in shorter limbs and smaller heads, and both of these factors appear to be markers for a raised risk of later dementia.[30] (As with the risk conferred by ApoE4, that does not mean that an unlucky start in life condemns you to inevitable senility, but you may have to work harder to avoid it.) Conversely, healthy eating patterns seem to go with better heart, cardiovascular, and brain health. As a recent review puts it:

Can we say what diet is best for health? If diet denotes a very specific set of rigid principles, then even this necessarily limited representation of a vast literature is more than sufficient to answer with a decisive no. If, however, by diet we mean a more general dietary pattern, a less rigid set of guiding principles, the answer reverts to an equally decisive yes.[31]

So what is that general dietary pattern? It was pithily summed up by journalist and food activist Michael Pollan as, 'Eat food. Not too much. Mostly plants.'[32] The review expands this apophthegm as follows:

The aggregation of evidence in support of (a) diets comprising preferentially minimally processed foods direct from nature and food made up of such ingredients, (b) diets comprising mostly plants, and (c) diets in which animal foods are themselves the products, directly or ultimately, of pure plant foods—the composition of animal flesh and milk is as much influenced by diet as we are—is noteworthy for its breadth, depth, diversity of methods, and consistency of findings. The case that we should, indeed, eat true food, mostly plants, is all but incontrovertible.

An example of a healthier eating pattern is the so-called Mediterranean diet. It includes plenty of fruit and veg, nuts, seeds, legumes (beans, peas, lentils), fish, whole grains, some dairy produce and wine, and not much meat. Other foods are not excluded, but moderation in all things is encouraged. Sweet treats and highly processed foods are not regarded with favour.

Healthy eating is associated with lower risk of diseases such as some cancers and heart disease. The specific case for diet having a role in preventing dementia is less strong. This may not be unrelated to the fact that, in the United Kingdom in 2010, total dementia research funding amounted to about £50 million, one-tenth of what was spent on cancer—and dietary research was a fraction of that.[33] Dietary studies are large, complex, and difficult to do well, especially when what is being investigated is the effect on late-life brain function of dietary intakes decades earlier.

Nonetheless, healthy eating patterns like the Mediterranean diet seem to have some protective effects (albeit people who eat well can still get dementia). In addition, good diets reduce the risk of conditions like cardiovascular disease, diabetes, and high blood pressure, which are themselves risk factors—or even possible causes—of dementia.

A healthy mind requires a healthy body. And that—in a world full of tempting, easy, and unhealthy food—is a challenging goal to achieve, and to maintain as you get older.

Caveat Lector—Reader Beware

One reason why research on obesity, and on diet and brain health, is not as clear and conclusive as you might think it should be is that doing such research on humans is difficult even when it does not involve dementia. Most people's diets contain a range of foods, and one person's range is rarely identical to another's, or exactly the same from week to week. Few adults are available, or willing, to go into seclusion for long periods and undergo intrusive measurements, so their intake cannot be strictly controlled. Instead, they must be asked about their eating habits. For example, the US national health survey NHANES includes questions about diet.[34]

Questions about diet, however, can open nasty cans of psychological worms. That fallible instrument human memory is especially prone to distortion when concerned with emotive topics like food consumption, even in people without dementia. Committed to the causes of science, honesty, and truth though we may be in principle, when faced with a food questionnaire we have a regrettable tendency to fib. To take one example, in 2013, a review of the NHANES stated that over the thirty-nine years it had been running, data 'on the majority of respondents (67.3% of women and 58.7% of men) were not physiologically plausible'. That is, humans could not survive on the energy intake these people reported.[35]

No wonder that some researchers think dietary measurements are not fit for purpose, and hope that new technology (e.g. smartphone apps) can solve some of the problems. Larger, better-designed studies are certainly needed. The current consensus, however, is clear: healthy eating patterns like the Mediterranean diet are good for your heart, and what's good for your heart is good for your brain as well. Conversely, some eating patterns, like so-called Western and junk food diets, are bad for you. So feel free to disregard media frenzies about new dietary fads. Our knowledge of the benefits and harms of eating patterns has considerably more research, of different kinds, behind it, and it is a better guide to a healthier brain.

16

Exercise

Another area where new technology may improve measurements that badly need improving is that of physical exercise, the output to diet's input. The Deckers review rated physical activity as the fourth most important modifiable risk factor for dementia.

Epidemiological evidence strongly links physical inactivity—in midlife or earlier as well as in later years—with increased dementia risk. For instance, a large Swedish study of army recruits found that low (versus high) cardiovascular fitness at age eighteen more than doubled the risk of early-onset dementia.[1] Exercise earlier in life has been linked to less cognitive impairment later. Recent studies using more accurate methods of measuring activity have found that those who exercise more, even in their eighties, tend to have better cognitive function. There is debate, however, about how beneficial physical activity is for people already suffering from cognitive impairment or dementia.

Moving is Good for You

Nor is it fully understood how physical exercise provides its benefits. Likely mechanisms include its positive effects on heart and vascular health: as well as boosting blood flow around the body and brain, regular exercise seems to help ageing blood vessels stay more elastic. Research suggests that in people carrying the ApoE4 gene variant, maintaining high aerobic fitness can reduce the risk of arterial disease, and cognitive decline, to levels comparable to those of non-carriers. Exercise is thought to affect the function of the sympathetic nervous system, and hence the stress response. And here again hormesis may apply, with moderate exercise exerting a mild stress on cells, enabling them to adapt their chemistry to be more stress tolerant, and therefore better protected against future stressors like those induced by ageing. (Extreme exercise, by contrast, can do considerable damage, which is why any sensible exercise programme starts gently and builds up the exertion gradually.)

Regular exercise also alters immune function, notably by reducing levels of pro-inflammatory cytokines. This may be why it seems to help treat mild to moderate depression, and also why overweight but physically fit people tend not to show the increased inflammation that is a risk factor for chronic disease.

Exercise may in addition specifically benefit the brain, increasing synaptic plasticity and improving connectivity between brain regions in humans. Animal studies suggest it achieves this by encouraging production of neurotrophins like BDNF.

The Killer Sloth

There may be continuing discussion of the mechanisms, but many researchers agree on one thing: people don't do nearly enough exercise, and modern lifestyles don't encourage them to do so. Modern governments have been much exercised by obesity, but physical inactivity is at least as big a problem.[2] Western populations are often said to be less active than their ancestors even a few generations ago—let alone the modern hunter-gatherer peoples whose lifestyle is the closest existing equivalent to that of our more distant ancestors.

And why wouldn't we be less active? If you travel to work, you may well find that it is easier and pleasanter to take the car than walk or cycle on a cold or rainy morning (and perhaps on other days too). Walking and cycling are good for you, but you and your daily occupation may be too far apart, or the route between too dangerous, the buses or trains too unreliable, or the daily grind too long and grinding, to make them realistic options. And if you are out of the exercise habit, it's painful, often boring, hard work.

As the fierce debate about the causes of obesity shows, there is immense controversy over the relative contributions of excessive food intake, food quality, lack of exercise, work patterns, overweening industry, supine government, and personal vice.[3] The complexity and incompleteness of the science leaves plenty of room for ideology, with consumers blaming industry and government, and *vice versa*. Both sides, however, focus simplistically on inputs and outputs: food quantity and quality, and exercise. The problem is that these affect the bit in between: the way our bodies handle food and respond to exercise. Bodies and brains adapt to poor diets and inert lifestyles, up to a point. Thus unhealthy people respond differently to changes—and may find it less easy to make them than they would if they were healthier.

Pollution, dietary changes like more highly processed food, differing sleep patterns, financial stress, and social isolation may also have affected our metabolism.

As I have noted repeatedly, these are not independent in their effects. They are also all thought to be risk factors for Alzheimer's.

With respect to obesity, we must await the results of better measurement and larger, longer, more rigorous studies before ruling it in, or out, as a risk for dementia. Exercise, however, has benefits beyond any effects on weight, and lack of exercise does a lot of harm. In 2004, according to the WHO, physical inactivity was responsible for about five per cent of all deaths on planet Earth: 3.2 million.[4] This makes it the fourth most deadly of their global health risks, after high blood glucose (3.4 million), tobacco use (5.1 million), and high blood pressure (7.5 million). Too much weight is fifth on the risk list, linked to 2.8 million deaths. We often think of these five killers as conditions affecting the developed world; and indeed, they are the top five health risks in high-income nations.[5] But they are also all—except for excess weight—in the top ten for low-income nations.

What the Experts Think You Should be Doing

In 2008, the US government issued guidelines for physical activity.[6] For adults, the recommendations are:

- Aerobic physical activity: do at least 2½ hours per week of moderate-intensity exercise (e.g. brisk walking), or 1¼ hours per week of vigorous-intensity exercise (e.g. running).[7]
- Muscle-strengthening activities: do moderate- or high-intensity exercise at least twice a week.

Yet the CDC reckons that fewer than half of American citizens do enough exercise to meet its guidelines (which are minimal amounts), and they are not alone. The WHO, in a 2015 summary statement, puts the proportion of insufficiently active adults at twenty-five per cent, globally, and gives the figure for adolescents as more than eighty per cent.[8]

The guidelines plead with readers to do as much as they can manage, because 'Some physical activity is better than none.' Regular exercise reduces the risk of early death and of numerous diseases, including heart disease, diabetes, stroke, some common cancers (e.g. breast and colon cancer), and depression. It also benefits hypertension, blood fat and sugar levels, and bone density, and helps prevent weight gain. High activity levels are thought to be one reason why some populations, such as the Tsimane of the Amazon, look like prime candidates for cardiovascular disease (they have low HDL, high blood triglycerides, and high levels of infection and inflammatory markers like CRP) but don't seem to get atherosclerosis.[9]

Keeping active is part of a pro-brain lifestyle. Yet even if you aren't concerned about dementia, there are clearly many other good reasons to take exercise.

In Chapter 15 we considered food. Now we return to consumption, and to some of the other interesting substances we humans like to put inside ourselves.

17

Traditional Vices

In August 2007, a study was published in the *American Journal of Epidemiology* which considered research linking smoking with dementia and cognitive decline.[1] Nicotine was—and still is—thought to have beneficial effects on cognition via its activation of receptors for acetylcholine, and there was conflicting evidence as to whether smoking protected against dementia.[2] The study, by Kaarin Anstey and colleagues, was a meta-analysis, pulling together information from previous studies on 26,374 participants (for dementia) and 17,023 participants (for cognitive decline).

The Many Trials of Meta-analysis

This was not easy, because different researchers had done very different science. Some studies recorded 'dementia', others 'Alzheimer's disease'. Cognition and its decline were measured in varying ways. Smoking could be logged in terms of how many packs for how long, or whether the person smoked now or had ever smoked. The size, age, gender balance, backgrounds, and countries of the samples also varied, and people were followed up for different lengths of time.

Some studies were case-control—that is, they compared a group of patients and a group of controls—people judged to be very similar to the patients, except for being healthy. Other research used cohorts: a sample studied for years in the expectation that some will develop dementia. Case-control studies are seen as inferior to cohort studies because their design means that researchers already know who the patients are as the study begins, which may unconsciously lead to bias. Case-control studies are also often smaller than cohort studies.[3] In cohort studies only time will tell who becomes a patient; but cohort studies can last for decades and cost a fortune.[4]

What kinds of bias might be relevant? Case-control studies of smoking and dementia involve retrospective questions (e.g. about the person's education and smoking history). Often the only feasible way to learn about someone's past is to ask them, and human memory is a very fallible construct, especially for someone with Alzheimer's.

As well as this recall bias, there is survival bias. Dementia is a lethal disease. People who survive long enough, and in good enough health, to take part in studies may not be representative of the whole population. The gradual nature of diseases like Alzheimer's can also cause bias. A person abruptly breaks a leg, but dementia is stealthier. It must cross at least two thresholds for formal diagnosis: the one at which the person goes to their doctor and the one where the bad news is confirmed. Some apparently healthy case-control study participants may already be developing Alzheimer's, blurring the differences between patients and controls. Indeed, a study of older people (aged seventy-plus) which looked for signs of Alzheimer's, Lewy body dementia, or vascular dementia found that 'approximately 95% of subjects without dementia in this age group have some pathologic evidence of at least one of these three diseases'.[5]

Then there are problems of sampling bias—how the cases and controls are chosen in the first place. Patients referred from a memory clinic, for example, may have different characteristics from people identified as having dementia by a survey of the population.

Meta-analysis is a method which tries to overcome, or at least take account of, this variability. It offers statistical ways of extracting and combining data while taking into account the strength of the original research.[6] Meta-analysis is effortful and time-consuming: it can take six months to do one. Almost all of that is not the actual statistics but the systematic literature review which precedes them, which sorts through the research, removing unsuitable papers—like those without numerical data. The Anstey study identified 6,455 initial abstracts. It whittled them down to nineteen it could use.[7]

Smoking and Dementia

And what, after all their labour, did Anstey and colleagues conclude about smoking and dementia? That 'elderly current smokers are at increased risk of dementia and cognitive decline compared with those who have never smoked but that there remains insufficient data to determine how past smoking affects risk of both cognitive decline and dementia'.

And yet earlier studies and reviews had found clear reduced risk for dementia among smokers. Lee (1994), for instance, found 'a highly significant (p < 0.001) negative association', with never-smokers at close on twice the risk of those who had ever smoked.[8] Could the nature of the relationship have changed in the decade between

1994 and 2005, the cut-off date for the Anstey analysis? Or could both findings be statistical hallucinations?

A 2010 publication by Janine Cataldo and colleagues offered an alternative explanation.[9] Another meta-analysis, it combined data from forty-three case-control and cohort studies on the link between smoking and Alzheimer's disease. Pooling all the resulting data gave no significant result—no apparent link. But Cataldo and her colleagues did something more interesting: they split the studies by type (case-control versus cohort) and by whether the authors were affiliated to the tobacco industry. Eleven studies did have such affiliations, of which three had said so.[10]

Cataldo *et al.* found that for case-control studies (favoured by the industry), pooling the data from the eight studies with tobacco industry affiliation gave a lower likelihood of Alzheimer's for smokers. The eighteen non-affiliated studies found no statistically significant effect. For cohort studies, the three with industry links found a reduction in risk, but it was not significant. The fourteen without industry affiliation found that smoking increased the risk of Alzheimer's significantly, by nearly one-half.[11] A 2015 meta-analysis has confirmed this, with a proviso: the effect depends on which ApoE gene variant people have.[12]

Scientific journals' policies on declaring conflicts of interest are tighter now than they were in 1994, but many still place the declarations within the paper, rather than upfront with the more widely read abstract. By highlighting the differences between industry-affiliated and other research, Cataldo and colleagues' publication was a useful contribution to the debate about smoking and dementia.

Nicotine may be good for concentration, but cigarettes contain a good deal more than just nicotine. A recent study on a large and well-characterized sample from the Lothian Birth Cohorts found significant brain differences between those who still smoked, or had smoked, and those who did not. Smokers had thinner cortex, especially in prefrontal areas.[13] Given the damage smoking is known to do to other areas of the body (like the heart and vascular system), and given the brain's reliance on its blood vessels, concerns about getting dementia are just one more reason to switch to e-cigarettes or patches, or give up entirely.

Drinking and Dementia

Annoying though it is of nature to have evolved human bodies which cope so badly with long-term poisoning, not all vices are equally bad for you. One poison for which the evidence of harm is less stark than it is for breathing in tar and heavy metals is alcohol. (Current evidence for other recreational drugs is meagre, so I will not be discussing them here.)

Drinking too much for too long is undoubtedly harmful. It costs the NHS about as much as smoking and has wider social costs, like policing and domestic violence. Apart from its well-known effects on the heart, liver, cardiovascular system, and dignity, it can do great damage to the brain.[14] Alcoholism can deplete levels of vitamin B1, *aka* thiamine; it can kill neurons and severely affect white matter. In extreme cases it can lead to confusion and psychosis, as in Wernicke encephalopathy and Korsakoff syndrome. (These can be treated by giving patients the B vitamin.)

Smaller quantities of alcohol, however, do not seem to have especially dire effects. Indeed, it has been suggested that light-to-moderate drinking may protect against cognitive decline and dementia, perhaps because it benefits the cardiovascular system.[15] Two meta-analyses, in 2009 and 2011, found protective effects against dementia. The second suggested that these effects came from drinking wine, not beer or spirits.[16] So, is it time to break out your favourite red?

Before you settle back with an extra glass—or, if you're not a drinker, resolve to add wine to the shopping list—I should sound some notes of caution. First, any benefits apply to social drinking only, up to fourteen units (six glasses of wine or pints of lager) per week, and may only apply to older women.[17] Often, 'light-to-moderate drinking' turns out to be heavier than the drinker reckons, and even the lower end of alcohol consumption can bring problems. Secondly, health authorities don't advise the abstinent to start drinking, whether to reduce dementia risk or for other reasons. There are lifestyle changes which are better for you and less expensive than a wine habit, regular brisk walks being one example. Thirdly, as a 2016 UK government review pointed out, drinking alcohol brings other risks, such as a higher likelihood of getting certain cancers (e.g. of the liver, female breast, large bowel, mouth and throat, and perhaps pancreas). The review estimated that '4–6% of all new cancers in the UK in 2013 were caused by alcohol consumption'. It put the lifetime risk of dying from an alcohol-related condition at around one per cent, comparable to the risk from routine driving, for people who drink fourteen or more units per week, which outweighs any likely health benefits.[18]

My final caveat relates—yet again—to covariates. Alcohol has multiple effects on the body, including the delivery of calories. Some of its harmful effects may be due to interactions between drinking and diet. For example, a healthy diet may protect against vitamin deficiencies like lack of thiamine, making diet an important, but often neglected covariate.[19] There is also a technical problem: objective measurements of both diet and alcohol intake are not easy to obtain. Furthermore, human beings still eat mostly foods, which contain multiple chemicals, rather than purer formulations like supplements or medicines—with the obvious exception of sugar. This makes it even more difficult to determine which ingredients may be providing any benefits.

Furthermore, both eating and drinking can vary a lot depending on the social conditions surveyed. These include both an individual's socioeconomic status and that of their neighbourhood, with residence in more deprived areas generally linked to more drinking, poorer diet, and more harmful drinking patterns such as bingeing. These social variables also affect people's readiness to visit doctors and participate in research studies. A typical volunteer tends to be well educated and middle class, already interested in looking after his or her health and already doing plenty to maintain it. One wonders, therefore, how much of the alcohol advantage is really down to the alcohol itself.

Minor Vices: Coffee, Tea, and Dark Chocolate

Nonetheless, there is little evidence that a glass of wine now and then will do you any harm, as long as the nows and thens are not too close together and the glasses not too large. The same seems to apply to both coffee and tea. Indeed, meta-analyses of caffeine consumption suggest potential protection against both Alzheimer's and Parkinson's. Cocoa and dark chocolate have also been found to be beneficial to cognition.

All of these contain phytophenols: compounds such as quercetin (found in onions) and catechins (in tea) which plants produce to protect themselves from dangers like infection or ultraviolet light.[20] Phytophenols are one reason why a food's unpleasant taste is no guarantee that it will be bad for you, and *vice versa*. They give dark chocolate its exquisite bitterness, yet this—to novices—foul-tasting substance is much healthier than the sweeter, milky version.

Chemically, phytophenols seem to act as anti-oxidants and anti-inflammatories. They also benefit the vascular system by reducing blood clots, atherosclerosis, and hence the dangerous blockages which, in the brain, can lead to strokes. Some, like quercetin, appear to be helpful in diabetes too.[21]

Many plant-derived chemicals may benefit health, but not all do. Some, like the phytoestrogens in soy, may interfere with the body's own hormones, although the science of soy's effects on humans remains uncertain.[22] Some, like the alkaloids in deadly nightshade, are downright poisonous. Some, like caffeine, are toxic only at very high—though feasible—doses.[23] This is unsurprising given that phytophenols are mild toxins which evolved to kill microbes. It is perhaps more surprising that many seem to be so good for us.

Why plant poisons do us good is not clear. They may act through hormesis, toughening up cells without being nasty enough to damage them. Some, such as the catechins in green tea, are known anti-oxidants. Another possible mechanism is that phytophenols increase production of nitric oxide, a key vascular regulator which affects endothelial cells, and thereby blood vessels. Nitric oxide is an extremely versatile molecule, with roles in the immune system, and as a cellular messenger in the brain, as well as in the control of blood pressure. It too obeys the principle of hormesis, being beneficial in small doses but dangerous in large ones. Genetic variants which affect nitric oxide levels influence the likelihood of getting coronary artery disease and have also been linked to Alzheimer's, not least since Aβ can influence nitric oxide production.

One last note of caution. Much of the work to date on phytophenols—and indeed on diet more generally—has been on animals, or comes from epidemiological studies rather than from large-scale, long-term clinical trials.[24] (Of course, we may lack evidence for an idea because people have looked and not found it, or because they haven't yet thoroughly looked.)

All in all, you might want to switch from milk chocolate to a darker variety, but the science doesn't currently support forcing yourself to drink coffee if, like me, you can't abide the stuff.

Diet, exercise, and smoking are among the lifestyle factors which are often thought to be under personal control. There are some aspects of the way we live, however, which even the most vehement individualist might admit are not altogether up to us. Those less modifiable environmental risk factors are our next topic.

Unhealthy Environments

Where you live and have lived, and what environments you have been exposed to, appears to have an impact on your chance of a healthy old age. The Industrial Revolution and its continuing aftermath brought many improvements, but also placed novel stresses on fragile brains.

Industry is not the sole culprit, however. Some studies suggest that living in rural areas is associated with higher risk for dementia and cognitive impairment than urban living. Whether this is due to differences in the setting (e.g. greater exposure to pesticides and poor nutrition in the countryside) or to differences in the people (e.g. lower education levels or more loneliness in rural populations)—or of course both—remains to be fully understood.

Chemical Poisoning

Modern life is full of poisons, but only some of them have been linked to increased risk of dementia.[1] Among the prime candidates are metals such as lead, arsenic, nickel, cadmium, iron, aluminium, and mercury.[2] Lead, for example, has long been known to be damaging to brains and their cognitive capacities, and high lead exposure is linked to low IQ, impulsivity, and violence. Studies of lead exposure as a risk factor for dementia are, however, few.

Extensive research into whether you can get Alzheimer's from either aluminium cooking utensils or mercury in your fillings has not found enough evidence to confirm either proposition. High exposure to air pollution—from second-hand cigarette smoke, traffic fumes, or industrial processes—is another matter. As well as metals, the emitted particulates contain high levels of carbon, carbon monoxide, nitrogen dioxide, and other toxins. These stress the heart, lungs, circulation and, it seems, the brain.

That stress may be exerted directly and via effects on other organs. Particulates are known to activate the transcription factor NFκB, increasing inflammation; and they can also raise oxidative stress. They worsen chronic conditions such as heart disease and diabetes, and they can raise levels of Aβ. A 2015 preliminary study in mice found changes in cytokines and amyloid build-up with prolonged exposure to particulates. Worryingly, particulates at levels that met national air quality standards were able to cause these changes.[3] Another study, in rats, of the effects of air pollution found that it was able to activate microglia and damage or destroy cortical neurons.[4]

If it were only rats who suffered from living in highly polluted cities, most people might be prepared to tolerate the situation. However, epidemiological research also suggests a link between higher pollution levels, poorer cognitive function, and signs of early neurodegeneration in human residents. I have already mentioned (in Chapter 6) research from Mexico City which found amyloid building up in children.[5] One population-based cohort study from Taiwan (of almost 30,000 people) found that those living in the most polluted areas, compared with the least polluted, had about a fifty per cent higher risk of dementia.[6] Studies on the effects of second-hand smoke also point to increased risk in those extensively exposed.

Organic compounds such as pesticides have been implicated too. They have been linked to neurodevelopmental disorders like autism and attention-deficit hyperactivity disorder, perhaps via effects on thyroid function. Much more research is needed to assess their roles, if any, in ageing and dementia. For example, a small study found that exposure to the pesticide DDT was associated with higher risk of Alzheimer's, especially in ApoE4 carriers.[7] Studies of US military exposure to chemicals in wartime—for example, Agent Orange in Vietnam and Gulf War illness—have suggested that these also raise the risk of dementia. A study of nearly 25,000 workers exposed to polychlorinated biphenyls (PCBs), however, found no increased risk of dementia, although PCBs have been repeatedly linked to effects on neurodevelopment.[8]

Electromagnetic Poisoning

Again, research is limited. However, what data I have been able to find suggest that living close to power lines is not linked to getting dementia.[9] Neither is being exposed to radiation from an atomic bomb. Although ionizing radiation—for example, repeated X-rays—might in principle be a risk factor for patients, evidence is lacking that the risk outweighs the benefits.[10] Governments minded to improve population health might prefer to concentrate their efforts on air pollution and leave the phone masts alone.

Being Poor

One of the major determinants of where you live is how much money you have. Being poor is thus a big contributor to living in an unhealthy environment.[11]

In the West, social mobility has been congealing for decades. It is now so ossified that most people's fates can be predicted from their parents' socioeconomic status. Economic inequality, meanwhile, has risen, and research suggests that both inequality and poverty can have profoundly detrimental effects on health and educational success, especially in young children. This is relevant to dementia because an increasing theme in neuroscience is that severely adverse events in early life may have lifelong effects—raising the risks for chronic disease and poor ageing.

Studying these potential effects of early life on old age is extremely difficult unless a large number of people has been followed from birth (or even before). Large age-matched groups like the ALSPAC cohort, started in the 1990s, are now being investigated, but will have to wait decades before their participants become vulnerable to dementia, though they could be invaluable for detecting its very first signs, in midlife or younger, if the funding lasts that long.[12] Older cohorts, like the Lothian Birth Cohorts—comprised of Scottish people who took a cognitive test while at school in 1932 or 1947 and were then followed up by later scientists—are proving immensely useful now, but lack access to the kinds of detailed early data that researchers crave.[13]

Evidence relating to poverty, therefore, is still being collected, especially as poverty and inequality have many potential mechanisms through which they can damage brains, whether young or adult. Financial deprivation brings many stresses: unhealthy environments, poor diets, a greater threat of violence, addiction, and abuse, and sometimes poor or non-existent education, recourse to justice, and health care. Drugs for dementia, for example, may be unaffordable. Poverty can thus be a major source of preventable health and social problems, especially in states with inadequate or non-existent welfare provision.[14]

Being at the unlucky end of the income scale also worsens the impact of other stresses. For instance, a large meta-analysis of the relationship between long working hours and diabetes found that the one does appear to be linked to a greater risk of developing the other—but only in people with low socioeconomic status (SES).[15]

The quality of evidence linking dementia to many of the risk factors I have been discussing is not ideal.[16] For financial status it is parlous because little research has yet been done. A small study in 2014 found evidence that poorer people wait longer before attending a specialist memory clinic, so that they are more likely to have gone beyond mild cognitive impairment to dementia.[17] In 2007, a larger, long-term study of civil servants reported that 'Those at the lowest SES ranks exhibited estimated

3-fold and 6-fold [higher] dementia rates', but noted potential biases.[18] In 2009, a study at an inner-city memory clinic found some support for low annual income being a predictor of dementia.[19] And in 2011, a cohort study of 1,789 people found that high SES persisting through childhood and adulthood was associated with about half the risk of dementia or cognitive impairment compared with low SES.[20]

These are mainly studies of adult income. Whether childhood poverty has an effect is not clear, although higher parental SES has been linked with better cognitive function in the grown-up children, and lower childhood SES has been linked to faster late-life cognitive decline.

The effects of poverty do, however, appear to be reversible if treated early. A 2008 study from Mexico found that poor children's cognitive skills could be improved by the simple expedient of giving their parents more cash, conditional on good behaviours like regular medical check-ups and school attendance.[21] The possible savings are huge. It has been estimated that if the health status of US citizens without a college-level education could be improved to match that of more highly educated Americans, the benefits would be worth around a trillion dollars a year.[22]

Sleep Debt

I have already mentioned sleep problems in the context of Alzheimer's, and the idea that sleep may allow the washing away of proteins like Aβ which would otherwise build up and damage the brain. Sleep proverbially knits up the ravelled sleeve of care; might it help unknit amyloid fibrils? Living in unhealthy environments unravels the sleeve, and poor sleep is often part of the problem.

The link appears to work both ways. Poor sleep leads to less Aβ clearance, while the build-up of Aβ can disrupt sleep, particularly the kind of sleep needed for memory consolidation.

Sleep deprivation—for example, due to shift work—is a risk factor for numerous age-related brain conditions, including Alzheimer's and stroke. Shift work also increases the risk of chronic diseases like diabetes.[23] A recent UK government report estimates that among workers '33% of men and 22% of women', mostly young, do shift work, so the potential health effects are considerable.[24] As well as age, there is also an interaction with poverty, as shift workers with the lowest income are more likely to report worse health than those with the highest income.

Poorer quality, rather than quantity, of sleep has also been proposed as a risk factor. Sleep quality may be affected by many things: eating patterns, noise and light pollution, temperature, anxiety and stress, late-night screen use, hormones, and so on. One hormone of interest to researchers is melatonin, which regulates the circadian rhythm, the daily, light-entrained cycle which governs many body processes and which is known to decline with age. Melatonin and similar drugs are used to treat insomnia and circadian rhythm disturbances like jet lag. Alzheimer's, like many diseases, varies in its intensity and the likelihood of mortality according to a daily rhythm, with symptoms tending to worsen towards evening ('sundowning').[25] Researchers giving melatonin treatment to dementia patients report that it eases these symptoms, while animal work suggests melatonin may contribute to healthy ageing.

Clinical conditions can also have an impact (likewise, poor sleep affects pre-existing illnesses). One common problem is sleep apnoea, estimated to affect between three per cent and seven per cent of people, in which the sleeper's airways relax so much that they collapse, restricting breathing and dragging the person back towards wakefulness.[26]

Finally, genes surely play a role in the human variability which leads us to react so differently to food and other stimuli. My flatmate can drink strong coffee and eat cake after dinner and then sleep placidly, undisturbed by drunken passers-by. I have on occasion semi-dismembered a bedroom in the effort to silence a tiny electrical hum, and if I drank coffee—at all—I'd be wide awake at three in the morning.

To acknowledge the influence of genes, however, is not to argue against the importance of studying environments. Both matter. And environments, given the will, can be improved.

The Western world faces many converging problems, the harmful legacy of our espousal of industrialized consumerism. The drive for profit—in some cases irrespective of whether the product kills people—is creating a 'bulge' of increased ill health in populations. This is already putting terrible pressure on Western health-care systems, and the rest of the world is starting to feel the pressure too.

Some of the problems, like physical inactivity and poor diet, worsened in the twentieth century, but may now be improving in the West. Others, like pollution and smoking, have clearly improved in the West in recent decades, driven by state action and vigorous media campaigns, but are worsening in parts of the developing world. Often the risk has been known for decades, but governments have struggled to make change happen. Even when risks are publicly discussed, however, those discussions are frequently incomplete—and far too short-term in outlook.

Some of us can, after all, smoke, eat appallingly, and take no exercise for years—lucky genes permitting—before the damage becomes incapacitating, especially if we can't or won't access health care. Unless we die of something else, however, we are likely to face a reckoning sooner or later. And despite those cheery stories of smokers reaching their centenary (which make the news because they are unusual), it is mostly sooner. The choices we make—now, today, whatever age we are—can affect not only how fast our bodies fall apart but when our minds succumb to the challenges of old age. If we can reduce as many risks as possible now, the swelling bulge of ill health in our societies will be less prolonged. Our governments will have a better chance of managing the finances without either abandoning all attempts at welfare or taxing us into collective ruin—or riot. And we will boost our chances of feeling better, and thinking better, for longer. It's a win–win situation. If only it weren't so hard to bring about.

The final set of risks I want to consider relates to how we use our brains. Such risks illustrate the themes that have emerged from our discussion so far: the intricate conversations between genetics and environment, body and history, and the social and individual forces that shape each person's arc from birth to death. Everything comes together at that extraordinary nexus we call the brain. There, external factors and personal choices mesh in the welter of chemical reactions and electron exchanges that underlie successful ageing—or synaptic failure and neuronal death.

Dementia is a brain disorder. Unsurprisingly, how we use our brains has much to do with our risk of getting dementia.

19

Use It or Lose It

One of the best-known findings in dementia research is that education is good for you; or at least, not having much education may be bad for you. And not just formal education, but brain employment in general: hobbies, lifelong learning, even just talking to other people. Multiple studies, reviews, and meta-analyses have found that people who keep their minds active seem to be at lower risk of cognitive impairment, illness, and death as they age. Education has been reported to offset about half of the risk imparted by having ApoE4, which should give pause to anyone inclined to the fatalistic view that genes are destiny.[1]

In the classical and mediaeval eras most writers who opined on old age fell under the influence of Aristotle. For him it meant inevitable loss of faculties: 'second childishness and mere oblivion, Sans teeth, sans eyes, sans taste, sans everything', in Shakespeare's memorable words.[2] Aristotle was one of many: cognitive failings in old age have been recognized at least since Pythagoras in the seventh century BC.[3] According to the fourth-century Athenian orator Demosthenes, for example, a man without male heirs could leave his assets where he pleased unless 'his mind be impaired by one of these things, lunacy or old age or drugs or disease, or unless he be under the influence of a woman, or under constraint or deprived of his liberty'.[4] (Yes, ladies, back then you were about as welcome as dementia, unless you kept quiet and stayed at home with the kids. So much for the glory that was Greece.)

A few thinkers, like the Roman lawyer Cicero, disagreed. Cicero thought that senility was not a certainty. In his remarkable *De Senectute* (whose arguments still echo in today's scientific literature) he argued that keeping mentally active could stave off the decline of old age.[5]

Cicero lacked Aristotle's authority on matters biological, and for centuries old age was considered a fateful biological catastrophe. Modern neuroscience, however, supports the idea that Cicero was an extremely clever man (and Aristotle was wrong about many things). Although debate continues over whether dementia is a disease or simply unavoidable in those who live long enough, maintaining an active mind—in the hope that your brain will last longer than some other part of your body, thereby granting you a quicker and easier death—is currently a well-recommended strategy for reducing your risk of Alzheimer's. (There are other benefits too. A finely honed brain gives you more things to do once you're judged too old to be playing the mating and career games which keep so many younger people busy.)

When highly educated people do get dementia, they often seem to get it later in life and to decline faster once diagnosed.[6] (An oft-cited example in the United Kingdom is the novelist Iris Murdoch, born in 1919, who was diagnosed with Alzheimer's in 1997 and died only two years later.[7]) Whether the illness is indeed more severe for having been delayed—squeezed into fewer years, as it were—is unclear, since earlier research supporting the idea has been challenged by work which controlled for more biases.[8] Even if the rate of decline is no different, however, having more education still seems to delay the onset of dementia.

This squeezing of illness into a shorter timespan, or 'morbidity compression', is one of the great aims of modern preventative medicine. For dementia and other age-related conditions, the hope is that people can live as well as possible for as long as possible. The assumption is that having a terminal illness for less time—but with symptoms that get worse faster—is preferable to lingering for years. It is certainly cheaper.[9]

Boredom and Loneliness

Mental activity doesn't just include worthy self-improvement. It means being with friends, talking to people, and doing stimulating things. Those need not be intellectual. One study suggested that since 'music, drawing, meditation, reading, arts and crafts, and home repairs, for example, can stimulate the neurological system and enhance health and well-being', it might be worth encouraging such activities.[10] So if you have ever been criticized for spending time and money on a hobby or DIY...A study of 396 elderly US residents assessed their school-age activity levels and IQ, and then looked at their current cognitive function. It found that higher scores on both youthful IQ and activity independently predicted the degree to which the seniors, aged on average seventy-five years, had escaped impairment.[11] The Deckers review of research on dementia prevention reckoned that low cognitive activity was the third most important modifiable risk factor.[12]

Socializing matters. Having larger social networks was found to reduce the risk of dementia in elderly women by one-quarter.[13] Smaller networks are often associated with loneliness, albeit one can feel lonely in a crowd of friends. Loneliness is bad for mental and physical health, boosting levels of cortisol and cytokines. Some researchers think that chronic loneliness accelerates ageing.

Whether this is because being alone deprives you of necessary mental stimulation, or because it reduces the feeling of being cared for, valued, and useful, I know not. Both may be important, though my guess would be that lack of stimulation is less of a problem than lack of love. A review by Age UK states that 'having friends is a more important factor in warding off loneliness than frequent contact with these friends', and that 'having children but not feeling close to any of them is associated with higher rates of loneliness than being childless'.[14]

Conversely, chronic illnesses like dementia often lead to isolation. If you're too ill to work or to go out, it's hard to stay connected with more active friends, especially if you don't have—or don't like, or can't cope with—the Internet. Apart from anything else, illness marks you out as different. It forces you to focus on your health—a topic less interesting to others—while reducing your interest in topics dear to them. Unsurprisingly, one study found that older people with chronic illness became more lonely over time than those in better health.[15]

Complacency

Data are limited, but a study of nearly 10,000 male civil servants found that those who were not striving for promotion because they were happy with their job status were nearly twice as likely to have dementia decades later as those who thought advancement was possible and were trying to achieve it.[16] Another sizeable study of twins (just over 10,000) found that those with more challenging jobs—especially jobs working with people—were less likely to develop dementia.[17] Mental stimulation, it seems, should be cultivated in the workplace as well as at the weekends.

A further report on the civil servants found that whether they defined themselves as secular or religious in midlife was associated with an altered risk of later dementia, as was the nature of their education. The proportions later diagnosed were 27.1% for the religiously educated and 16.1% for those with a secular education. For self-definition, the authors reported proportions diagnosed of 9.7% for the least religious, 28.8% for the most religious. Intriguingly, that study also reported that men with a mixed secular and religious education had a slightly lower risk than men with a purely secular education—and both had notably lower risk than the religiously educated.[18] (The cohort is from Israel, a state in which religion has considerable political as well as intrinsic importance.) We do not know why this might be: to quote the authors, 'Mechanisms underlying these associations remain elusive.'[19] The work provokes fascinating speculations about the potential effects of different belief systems—ideologies—on the believer's chances of ageing well.

Most such speculations have not a shred of evidence to support them as yet, but in the age of Big Data—and of ideology as a resurgent political force—the role of beliefs in human health is likely to be extended far beyond work on the placebo effect.[20] Of course, the implied analogy (that certain passionately held convictions could be a risk factor for brain health, like diet or depression) carries with it extremely difficult ethical and social implications. At the moment, however, all we can say—and that only provisionally—is that the unexamined life in which convictions are never challenged, whether or not it is worth living, may not be the most helpful approach to ageing.

Those Covariates, Again

There are, inevitably, caveats to the mental stimulation narrative. Some studies query the way cognitive abilities are measured, and not all have found benefits.[21] In some cases this may be because the studies sample very similar people; the statistical methods used need some variation in order to work.[22] There is also the usual covariate caveat.

Take IQ, for example. Higher IQ, even measured early in life, seems to predict a lower chance of cognitive decline later on. A study of over a million Swedish army conscripts found that poorer cognitive performance at age eighteen was linked to both late-life cognitive impairment and a greater risk of early-onset dementia.[23] Yet cognitive performance may be affected by motivation and life events as well as by IQ. And IQ may affect a person's trajectory through life in multiple ways, which often in turn affect each other. A brighter child may find school more rewarding, and bright parents may reward a bright child more. School rewards may set up the expectation of success. That confidence may help the young adult land a good job, and so on.[24]

Genes matter. Good early health, decent nutrition, and a supportive family environment also make a big difference. All of these can influence a child's intelligence and how that intelligence is applied, in school and beyond.

Building Up Reserves

Why would education and IQ help protect against dementia? In 1988, Alzheimer's researcher Robert Katzman and colleagues introduced the idea of reserve.[25] They invoked it to explain the puzzling finding that some elderly people may score poorly on a test of cognitive function, and others do well, despite their brains showing similarly extensive signs of neurodegeneration. The reserve hypothesis proposes that human brains vary greatly in their ability to withstand damage and disease, and that some features of human lifestyles, like education and keeping active, enhance this ability, providing a buffer against damage and the effects of neurodegeneration. The concept applies beyond dementia. Studies suggest that reserve-boosting, pro-brain lifestyles may also reduce the clinical effects of other damage, such as that inflicted by head injury, multiple sclerosis, and Parkinson's.

What is Reserve?

But what is reserve? What is it about the human brain that enables some people to age successfully? The concept is intuitively appealing, and highly influential: the search for pharmaceuticals to boost reserve is one of the most intense in biotechnology. But as with many exciting scientific ideas, questions bubble up once you start unpacking the details.

For a start, researchers distinguish cognitive and brain reserve. Cognitive reserve is about the networks of associations you hone over time, how accustomed your brain is to mental exercise, the range of new stimuli to which it is exposed. As with muscles, so with mind: more activity makes being active easier. Cognitive reserve may be influenced by genes, intelligence, and early experience, but it can to some extent be changed throughout life.

Brain reserve is about the underlying structures and processes that make some brains especially resilient. One obvious candidate is the number of cells: resilient folk may simply have more brain tissue to lose.[26] In support of this idea, male brains, which tend to be larger, seem to be slightly less at risk of dementia, especially at older ages. As noted earlier, head circumference, which reflects how well nourished the person was in childhood and how well their brain was able to grow, has also been linked to dementia risk, with very small values increasing risk. Another proxy measure, overall brain volume as measured by the size of the skull vault, has also been found to influence dementia risk, independently of education.

Brain size cannot be the only contributor to reserve, though, because accounting for variation in brain size does not explain all the variation in resilience among people with markers of neurodegeneration. It is therefore likely that connectivity can also make a difference to how long brains can keep functioning. Connectivity means more than the number of synapses, however.[27] It can also relate to how quickly brain networks transmit signals, and how adeptly brains cope when a synaptic pathway is damaged.

The type of link also matters. Neurons have both local connections and more distant ones, and long-range connections seem especially vulnerable to damage and energy stress, especially if they are not coated in myelin. Many of the great regulatory swathes of connections from subcortex to cortex—such as the noradrenaline, acetylcholine, and dopamine pathways—lack myelin sheaths. They must therefore use more energy to send signals, and so have less in reserve for emergencies. Such pathways may function well until some stress impairs them, but then they will be early casualties—as happens with dopamine neurons in Parkinson's disease and acetylcholine neurons in Alzheimer's.

A healthy brain maintains a balance between efficiency (fast, well-honed pathways), redundancy (multiple routes in the network), and flexibility (for swift adaptation to new situations). So whatever brain reserve is, it must involve the ability to create, delete, maintain, and repair synapses. That links it to levels of synaptic proteins and neurotrophins, the flexibility of neuronal membranes, mitochondrial function and distribution, and the amounts of neurotransmitters and receptors.

As yet, however, neither brain nor cognitive reserve is directly measurable. Instead scientists rely on proxies such as brain volume or glucose metabolism (for brain reserve) and measures of IQ, processing speed, or executive function (for cognitive reserve).[28] More clarity is needed about what reserve is.[29] The same is true of those other key concepts in dementia, cognitive function, decline, and impairment. Cognition has many aspects, and these change in different ways as we get older. For example, a large-scale study using Internet games to assess people's cognitive skills found that short-term memory for images is greatest from the mid-twenties to the mid-thirties, whereas the 'theory of mind' capacity to understand other people's feelings continued to improve into the forties and fifties.[30] How you think cognition changes with age depends on how you define it.

Nonetheless, researchers find the idea of reserve immensely useful, and numerous studies have supported the power of education to boost it. IQ also contributes, as do other lifestyle and health factors, but accounting for these does not fully explain the statistical association with dementia. That is, education seems to be protective however clever, rich, and healthy you are.

Your brain is an amazing gift—from God or chance, depending on your viewpoint. Use it well, and you boost your chances of an enjoyable old age.

20

What are Your Chances?

These are the only ones of which the news has come to Ha'vard,
And there may be many others, but they haven't been discavard.
Tom Lehrer, *The Elements*

The immune system. The heart and vascular system. The pancreas and glucose regulation. Fat and cholesterol. Kidneys. Metabolic problems like fatty liver disease. Lung problems. It's beginning to look as if most of the body could be involved in neurodegenerative disorders. Indeed, some researchers have made a general argument for metabolic stress as a contributor to dementia.[1] Even bones have been implicated, with osteoporosis (brittle bone disease) linked to later dementia, low vitamin D (which can cause brittle bones) likewise, and osteopontin, a key bone protein, turning out to be a pro-inflammatory cytokine.

And if you're thinking that bones seem unexpected players in Alzheimer's, try ears and noses. Problems with hearing and smelling have both been proposed as markers for the disease.[2] Had I but cash enough and time, I'd offer a prize for any enterprising researcher who could prove that there exists a body system *not* linked to Alzheimer's.[3]

In this book I have tried to give you a glimpse of the immense complexity that underpins each of the roughly 50,000,000,000,000 cells which, at a rough estimate, make a human being—including the roughly 170 billion cells, and trillions of synapses, in the brain. It is this fearsome entanglement that makes dementia research so extremely difficult. This is why, after years of funding, researchers have still not found a cure for dementia, although progress has been made and is accelerating.

Complexity allows for redundancy. There are so many pathways that if one fails others can compensate—at least in the early stages of a disease. And complexity provides robustness. Mild disturbances of the system are unlikely to tip it over into seriously abnormal functioning—unless they persist for long periods.

Complexity also, however, means many ways in which small imperfections can affect the cell's efficiency. Over time, those flaws can mount up until—perhaps quite suddenly—the system fails: it begins to operate abnormally, or it dies. For researchers, this can make it extremely difficult to work out what is causing a given problem. For clinicians, intervening in such a complex system runs a big risk of unintended consequences, as drug trials for Alzheimer's have discovered.

Alzheimer's is one of the most intensively studied brain disorders, but this is an investigation in its very early stages, and there are multiple suspects. Mitochondrial dysfunction and lower glucose metabolism, damage to blood supplies, disrupted calcium signalling and excitotoxicity, problems with protein production and folding, faults in cells' waste disposal systems, membrane or other damage due to oxidative stress, inflammation, epigenetic changes, problems with the cell cycle and premature senescence, and damage to DNA: all these and more are suspects in the death of brain cells during dementia. The most challenging crime novels have a pitiful range of potential culprits in comparison.

Nonetheless, these are the intricate details which scientists will have to grasp if there is ever to be the kind of treatment people working on Alzheimer's dream of in their softer moments: a quick, cheap, safe way of halting the slide towards cellular destruction and the slow mental fragmentation of dementia.

And, of course, studying each detail in isolation takes the science only so far, because our body systems are so well integrated. Particulates in air do not just affect our lungs and heart, they also worsen our ability to regulate blood glucose levels. Clogged up blood vessels can damage multiple organs. So can impaired regulation of salt and water balance, or micronutrient deficiency, increased inflammation, or oxidative stress.

And the physiological failures and imbalances are in turn affected by many aspects of our lives. Some of these, such as diet, exercise, and smoking, are within our power to change, to an extent. Others, such as age, childhood IQ, genetic make-up, and personal history, are beyond our control (although how we interpret what has happened to us can be altered; this is the basis of many forms of psychological therapy). Many factors, like our economic and social status, the environmental hazards and learning facilities of our neighbourhoods, and our friendship and work connections, are less controllable than we might assume.

Here, as ever, viewpoint matters. Someone who has never had a serious illness or any financial worries is likely to underestimate the effect of developing a chronic medical condition on someone who lacks the knowledge to change their diet, the time to take more exercise, and the money to move to a better part of town. That would matter less if the decision making about where to spend public money

Table 4: Common risk factors for dementia

Risk factor	Compared with…	Average risk (minimum, maximum)
GENETIC		
No ApoE4 alleles	General population	0.63 (0.60, 0.68)
One or more ApoE4 alleles	General population	6.55 (1.20, 33.10)
PHYSIOLOGICAL AND MEDICAL		
Depression	Not diagnosed	1.89 (1.55, 2.52)
Diabetes	Not diagnosed	1.73 (1.21, 2.48)
High blood pressure	Not diagnosed	1.80 (0.97, 4.84)
Prior cancer	Not diagnosed	0.64 (0.57, 0.72)
FOOD AND DRINK		
Healthy diet	Other	0.74 (0.36, 1.12)
Drinking coffee	Non-drinker	0.76 (0.70, 0.84)
Drinking alcohol	Non-drinker	0.77 (0.53, 1.12)
WEIGHT AND FITNESS		
BMI—underweight	Normal range	1.66 (1.36, 1.96)
BMI—overweight	Normal range	1.21 (0.88, 1.35)
BMI—obese	Normal range	1.69 (1.42, 2.04)
Low physical fitness	General population	2.84 (1.50, 4.40)
High physical fitness	General population	0.53 (0.32, 0.64)
SMOKING		
Smoking (at baseline or ever)	Smoking (former or never)	1.44 (0.91, 1.79)
OTHER		
Low or medium education	General population	4.08 (1.23, 16.70)
High education	General population	0.50 (0.50, 0.50)
Low socioeconomic status	General population	3.41 (1.16, 3.09)
High socioeconomic status	General population	1.05 (0.49, 1.39)

Table 4 shows 'ballpark' risk estimates for some of the common risk factors for dementia (see the main text for details). The estimates are shown in the right-hand column as averages with the range given as (minimum, maximum). The data were obtained from a search of the literature on risk factors and dementia, from which odds ratios or equivalent measures were extracted, tabulated, and averaged. The sources from which the data were taken are given in Chapter 20, note 4.

were not done mostly by the healthier and better off, rather than by the poor and ill.

In Part 2 I have looked at many of the risk factors associated with dementia. What does all the research mean if you want to know your likelihood of getting the disease? Of course I cannot possibly tell you, first because *The Fragile Brain* offers information, not instructions, and secondly because your precise combination of risk factors is yours alone. However, I can provide a general view of some of the common dementia risk factors discussed here. From a search of the literature, it is possible to estimate—very approximately—a 'ballpark' risk for these factors.[4] Table 4 lists the results. A value higher than 1 suggests a risk; lower than 1 suggests a protective effect.

Table 5: Estimated risk of dementia at ages 65–69 and 85–89 for common risk factors

	Age 65–69		Age 85–89	
	Male	Female	Male	Female
NUMBER EXPECTED TO GET DEMENTIA (PER 1000 PEOPLE)				
	15	18	151	202
GENETIC RISK FACTOR				
No ApoE4	1	2	13	18
One or more ApoE4	14	16	138	184
PHYSIOLOGICAL AND MEDICAL RISK FACTORS				
Depression	10	12	99	132
No depression	5	6	52	70
Diabetes	10	11	96	128
No diabetes	5	7	55	74
High blood pressure	10	12	97	130
No hypertension	5	6	54	72
Prior cancer	6	7	59	79
No prior cancer	9	11	92	123

(continued)

Table 5: Continued

	Age 65–69		Age 85–89	
	Male	Female	Male	Female
FOOD AND DRINK				
Better diet	6	8	64	86
Other diet	9	10	87	116
High caffeine	6	8	65	87
Low caffeine	9	10	86	115
Drinking, overall	7	8	66	88
Non-drinking, overall	8	10	85	114
WEIGHT AND FITNESS				
BMI underweight or normal	7	8	72	97
BMI overweight or obese	8	10	79	105
Poor physical fitness	13	15	127	170
Good physical fitness	2	3	24	32
SMOKING				
Smoking, all (non-industry)	9	11	89	119
Non smoking (non-industry)	6	7	62	83
OTHER RISK FACTORS				
Low education	13	16	135	180
High education	2	2	16	22
SES, low	11	14	115	154
SES, high	4	4	36	48

Table 5 shows the estimated number of people (per thousand, in order to show whole numbers) who might be expected to get dementia at ages 65–69, and 85–89, if they had the common risk or protective factors listed in the table. Data are shown separately for men and women and were derived by combining data on the prevalence of dementia in the UK from the Alzheimer's Society (see Table 3) and data about common risk factors (as shown in Table 4). The numbers illustrate the impact of age, the gender differences, and the differences made by education, SES, physical fitness, and genetics (ApoE status), compared with other common risk factors. SES: socioeconomic status. As noted in the main text, these are rough estimates and should not be taken as definitive.

The next step is to combine these extremely rough estimates with data on the prevalence of dementia (I used the figures from the Alzheimer's Society cited in Chapter 11). This gives us some idea of the likelihood that—for instance—someone who takes no exercise will have dementia at ages 65–69 or 85–89. The results are given in Table 5. They suggest that, for example, men who are physically inactive have a nearly thirteen per cent chance of dementia by age ninety; for active men the chance is 2.4%. For unfit women, the risk is seventeen per cent; for highly active women it is around three per cent. The data imply that lifestyle factors can make quite a difference to your risk of dementia.

I have already mentioned some caveats concerning these estimates—which should on no account be taken as definitive—and here is one more. If you are, for example, a man wanting to lower your chance of having dementia at age 65–69 (overall, around 1.5%), and you have had both cancer (which supposedly lowers your risk to 0.6%) and an excellent education (0.2%), you might reason as follows. 'Risk factor estimates are probabilities, and probabilities are combined by multiplying them together. So if I maintain good physical fitness (0.2%), eat a healthy diet (0.6%), and drink regular coffees (0.6%) and glasses of red wine (0.8%), I can reduce my overall risk to only 0.01%!'

Alas, no. That mathematical trick only works for independent probabilities; and even if the estimates are in the right ballpark, these risks are not independent. Diet affects fitness; education affects earnings and hence your capacity to eat good food, and so on.

What Can We Do about Dementia?

If you'd like a moral, it is obvious and unoriginal: healthy brains need pro-brain lifestyles. If you don't want either to die before you reach retirement or spend your last years in the shadowlands of dementia, don't smoke, don't drink heavily, keep fit (i.e. don't work all the time), and eat well instead of relying on packaged dinners and food supplements. (The trouble with taking the alternative approach of loading your system with alcohol, toxins, and flab is that while it may deliver a quick, easy, heart attack exit, it may not, and then you will be left with a thoroughly miserable existence.) Try to keep your waistline, blood sugar, and blood pressure under control; this may be easy or difficult, depending on your genes. If you live at high latitudes, check your vitamin D levels. Avoid situations likely to give you head injuries.

Keep active. Make sure to keep up the hobbies, preferably in company. Practising kindness, forgiveness, and gratitude, and not being angry, might be no bad thing either; anger and aggression strain the arteries. If possible, spend life with someone who loves you dearly and whom you love. Work at your friendships as much as, or more than, your physical health and your work or other interests. All are required for a good old age, but we—and our employers—often prioritize work at our own expense; being keen to work hard and get promotion should not imply the kind of body-and-soul commitment seen in cults. (Remember, your employer has little incentive to worry about what happens to your health after you retire.) Avoid poverty if you can, but don't get too stressed about chasing wealth.

Easy, yes? Having myself been compelled by ill health to make big lifestyle changes, I know it isn't easy, not at all. And I am lucky, born into a rich Western country, with help from family, friends, and the National Health Service. It took me years even to accept that change was needed—that my work–life balance was dreadful, my 'OK' diet wasn't OK, and my draw in the genetic lottery was suboptimal. Better ways of exercising, eating, and sleeping, less stress, and above all, healthier work patterns were imperatives, not luxuries. Some changes, like cutting stress and sorting out my vitamin D deficiency, had to wait until conditions made them possible. Vitamin D testing, for example, has only recently become available where I live.

Making even a few changes, however, makes it easier to achieve other, more challenging ones. Someone who is physically inactive will feel better taking even a very short walk each day, and can then stretch the length gradually, say by a tenth every week or two. Someone who is vitamin D-deficient will feel better for supplementing. Both may then find they have the energy, improved mood, and motivation required to face the task of getting their blood sugar down, or quitting smoking, or whatever it is that they need to do to lower their risk of dementia.

This is not a self-help book, and it certainly carries no self-satisfied message about my current glorious state of super-fitness, because I don't have one and I never will. Nor do I know whether the changes I've made will stave off dementia; the answer to that question must be left to that great researcher, time. But the science as we currently understand it suggests that the kinds of changes I have made bring many benefits apart from less risk of dementia. And I can testify to one thing about them: they do make you feel better.

Part 2 asked the question: 'What factors raise the risk of getting dementia?' The next and final Part 3 brings together the science of risk and the science of neurodegeneration, asking, 'Could we have a theory of dementia that can explain the risks and give us new and more successful treatments?' The answer is probably yes, but we're not there yet. To see why, we must return to the dominant contender: the amyloid cascade hypothesis.

PART 3

Mechanisms

…all the most acute, most powerful, and most deadly diseases, and those which are most difficult to be understood by the inexperienced, fall upon the brain.

Hippocrates, *On the Sacred Disease*[1]

21

The Puzzle of Amyloid

The amyloid cascade hypothesis argues that changes leading to increased levels of Aβ in the brain trigger a swathe of other changes that lead to the neurodegeneration seen in Alzheimer's disease. Although the exact nature of the proposed cause has changed over the years, with amyloid plaques giving way to soluble oligomers, this hypothesis still dominates Alzheimer's research.

The hypothesis implies three stages at which, potentially, interventions could stop or slow the processes of neurodegeneration. First, something must cause the changes in Aβ. Genetic mutations are thought to be the main culprit in familial forms of the illness, and a contributor in sporadic dementia. Other factors play a larger role in sporadic dementia, but probably also affect the familial disease.

What factors? As we have seen, there are many suspects, including:

- *diet*: the proportions of processed food; the quantities and variety of food eaten; intake of carbohydrates, proteins, fats, vitamins and minerals, or other dietary components such as polyunsaturated fatty acids;
- *genes*: genetic variations in APP and Aβ processing, or in the systems regulating lipids like cholesterol, hormones like angiotensin and insulin, neurotransmitters like acetylcholine and glutamate, neurotrophins like BDNF, or other signalling molecules like nitric oxide;
- *over-use*: for example, excitotoxicity, or the reduction of insulin receptor numbers due to overstimulation of insulin production by high blood sugar;
- *bodily ills*: for example, diabetes, heart disease, inflammatory and infectious diseases; vascular problems like atherosclerosis;
- *environment/wear and tear*: environmental levels of metals, particulates, or other toxins; UV exposure, etc.

Secondly, there is the amyloid protein itself. Its amounts, formats, and behaviours are directly affected by some environmental and genetic factors (e.g. dietary iron levels, variants in the gene for APP), and less directly affected by others (e.g. poor diet). In turn, they affect many other cellular systems.

Thirdly, there are those systems: the various physiological mechanisms that underlie the neurodegenerative process. These include:

- *oxidative stress* causing damage to DNA, proteins, lipids, cell membranes, and organelles such as mitochondria;
- *inflammatory stress* due to increased/prolonged production of pro-inflammatory cytokines and/or weakening mechanisms of inflammation resolution;
- an age-related *reduction in efficiency* of many biochemical and physiological processes, including those supplying nutrients to the brain and maintaining its cells, as errors mount up;
- *changes in receptor numbers* in response to altered stimuli, leading to changes in intracellular signalling and in cell functions such as glucose uptake or clearance of Aβ;
- *excitotoxicity*: cell damage and death due to excessive calcium influx;
- *mitochondrial dysfunction* impairing energy production;
- cellular *senescence* and impaired regulation of the cell cycle;
- *failures in cellular maintenance and repair* systems, such as the superoxide dismutase anti-oxidant enzymes;
- *disrupted regulation of protein folding* and cellular waste disposal systems.

Note that these processes occur in healthy ageing to some extent, and that they can also 'feed back' to influence amyloid production, as well as other aspects of bodily function. Inflammation, for instance, can both increase Aβ secretion and worsen vascular disease. The amyloid hypothesis proposes that Aβ exerts its deleterious effects by either triggering or boosting neurodegenerative mechanisms to such a degree that synapses and cells die off unusually quickly. As the doyen of amyloid John Hardy put it, 'Our hypothesis is that deposition of amyloid β protein (AβP), the main component of the plaques, is the causative agent of Alzheimer's pathology and that the neurofibrillary tangles, cell loss, vascular damage and dementia follow as a direct result of this deposition.'[1]

Amyloid Hypotheses

The amyloid cascade hypothesis is what is known in the jargon as a 'high-level' hypothesis. In other words, the devil's in the detail. How exactly do the environmental triggers interact with amyloid processing? Which mechanisms does Aβ stimulate, and

(1) Amyloid as the sole cause of effects which then cause neurodegeneration; simple linear pathway shown by black arrows

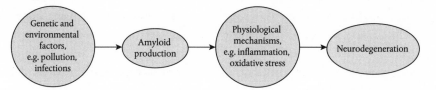

(2) Amyloid as the sole cause, both acting directly and triggering other causes of neurodegeneration; grey arrows indicate feedback pathways

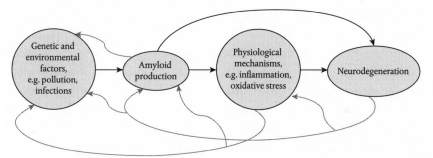

(3) Amyloid as one among many causes of neurodegeneration

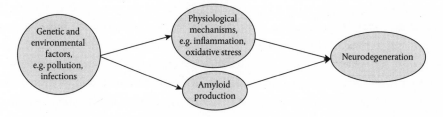

(4) Amyloid as a reaction to neurodegeneration and its causes

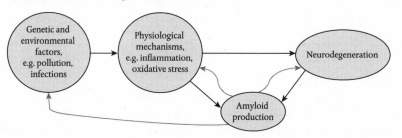

FIGURE 9: Amyloid hypotheses.

how much does that add to the normal changes of ageing? That is, how big a contribution do amyloid-driven mechanisms make to neurodegeneration, and how much would happen anyway by other means if the person were to live for long enough?

The amyloid hypothesis can be interpreted in various ways. Figure 9 shows four examples. The first example represents the strongest and simplest version of the hypothesis. Here, Aβ is the sole cause of neurodegeneration, and it acts by triggering other mechanisms. The second example in Figure 9 amends the first to take account of a) evidence that Aβ oligomers can directly damage cells; and b) evidence that neurodegenerative processes can affect their triggers (e.g. cell damage can activate microglia). Once neurodegeneration has begun, it may also increase vulnerability to environmental factors such as toxins.

Many commentators, however, interpret the amyloid hypothesis more weakly, accepting Aβ's key role but emphasizing other factors too (as shown in the third example in Figure 9). For example, in the high-profile journal *Nature Neuroscience* Karl Herrup agrees that Aβ is an important part of the Alzheimer's story, but argues against the idea that Aβ is 'the causative agent', with a tidy linear path from cause to neurodegenerative effect.[2] Listing thirteen potential contributors to the disease (all of which are mentioned in *The Fragile Brain*), he says, 'We can assume that there is a common final path to AD and still entertain the notion that there are many ways to access that path.'[3] Herrup is not alone. John Hardy himself has called for a 'critical reappraisal' of the amyloid hypothesis to reconsider the physiological role of APP.[4]

Some critics of the amyloid hypothesis go even further, as shown in the fourth example of Figure 9. They argue that amyloid production does not cause neurodegeneration either directly or indirectly (at least not to begin with or to a significant extent). Rather, it is a reaction to pre-existing problems. To return to our crime metaphor, imagine you come across a person dying in the street, with someone else crouching over them. Your first thought is that this is the murderer caught in the act, but then you see the desperate attempts at resuscitation. On this view, Aβ is not a cell-killer but a helper. (A detective novel might hint at this point that amyloid had been wickedly framed by some other suspect, like tau, but we have enough twists and turns in the amyloid story without giving our proteins motives as well as means and opportunity.)

When the brain is exposed to challenges like hypoxia, low glucose, toxins, or oxidative stress, could it be that cells react by switching from a 'grow-and-maintain' production of sAPPα to a more defensive pathway, producing Aβ? Furthermore, the multiple levels of control around the biochemical switch from sAPPα to Aβ imply that the switch itself is important—and that suggests that Aβ, as well as sAPPα, has a useful cellular function. So could it be that only Aβ *over*production is toxic?

This question is key to treating Alzheimer's. If Aβ production is, like cancer, a biological error, then effective treatments need to stop Aβ being made—for example, by targeting γ-secretase. If, on the other hand, Aβ build-up is due to normally useful molecules, Aβ monomers, being produced in an attempt to repair the brain and then forming dangerous aggregates—either because there is too much of the stuff or because it is not being adequately cleared away—blocking Aβ production could have dangerous side effects. In that case, treatments should instead target Aβ aggregation, or its more harmful effects, for example, by using ultrasound to open up the blood–brain barrier or heat shock proteins to disentangle Aβ.

As noted earlier, Aβ-blocking treatments have been attempted—for example, with antibodies. So far the results have not been promising and in some cases patients have been harmed, although new, more precise therapies are being developed.

What other systems deliberately pump out molecules that are dangerous in high doses? Two obvious answers are immune cells—which produce pro-inflammatory cytokines and ROS in response to pathogens or damaged cells—and mitochondria, whose production of ROS increases under stress. As with Aβ, both are normally tightly regulated, but controls weaken, especially as the body ages. By analogy, could Aβ too be part of neurons' defensive reactions to stress? It makes sense, since cells can switch from making sAPPα to Aβ, that if one pathway promotes healthy neurons the other acts when they are threatened, for example by hypoxia.

Neurons' ROS levels rise when their energy production goes wrong; they release cytokines when synapses are damaged. Perhaps rising Aβ levels might indicate another failure: of protein packaging, transport, and recycling systems. Like cytokines and ROS, Aβ can activate cell suicide pathways or damage membranes, resulting in cell death; it can also prompt microglia to clean up debris and remove unhealthy cells.[5] Thus low levels of Aβ, ROS, and cytokines may help to maintain neurons, not least by signalling that the cells are healthy, while higher levels stimulate immune defences.

Alternatively (or as well), as we noted in Chapter 15, Aβ is a potent mopper-up of highly reactive metal ions. Maybe it evolved as part of the body's defences against blood-borne toxins. We think of metal pollution in relation to modern industry, but humanity's relationship with metals is far older, not least because they are in the soil—especially in soils enriched by volcanic emissions—and thereby in the plants and animals we eat.

Like cytokines and ROS, amyloid could be part of the brain's reaction to trouble—a reaction that may, if prolonged, proceed to cause trouble itself. In support of this idea, Aβ shares features with innate immune components like complement and pro-inflammatory cytokines (it has been suggested that its origins may lie in evolutionarily ancient wound-healing mechanisms).[6] All three increase early in Alzheimer's disease.[7] Aβ, like complement, can form membrane-puncturing pores, and it can activate microglia, astrocytes, and complement. Activated microglia increase production of ApoE and Aβ-degrading enzymes, helping to restrain Aβ, rather like the way in which some complement proteins rein in others. Aβ's activation of complement, meanwhile, might promote synaptic pruning and the synapse loss of dementia.[8] And just as Aβ can activate innate immune responses, so their activation—for example, by infection—can lead to late-life Aβ pathology.

As always in the immune system, timing and duration are crucial. Low levels of Aβ may be useful, as noted earlier; and in early life they may easily be controlled. But if the stimulus persists, and Aβ keeps being made, then oligomers and fibrils will build up and begin to do damage. Furthermore, research suggests that over time, prolonged high levels of cytokines may impair microglial function—including microglia's ability to clear Aβ. If neurons start to die, furthermore, they will be releasing pro-inflammatory molecules into their environment while reducing the restraining influence of molecules which damp down microglial activation.[9] While inflammation may increase with ageing, the ability to heal damaged tissues diminishes. Thus while acute inflammatory processes could work in tandem with APP–Aβ processing to resolve brain problems, chronic inflammatory stress could exacerbate amyloid build-up. (A similar relationship may hold between amyloid and oxidative stress.)

If amyloid production is a response to damage, we should expect to see more amyloid and APP in injured brains, even if the brain's owners are not suffering from dementia. I have already mentioned the studies in mice and children which found evidence of increased amyloid after exposure to air pollution. Another set of cases comes from severe brain injuries, for example due to traffic accidents or combat exposure. Victims are typically comatose for some time, and show widespread damage to neurons—in particular, to their axons. They also show inflammatory changes and microglial activation, as well as changes in levels of APP.

APP is concentrated in axons, and after injury its levels rise and then fall.[10] It is so good a marker for axonal damage that APP staining is one of the diagnostic criteria for this kind of brain injury. Along with APP, other proteins also collect in axons after injury, including enzymes that can convert APP to Aβ. APP changes—and Aβ deposits—are found in TBI sufferers who do not have either pre-existing dementia or Down's syndrome. This may help to explain why severe head injuries increase the risk of later cognitive decline.

As we saw in Chapter 5, small holes in white matter increase with age. They are also a feature of cerebrovascular disease before it becomes clinically apparent, and cerebral microbleeds are more common in people with a heavier amyloid burden.

This all implies that too much amyloid may cause particular damage to axons. It is tempting to speculate that one of the differences between healthy ageing and sporadic dementia lies in whether the decline involves the gradual loss of synapses, followed eventually by axonal and then neuronal death, or whether early axon damage results in a much more rapidly spreading dysfunction.

A 2010 study which sampled human brain extracellular fluids directly after TBI revealed two intriguing findings.[11] First, by about a day after injury—when the catheters used to take the samples were installed—Aβ levels dropped considerably. In Alzheimer's, a similar finding has long been a puzzle: levels of $A\beta_{42}$ in CSF are lower, not higher, than in controls. If Aβ were causing the damage, why would there be less of it in patients?

Aβ is produced by active neurons, and its levels were higher in patients' brains when more glucose was being used, so the study's authors propose that reduced Aβ could be due to the fact that many neurons stop firing temporarily after TBI. And yet, it is then that the cellular damage is done, so how can excess Aβ be the cause? Other researchers have suggested that the reason $A\beta_{42}$ levels drop in Alzheimer's CSF is because the stuff has been hoovered up into plaques—presumably having done its harmful work. Yet the timing again seems odd if Aβ is killing cells, since amyloid plaques do not necessarily become more numerous as brain tissue dies (and a 2015 study of middle-aged, cognitively healthy volunteers found $A\beta_{42}$ levels dropping years before plaques could be detected).[12] Of course, plaques could be damaging sources, rather than safe repositories, of toxic protein (or perhaps they could be safe in the short term, toxic in the longer term). But this doesn't explain the drop in Aβ levels. If, on the other hand, Aβ is part of an early cellular defence mechanism that is eventually overwhelmed by too much stimulation, the timing makes more sense.[13]

The second finding of interest from the 2010 study was that higher Aβ levels correlated with better outcomes and with a better neurological status (e.g. lighter coma) for patients. Which is also odd if Aβ is directly neurotoxic, but fits if it is in fact part of the brain's attempts at self-repair.

Instead of a single protein whose abnormal production causes Alzheimer's, therefore (as in the case of genetic cases of the disease), perhaps what we have is multiple defensive mechanisms, including Aβ, being over-activated by chronic stimulation, and gradually wearing out.

The Hole at the Heart of the Hypothesis

One reason why we cannot yet definitively rule on which interpretation of the amyloid hypothesis is best is that we lack one crucial piece of information. Researchers still aren't sure what Aβ is for, and what evolution was playing at, installing such a problematic protein in a vulnerable organ like the brain.

The facile answer to that is that evolution wasn't playing at anything. Play requires intelligence, design even (and science writers should be careful with their metaphors).

Another answer is that perhaps evolution doesn't apply. After all, dementia is a disease of old age, not parenting age, so how could it affect reproductive fitness? That is evolution's basic measure of success: if a disease has no impact on the capacity to have babies it is invisible to natural selection.

Maybe. But some cases of dementia strike before the age of child-bearing is over, and besides, dementia imposes considerable costs on families.[14] Healthy elders can provide extra child care and labour as well as accumulated wisdom. Unhealthy elders can require resources that might otherwise be expended on the children. Caring for someone with dementia can be an exhausting strain on mental and physical health.

Even if dementia has exerted only minor costs in terms of reproductive fitness, one might still expect evolutionary pressures to have worked against the persistence of contributing genes—unless those genes bring benefits that outweigh the costs. This is antagonistic pleiotropy: the idea that late-life dementia and some—presumably cognitive—advantage have been traded off during human evolution. Potential benefits include bigger brain size, greater synaptic plasticity, and extended longevity, with all the consequences that have flowed from these.

It is possible to make this case for at least some of the genes linked to dementia, not least APP itself, given its apparent benefits for neural health. Chopped up by α-secretase, it forms sAPPα, another good thing. But why would evolution maintain at least one, and possibly more, alternative pathways which produce a slew of apparently harmful proteins, most notably Aβ? Is this small protein (with the enormous literature) just an unavoidable quirk of the biochemistry? Is it an error that evolutionary forces have not yet erased because, to put it crudely, until modern industrialized societies pushed up average life expectancy there was insufficient pressure for them to do so?[15] Or could Aβ be doing more than just damage in the brain?

After decades of research, we still do not know. Why not? Media headlines about genetics research, and the way gene science is shown in the movies, can give the impression that once researchers have the DNA the hard part is over. Yet the DNA for Aβ's precursor protein was identified thirty years ago, and we still don't have a cure for Alzheimer's. The reasons for this disappointing situation lie partly with the science itself, and with its funding; but also with us, the public, and our expectations.

Expectations 0, Reality 1

Modern medicine has wrought innumerable marvels. I owe my life to its genius; quite likely you do too. Science has brought so many wonders that it has raised our expectations of its powers to a degree formerly reserved for supernatural entities. Egged on by a media which depends on constant novelty—or the appearance of novelty—we have become used to the idea that, whatever the problem, scientists can solve it, given enough time and money. And in many cases this is true.

Unfortunately, even some scientists—let alone journalists ignorant of science but deputed to report on its latest 'breakthrough'—have repeatedly underestimated the scale of the challenge. We all pay lip service to the notion that human brains are immensely complicated, but there's a world of difference between mouthing the words, or even considering them intellectually, and intuitively grasping their implications. Some of the wisest scientists get the point. Here's Nobel Prize winner David Hubel advocating humility in 1979:

> How long it will be before one is able to say that the brain—or the mind—is in broad outline understood (those fuzzy words again) is anyone's guess. As late as 1950 anyone who predicted that in 10 years the main processes that underlie life would be understood would have been regarded as optimistic if not foolish, and yet that came to pass. I think it will take a lot longer than 10 years to understand the brain, simply because it is such a many-faceted thing: a box brimful of ingenious solutions to a huge number of problems.[16]

Evolution has had four billion years to come up with those solutions. Modern neuroscience approached the brain with the confidence born of success elsewhere; but so far Hubel's reality check still applies. Not that you'd know it from the way science is reported in some media outlets.[17] Many researchers detest the way their work is represented to the public precisely because it raises hopes that cannot possibly be met— and it is the scientists who feel the weight of the public's agonized disappointment.

I hope that *The Fragile Brain* has given you a glimpse of why progress has been so slow, and what researchers working on dementia are up against. If amyloid proteins came in just one variety and format, the task would be much simpler; but APP has three varieties in humans and $A\beta_{40}$ and $A\beta_{42}$ are not the only lengths available. As for formats, $A\beta$ can form oligomers, fibrils, plaques, tubes, and even spheroids. No one has yet discovered that it can gather itself into pairs and do the tango up and down cell membranes, but there are undoubtedly other things it can do that we don't yet know about.

Progress would also have been considerably faster if this shape-changing protein were less of a biochemical libertine: it interacts with far more molecules than any decent protein should. Or to put it more respectably, as neuropathologist Robert D. Terry did, 'A textbook of cell biology could well be written utilizing Alzheimer disease as the paradigm around which nearly the whole of cell metabolism could be described.'[18]

It would also be easier if APP gave rise to a smaller range of active products. I have mentioned sAPPα and Aβ, but there are others. Indeed, as I was revising this book in September 2015, a paper in *Nature* announced 'a new physiological APP processing pathway', involving APP's cleavage not by α-, β-, or γ-, but by η(eta)-secretase.[19] The products of this pathway are not merely decorative additions to the biochemical landscape; they appear to reduce the activity of hippocampal neurons, making them potentially relevant to dementia. We have much still to learn about APP processing.

Given these obstacles, it is a remarkable achievement to have any viable hypothesis of dementia, let alone one as theoretically fruitful—if not, so far, clinically fruitful—as the amyloid hypothesis.

Methods

Another reason for the slow pace of progress is technical. Amyloid, as befits a top suspect, is a slippery customer, hard to pin down in the lab. Apparently small differences in experimental technique—for example in pH, or the amount of detergent used in extraction— can affect its tendency to shift between forms, and hence its behaviour.[20] Detecting amyloid plaques in living human brains has only recently become possible, and more precise techniques, capable of measuring smaller amounts and different conformations of the protein, are still needed. As Figure 9 implies, to distinguish between rival interpretations of the amyloid hypothesis, scientists need much more detailed information about the timing of changes in Aβ's production, clearance, and format. They also need far greater knowledge of how those changes relate to other alterations in, for example, microglial activation, DNA errors, cell cycle re-entry, oxidative stress, inflammation, and glucose uptake.

At the moment we simply do not have the tools to accomplish all of this. As I described in *The Brain Supremacy*, however, neuroscience methods are rapidly advancing, and many new ways of tracking neurodegeneration are becoming available. Ideally, multiple simultaneous measurements of different mechanisms—in individuals with the disease, and at high or low risk for it—would soon be possible. Taken repeatedly over many years, these would be combined with genetic and epigenetic analyses, life history data (including major stresses and environmental and dietary exposures), and detailed biochemical studies done on stem cells generated from the volunteers. But that is for the future, though hopefully not the distant future.

It may be that when the methods arrive and the science is done, we will find that there is no single 'right' interpretation of the amyloid hypothesis. We already know that dementia is multiple diseases, and there may be many forms of Alzheimer's, many vascular dementias, and so on.[21]

Much of the work on amyloid has been done *in vitro*—in cells or slices—and this too has cons as well as pros. Many studies identify their target cells (e.g. microglia) or molecules (e.g. NFκB) using antibodies that bind to the molecules in question or to a cell surface marker—a molecule thought to be unique to that kind of cell. Unfortunately, markers may turn out not to be unique, and antibodies may also bind to other molecules. Or the markers may simply not exist. For example, as noted earlier, distinguishing the brain's resident microglia from invading monocytes has not been feasible until recently.

Then there is the question of tissue: the raw materials.[22] Where do researchers get the living cells they study? As an instance, human microglia come mainly from two sources: abortions and samples removed during surgery. Neither is ideal, since in both the extraction procedures may damage or alter the chemical state of the cells. Worse still, it seems that the process of culturing microglia affects their properties, as does the donor's sex and age and the area of brain from which the cells are taken.[23]

An alternative source, animal tissue, yields cells in better condition; yet they cannot be assumed to behave in the same way as human microglia, either in culture or in a living brain.[24] Nonetheless, they are widely used. As you will have gathered, the amyloid hypothesis is heavily dependent on animal research. Whatever their view of this controversial topic, most people accept that there are some experiments we just don't do on human beings. Giving them Alzheimer's is one such. If science is not simply to give up on dementia, that means doing research on cells and cell groups (such as stem cells, slices, or lab-grown organs); but it also means using animals. Computing power can take us a long way—and we are only at the start of that fascinating journey—but computer models need to be tested against something. And dementia is, as we have seen, a disorder affected by many other body systems, so studying whole bodies will be essential.

Ethical issues aside, the problem with animal research is that Alzheimer-like symptoms are extremely rare in species other than humans. Left to their own devices, rats and mice don't get dementia. Not even in the lab, where they have food and shelter and no predators except humanely killing scientists. Neither do most other animals.

Studies have found amyloid deposits in aged captive primates—such as rhesus macaques and chimpanzees—and also in some other mammals, such as dogs and bears. But they found very few plaques, even in our closest relatives. (There is also the problem of how to assess dementia in an animal, since you can't usefully ask it what today's date is or what has recently happened in the news.[25])

Most animals—including the most common rodent research models—have a different version of the APP gene to ours. For rats and mice, differences in only three amino acids are enough to protect against amyloid deposition. To obtain rat or, mostly, mouse models of Alzheimer's, therefore, transgenic animals have been created with human-type APP, using mutations from familial Alzheimer's.

Controversies rage over how realistic these numerous models are with respect to sporadic Alzheimer's. As a 2013 article advancing a new rat model put it, 'faithful recapitulation of all AD features in widely used transgenic (Tg) mice engineered to overproduce Aβ peptides has been elusive'.[26] Animal models tend not to show the behavioural changes one might expect of a demented rat; nor do they develop the brain damage seen in humans. They do have memory problems, but those can be reversed with treatments (e.g. Aβ vaccines) which do not reverse human symptoms. Transgenic animals also produce much higher levels of amyloid than Alzheimer brains. And they are based on the gene variants we know cause dementia—familial dementia—that as we saw earlier are not the variants found in sporadic Alzheimer's.

Dogs and primates, which share the same version of APP as humans, increase the ethical tensions and are more difficult and expensive to study. Guinea pigs, which also have 'our' version, are not widely used in genetics research these days compared with rats and mice. The study of their genetics has been slower—their equivalent of Glenner and Wong's 1984 identification of APP came only in 1997—and this means that there are fewer tools and models for scientists to choose.[27] However, guinea pigs are already preferred for studying some conditions, like atherosclerosis and vitamin C deficiency. As long ago as 1991 they were being proposed as non-transgenic models for dementia; but growing criticism of other rodent models has renewed interest in alternatives, so this is an area to watch.[28]

Another technology where new advances could bring benefits for Alzheimer's research involves the culture of human cells, including stem cells. The tradition of the slab-in-a-dish is being replaced by 3D cultures, such as 'spheroids' produced from stem cells, which can spontaneously develop functional neurons, astrocytes, and cortical layers. These brainlets are still extremely simple compared with what's in your head, but they offer great promise for testing ideas about the mechanics of brain cell development, maintenance, and degeneration.

Facts

Another reason why the amyloid question remains unresolved is that the hypothesis has been a victim of its own success. The gigantic literature that has flowed from it includes findings that greatly complicate the initial picture of a single protein, albeit a chameleon of its kind, as the sole cause of Alzheimer's dementia. If neurodegeneration as a whole, not just Alzheimer's, is to be understood, then one protein is definitely not enough. In some age-related brain conditions, like vascular disease, Aβ plays a major role; but not in others.[29]

Aβ is not the only protein which can aggregate into oligomers, fibrils, and solid deposits. Since the idea took hold that dementia might be a 'proteinopathy', scientists have hunted down numerous proteins linked to neurodegeneration. Indeed, we have already encountered three of them. One is p53, cancer suppressor and regulator of the cell cycle. Another is the Josephin protein, cause of spinocerebellar ataxia. And a third is the cytoskeleton-supporting tau, whose tangles are one of the characteristic signs of Alzheimer's disease.[30]

Timing and Tau

If Aβ sets events in motion, as the original amyloid cascade hypothesis proposed, then one might expect tau tangles to appear after the onset of amyloid plaques. This has been found in familial disease, but it is not what seems to happen in sporadic Alzheimer's.[31] There plaques and tangles arise independently. Tangles are a better predictor of disease severity than plaques, and synapse loss correlates better with tau than with amyloid.[32] Moreover, plaques and cell damage do not begin in the same places. Plaques often emerge in frontal cortex, while cell loss initially afflicts limbic areas. Nor does plaque density necessarily reflect the severity of the dementia.[33]

Tau build-up begins in areas of the medial temporal lobe, hippocampus, thalamus, and in subcortical nuclei such as the cholinergic cells of Meynert the poet. Tangles then spread through the hippocampus, amygdala, and cortex, in six distinct stages. These 'Braak' stages, identified by husband-and-wife team Heiko and Eva Braak, are so characteristic of dementia that they are now used to assess disease severity.[34]

For amyloid deposits, by contrast, the Braaks were able to identify only three stages, because they found so much variation between cases.[35] Brains with a heavy burden of tau (inside neurons) tended to have plenty of amyloid deposits (outside neurons), but some with heavy amyloid did not have much in the way of tangles, and many had tau without detectable amyloid. Animal models with amyloid but lacking tau develop fewer plaques, lose fewer neurons, and show less severe memory problems. Furthermore, although both proteins often build up as brains get older, they don't inevitably do so.[36] And both have been found in young brains.[37]

Interestingly, a 2015 study suggests that higher brain tau levels are associated with one sign of Alzheimer's (cortical thinning), but not with another (hippocampal atrophy). Levels of $A\beta_{42}$, conversely, were linked to tissue loss in the hippocampus but not in cortex.[38] This suggests that tau and amyloid may work together to do their damage; but tau may also be an important contributor to neurodegeneration in its own right.[39]

How might tau do its damage? The theory is that, because tau helps build stable microtubules—and hence a sturdy skeleton for the cell—abnormal tau should wreck the systems by which essential supplies like proteins, cholesterol, and mitochondria are transported along axons to the synapses. Supporting this idea, a study comparing neurons from Alzheimer and control brains showed that microtubules were shorter and fewer in the diseased neurons.[40] Unfortunately for tau's advocates, the change bore no relation to the amount of tau present in the cells, suggesting that other cytoskeleton-disrupting mechanisms may be involved.

Nonetheless, many researchers think that tau is implicated in neurodegeneration—in it up to the very last twist of its tangles. There is evidence to support their view from animal research and studies of human proteins in blood and cerebrospinal fluid (potential biomarkers of dementia) as well as from post-mortem analyses. As with Aβ, it has been suggested that tau, which is thought to have useful functions in synapses, may form aggregates as part of a defensive response to cell stress. Tau tangles correlate with synaptic problems and cognitive impairment—in animal models as well as in human brains—but if they actually kill cells, they do so only very slowly. Much work remains to be done to clarify what exactly tau is doing in healthy, injured, and neurodegenerating brains.

Other Suspects

Many people already know of one other protein capable of causing neurodegeneration. It is the prion protein, infamously linked to mad cow disease and to the devastating human illnesses variant Creutzfeldt-Jakob disease and kuru.[41] These rare neurodegenerative disorders usually kill within a year of symptoms appearing, though they can take decades to reach that stage. They are caused by the consumption of prion proteins. These can survive cooking and standard sterilization procedures, which is why humans can, rarely, get vCJD from contaminated blood or other products (such as human growth hormone extracted from corpses), or by eating meat from cattle infected with the prion disease bovine spongiform encephalopathy (BSE).[42] Kuru was identified in Papua New Guinea among tribes with a tradition of ritual cannibalism at funerals, including the consumption of brain tissue. Because of the long incubation period, it was still afflicting people long after the tradition had been abandoned.

Prion protein gene mutations cause inherited forms of CJD; and which variant of the prion protein gene a person carries also affects their chance of catching the sporadic disease.[43] One variant—found, unsurprisingly, in populations ravaged by kuru—is protective against the disease, suggesting the possibility of future genetic therapies.[44] Even without such protection, however, the risk of catching CJD is very low—about 1,700 times smaller than the risk of getting Alzheimer's.[45]

Prions are thought to have normal roles in numerous physiological processes, but they can become abnormal and form aggregates which, like viruses, can spread from cell to cell.[46] One of the most fascinating—and potentially alarming—findings of dementia research has been that tau, amyloid, and other aggregating proteins may also do this.[47] Experiments in which human Aβ-containing brain tissue was mashed up and injected into marmoset brains showed that Aβ could take hold in the recipient, causing amyloidosis in the form of plaques and blood vessel deposits (angiopathy). If this happens in living human brains, dementia and CJD may have more in common than previously realized.

Note that as well as having a high yuck factor, such procedures are not a realistic model for the spread of Alzheimer's between people. Brain injections are rare, unless you have volunteered for a trial of stem cell transplants. Another potential entry route, direct oral consumption, is also unlikely, since most people are not in the habit of eating even the squishiest bits of their deceased elders (and hence risking kuru). That leaves two possible sources of contamination: meat products and medical procedures.

The former is exceptionally unlikely. We have seen that there is some (by no means definitive) evidence that eating a lot of red meat may raise the risk of dementia, but there is no evidence to my knowledge that this could occur by the transmission of amyloid proteins. For one thing, human brains are quite capable of forming their own aggregates. For another, the animal species we most readily consume, if they form amyloid deposits, do so only in extreme old age, and are usually slaughtered at a young age.[48]

As for medical procedures, there is now some evidence that Aβ might be transmissible by this route in humans. A post-mortem study of eight CJD patients, published in Nature just as I was finishing this book, found high levels of amyloid (as plaques and angiopathy) which they think came from the same contaminated human growth hormone which gave these unlucky individuals CJD.[49] The patients were very young to have so much amyloid, and did not have any major risk genes, not even ApoE4.

The study is small, however, and not definitive. It will undoubtedly generate much follow-up research.[50]

Meanwhile, it does seem that Aβ and tau may spread within a brain from region to region and cell to cell. This matches data from fMRI studies suggesting that Alzheimer's pathology spreads not from one area to its physical neighbours, but from one area to others linked by synaptic connections. The analogy with prions, however, is far from complete. CJD generally kills its sufferers quickly—in a (failed) drug trial the average time from clinical onset to death was under nine months— whereas people and their neurons can live for years with amyloid plaques, tau tangles, and dementia.[51] Moreover, prion-like proteins may not have all the characteristics of prions, such as being able to survive cooking and spread by infection. Nor is it clear why some cell types and regions show damage long before others, when these proteins are found all over the brain.[52]

Calling Aβ and tau 'prions', therefore, is alarming and inaccurate. Instead, some researchers use the term 'templating protein', reflecting these molecules' ability to act as templates from which copies of abnormal proteins are generated. How such proteins trigger their cascades of copies, infiltrating previously healthy neurons, is not yet understood; but bear in mind that their ability to do this has only recently been identified. Unravelling the details, and assimilating the templating hypothesis with the pre-existing evidence that some cells are more vulnerable than others, will take time.

Other templating proteins are also suspects in neurodegeneration. One is the DNA-regulating protein TDP-43, which is linked to frontotemporal dementia, ALS (amyotrophic lateral sclerosis, a form of motor neuron disease), traumatic brain injury, and other conditions, including Alzheimer's.[53] Then there is alpha-synuclein, most associated with Parkinson's disease and Lewy body dementia. Like tau, it is abundant, especially in synapses, where it is thought to help regulate the process of neurotransmitter release. It has also been shown to cross the blood–brain barrier in rats, and to produce different symptoms depending on which brain areas are affected and which forms of the aggregated protein predominate.

In Huntington's disease, meanwhile, an abnormal form of a protein was found to form damaging aggregates in neurons. The protein was named huntingtin, and mutant huntingtin too can be a template. For example, it has been shown to spread from neurons to microglia when the latter eat the former as part of their cleaning operations.[54]

In familial forms of ALS the abnormal, misfolding protein is the enzyme superoxide dismutase, an important player in the cell's defences against oxidative stress. In spinocerebellar ataxia, as we saw in Chapter 9, the problem is Josephin. There are, in other words, many amyloid-like proteins. Researchers are already classifying dementias as amyloidopathies, tauopathies, TDP-43 proteinopathies, and so on (while carefully avoiding the term 'SODopathies' for superoxide dismutase diseases).

Moreover, Aβ and its aggregation-prone colleagues not only exert independent effects on cells, they can interact, egging each other on to get together. Thus while some patients with neurodegenerative conditions may show changes in only one—a 'pure' tauopathy or synucleinopathy—it is common to find multiple proteins involved, especially in advanced disease.[55]

Furthermore, dementia of any kind is a clinical diagnosis, given to a person, not a brain. An obvious point, perhaps, but it has important implications, because it makes the protein problem a problem of quantity, not quality. The mere presence of amyloid, tau, or some other templating protein is not enough to guarantee dementia; it must build up to some threshold level. Just as dementia itself, in its earliest stages, can be indistinguishable from problems caused by overwork, sleep loss, or alcohol, so neurodegeneration is a slow and complex process which probably begins decades before we notice the first signs of ageing: the senior moments, the word slips, the feeling of fog after a bad night's sleep. While this extended timescale makes dementia research exceptionally challenging, it also offers hope that there may be many ways to slow, or even reverse, neurodegeneration. With luck, they may even spare us the need to take pills all our adult lives.

In Chapter 22, we look at what the science has taught us about the clinical possibilities for treating dementia.

22

The Promise of Amyloid

If doctors cannot cure an illness, they may still be able to delay its onset, ease its symptoms, or prevent so many people from falling ill. As I write in the autumn of 2015, doctors cannot cure dementia or reverse neurodegeneration, although there are drugs that can, to a modest degree, ease its symptoms—for a while. There are tantalizing hints in the literature that, as our understanding of brain cells improves, we may one day be able to tweak those cells' own mechanisms to stall the processes which eventually destroy them. If we could confirm, for example, that the destruction does indeed start in deep brain nuclei, we could in principle monitor those areas in people at high risk of dementia, and perhaps even intervene to save the cells. Alas, such treatments are, I suspect, unrealistic in the near future (though I would be delighted to be proved wrong).

At present, as this book has made clear, we already have enough information to be able to do more about preventing dementia, should we so choose. I have emphasized prevention because it seems the most immediately practical approach for most people. With respect to treatments, however, where the science offers most hope is in delaying the onset of the disease.

Unfortunately, drugs based directly on the amyloid hypothesis, such as γ-secretase inhibitors, were not the easy, early success proponents hoped. Their trials (and tribulations) have already been discussed, as have the prospects of newer approaches like antibodies specific for Aβ oligomers and drugs that specifically block protein aggregation. It may be that other strategies such as boosting Aβ clearance will prove more beneficial. (If Aβ is indeed a defence molecule, as some scientists think, we might even end up administering early stage drugs to boost its production, in combination with methods of clearing it more efficiently.)

Time and effort will bring us the verdict on amyloid-related therapies. For now, let us consider some of the other mechanisms implicated in neurodegeneration, which interact with amyloid processing and which may also have independent effects in dementia. It may be that a combination of treatments targeting multiple pathways will eventually be found to gain the best results. What might such combined treatments include?

Inflammation and Oxidative Stress

There is considerable evidence that inflammatory and oxidative processes have much to do with ageing, and perhaps with the unhealthy ageing of dementia, as well as with many other chronic conditions. One strategy that is being explored in dementia research, therefore, is to look for treatments that alter microglial activity or ROS levels, and/or ways of boosting anti-inflammatory cytokines and other repair molecules.

Yet again the direct approach has not been successful. I noted weak evidence that chronic use of anti-inflammatory drugs such as glucocorticoids might spare brain function later, but clinical trials of non-steroidal anti-inflammatory drugs on people already diagnosed with dementia found no significant benefits and some harms. The evidence for anti-oxidant supplements like vitamins C and E is also weak, although the evidence for eating plenty of oily fish, fruit, and vegetables, and maintaining vitamin D levels, is stronger. Clinical trials of anti-oxidant extracts from turmeric, green tea, and gingko biloba have also hinted at benefits, although more research is needed.[1]

However, research on microglia—and on other cells such as astrocytes which contribute to the brain's immune response—is a growth area, and with the development of more precise methods of marking, identifying, and tracking these cells in living brains we can expect more effective methods of controlling their behaviour. Whether simply suppressing microglia is a good idea is another matter. It may be that inflammation is not the cause of neurodegeneration but an early attempt to prevent it, which is then overwhelmed (perhaps as microglia become exhausted and senescent). So research on how to prevent or reverse senescence may be an important part of understanding 'neuroinflammation'.

As for oxidative stress, various lines of research could lead to viable treatments: work on mitochondria and why they age, the study of cell systems for repairing DNA errors and how they could be enhanced, and the biochemistry of the brain's own anti-oxidants, such as superoxide dismutase. Also of interest is the recent work, mentioned in Chapter 11, on assessing people's biological age, as opposed to their calendar years, which should help to identify people at high risk of developing dementia, the ideal participants for many experiments.

I have also mentioned the views of some researchers that specific infections (e.g. spirochaetes, herpes, or toxoplasma) may contribute to neurodegeneration. These are fairly speculative proposals at present, though they open up interesting possibilities for treatment.

Metals

As we have learned, some researchers believe that Aβ could be released as a reaction to external chemical threats. It is, after all, secreted into the extracellular spaces; and amyloid plaques form between cells, not inside them. One likely threat is oxidative stress, and sources of ROS include highly reactive transition metals like iron and copper, which are thought to accumulate in ageing brains and are enriched in amyloid plaques.

If this is the case, chemicals called metal chelators, which soak up excess metals and stop them doing damage, could be helpful in dementia. Some have already been shown to be beneficial in animal models. However, evidence from human trials is so far inconclusive and there are safety concerns. Whether altering other aspects of, for example, iron metabolism in the brain would be useful has yet to be determined, but iron pathways are notoriously complex, so the development of treatments is likely to be slow.

Insulin

Yet another possibility is that Aβ might be produced as a counterbalance when excessive insulin production in the body leads to increased insulin levels in the brain. Aβ oligomers can inactivate insulin receptors, potentially causing brain insulin resistance, and the degree of resistance correlates with the extent of amyloid plaques in human cortex and hippocampus. As noted earlier, therapies based on the insulin hypothesis are already being tested, so far with promising results.

Vascular Therapies

Drugs affecting the vascular system (e.g. blood-pressure-lowering treatments like angiotensin receptor blockers) are another possibility. Given the importance of the brain's blood supply, work on ways of boosting its efficiency—and hence supplies of glucose and oxygen—from midlife or earlier, especially in ApoE4 carriers, is an obvious research priority. It might also be possible to strengthen the ageing blood–brain barrier, for example by enhancing production of the proteins which control the tight junctions between its endothelial cells. However, there is also research suggesting that opening up the barrier is beneficial, because it allows for the greater clearance of amyloid. More research is therefore essential if the risk of treatments worsening the disease (as has been known) is to be minimized.

Given the role of ApoE4 in vascular disease and dementia, I would hope that a test for this risk factor soon becomes routine, enabling carriers—and their doctors—to be warned at an early stage that they may have to work harder to maintain good health.

Neurotransmitters

Work on the relationship of Aβ with neurotransmitter systems has mainly focused on acetylcholine and glutamate, since Aβ is known to bind to their receptors. The inhibitory transmitter GABA is thought to be more resistant to Aβ's harmful effects, but appears to have important interactions with other proteins in the amyloid pathway such as APP. Aβ also influences the activity of other receptors, notably those of neurotrophins such as BDNF. These are of interest because of research suggesting that the acetylcholinergic cells which die off early in Alzheimer's also have receptors for neurotrophins. This finding might help to explain why standard acetylcholine-boosting drugs have only modest and temporary benefits. Indeed, it may point us to an underlying principle of dementia science: if many factors are involved, then perhaps many need to co-occur before the disease takes hold. In which case, the failure of direct approaches that target one particular pathway becomes less baffling. Working out which combinations of factors can be targeted for the least cost and greatest benefit will, however, be a huge challenge.

Research on other neurotransmitters such as dopamine and histamine is less advanced, though there are again interesting ideas in the literature.[2]

Cholesterol

A further important player in amyloid's network is cholesterol, used for membrane repair and myelination, and transported to neurons by ApoE (less efficiently in ApoE4 carriers). Normally the build-up of cholesterol in membranes is inhibited by an enzyme called ACAT1, whose gene has been linked to Alzheimer's; blocking this enzyme in amyloid-bearing mice reduces the damage and lowers levels of Aβ oligomers.[3] We are used to thinking of high cholesterol levels as harmful, but this research suggests that low levels of brain cholesterol in cell membranes might contribute to amyloid build-up. ACAT1 blockers are currently being investigated as potential treatments for Alzheimer's.[4] Other participants in cholesterol metabolism have also been linked to the disease and are under investigation for potential therapies.[5]

Another possibility, given the prominent role of ApoE4 in dementia and other diseases, is that gene-therapy and gene-editing techniques like CRISPR could be used to replace the more risky variants with safer ones. At least one patent proposing this possibility has already been filed, but research publications to date are scarce, so we await developments.[6]

DNA and the Cell Cycle

Some research suggests that DNA damage and abnormal re-entry into the cell cycle may be early features of neurodegenerative disease. Oxidative stress causing DNA damage can enhance the build-up of amyloid. Moreover, research has found that changes in APP processing can trigger cell cycle re-entry. APP may also affect transcription factors, the master regulators like NFκB which can interact with DNA to control which proteins are produced. Greater understanding of cell cycle control and DNA damage could have many other benefits, most notably for cancer treatments, but also for dementia, and this is an area where increased interdisciplinary collaboration between neuroscientists and other specialists might be a relatively feasible and rapid way to gain results.

Calcium, Cytoskeletal, and Endoplasmic Reticulum Stress

Earlier I raised the possibility that, just as levels of cytokines rise in response to cell damage or the presence of pathogens, so Aβ levels might act as a signal of problems with protein control systems, from their production in the nucleus and folding in the endoplasmic reticulum to their transport via the cytoskeleton and their eventual recycling and disposal. If this were the case, then treatments addressing the causes of protein packaging and transport problems—causes like altered intracellular calcium and cytoskeleton dysfunction—might be useful. Experiments altering APP levels in cells affect calcium signalling, for example, and calcium-channel blockers are already being studied in human trials, although the evidence to date is inconclusive. Research into regulation of protein folding and disposal is also on-going, but again, it is early days.

This is a young science. I believe that, given the wealth of hypotheses it has already generated, and the remarkable and growing array of methods available to test them, we have a very good chance of finding more effective treatments for dementia in the next decade. In the meantime, it lies with us to use the knowledge already accumulated as best we can to reduce our risk of falling prey to the ravages of neurodegeneration. Prevention, after all, is better than a cure which may one day transform our attitudes to ageing, but whose arrival is unlikely to be imminent.

23

Probing the Frontiers

O f all the things we don't yet understand about dementia, what are the priorities for future research? What science do we need to know in order to reach the three great goals of preventing, delaying, or curing this and other neurodegenerative diseases?

Most obviously, we need a much clearer grasp of the brain's internal mechanisms. In particular, we need to know more about:

1. *Risk.* How—and how much—does a given dementia risk factor alter brain cells' ability to maintain homeostasis? How should we quantify the amount of risk of, say, high exposure to infection or having high blood sugar—both on a person's chances of later dementia, and on an individual cell's capacity for self-repair?

2. *Environments.* Some of the research on risk factors such as poor diet and pollution is frankly terrifying. But it is also preliminary and in serious need of more data. It would make sense for those in charge of research budgets to prioritize an intensive multidisciplinary effort to find out whether these preventable risks are indeed a major problem, and if so how best to reduce them.

3. *Funding.* Talking of research budgets, we need to spend a lot, lot more on dementia. How to achieve this is yet another hard question, but a political rather than a scientific one, and thus beyond the scope of this book.[1] Political questions are answered most successfully in the long term, however, when they are answered on the basis of evidence rather than ideology. Developing more effective treatments for dementia, and learning more about when those treatments need to start and who is most likely to benefit, are political as well as research priorities.

4. *Repair.* How can the body's own repair mechanisms be strengthened safely, i.e. without triggering unwanted side effects like cancer? To what extent can this be

done with lifestyle changes such as eating more fish or taking more exercise, rather than by using drugs?

5. *Neurons.* Which cells are most affected? If some neurons are especially vulnerable to neurodegeneration, is this because of the neurotransmitters they use, the length of their axons and how well those axons are myelinated, the neurons' size, their location near to ventricles and CVOs, the synaptic networks of which they are a part, or some other factor or factors?

6. *Other cells.* How are astrocytes, microglia, oligodendrocytes, and endothelial cells affected by risk factors, and what are their roles in neurodegenerative processes?

7. *Pathways.* Current research on dementia gives us an immensely complicated picture of possible mechanisms: brain cell death by a thousand cuts. Which of all the myriad biochemical pathways are significantly relevant to the problem of dementia, and which can be safely targeted by drugs?

8. *Timing.* When to intervene is a vexed—and potentially multimillion-dollar—question. In late-stage dementia so much goes wrong that the list of unaffected systems is probably shorter than the list of affected ones; so the aim is to catch the disease as early as possible. But how early is that? The answer will depend on the length of time between initial processes and clinical signs. In familial Alzheimer's and Down's syndrome dementia, assuming that brain Aβ build-up is an accurate marker of the underlying processes, that gap has been estimated at around a quarter of a century.[2] Whether this applies to sporadic dementia is not known. Nor are we yet certain, of course, that Aβ is the most accurate marker of disease progression.

9. *Neurodegeneration.* We do not yet know enough about this. More work is needed on the 'templating' hypothesis—the idea that dementia's agents can infiltrate neurons by spreading from synapse to synapse. If it is correct, then drugs to block the spread could potentially halt the disease. We also need to know more about how synapse loss occurs—is it, for example, due to overactive complement, excitotoxicity, mitochondrial or cytoskeletal problems, or something else? It is assumed that synapse loss is the starting point of neurodegeneration, but at least some neurons can survive reductions of around one-third in their synapse numbers, so how and when does the loss of its communications lead to a cell's collapse—and to cognitive problems? And is damage to axons a more potent trigger of neurodegeneration than synapse loss? If so, how can we best protect white matter?

10. *Methods.* Have we got the techniques we need to understand dementia, and are they telling us what we think they're telling us? The answer, as we have seen with the queries about antibody specificity, is unfortunately: not always. Methods are a widely underrated part of science, as I noted in *The Brain Supremacy*. Not only are they vital for discovery, they shape the questions scientists ask and their interpretations of the answers. Without the development of live-brain amyloid imaging, for example, the amyloid cascade hypothesis would be more secure on its foundations.

11. *Computing power.* Only in recent years has the number-crunching capacity needed to understand dementia and model its intricacies begun to be a practical possibility.

12. *Conceptual change.* As researchers find new ways of analysing massive genetic and biochemical datasets, the result is a new way of thinking about neurodegeneration. At the heart of the amyloid cascade hypothesis is the concept of a linear progression: a chain of events culminating in cell death. More and more, however, it seems that what happens in dementia is not so much a chain of events as a network, in which many slight happenings may, over time, reinforce each other until the entire system tips over into disaster. As with ecological collapse or the birth of a tornado, there may be no clear single cause. Neuroscience has benefited greatly from other sciences. No doubt dementia researchers are already raiding their colleagues' disciplines for models and techniques applicable to the ecology of the ageing brain.

Whatever they find, the next decade or so looks set to be transformative for the study, understanding, and treatment of dementia.

24

This End is Only a Beginning

Two decades on, the amyloid cascade hypothesis still dominates research into dementia. Its chief suspects, the proteins amyloid-beta and tau, were first implicated (as so often) by DNA evidence: in this case, from victims with familial forms of the disease. On a majority vote, the suspects would probably face conviction. However, a few voices have maintained that tau and amyloid are innocent, and rather more have queried the standard narrative of their crimes.

Authors, even science authors, are expected to express their point of view; so here is mine. As this book has shown, a crowd of other suspects is present in ageing brains and those stricken by dementia. My own feeling, after prolonged immersion in the most complex literature I have ever encountered, is that neurodegeneration is likely to be a gang murder—and by a large gang at that. Changes in mitochondria, insulin, and glucose, accumulating toxins and pollutants, DNA errors, blood–brain barrier and vascular damage, excitotoxicity, oxidative stress and inflammation, cell senescence, and problems affecting calcium signalling, membrane integrity, or protein synthesis, folding, and disposal are my major suspects, influenced for better or worse by genes. No doubt there are others. If pushed, I would have to say that I am not altogether convinced by the amyloid hypothesis: at least, in its claim that amyloid-beta and phosphorylated tau are the villains of the neurodegeneration story. We need to know more about their normal roles in healthy brains before we can be sure that is the case.

Only further investigation will unravel the complex realities, but I return to the basic fact about Alzheimer's, stroke, and other age-related brain conditions: *they are age-related*. Even familial Alzheimer's does not strike in childhood, but usually in mid-adulthood or later. (There are, dreadfully, rare cases of childhood and young adult dementia, usually due to severe genetic malfunctions; one afflicted family, for instance, has a mutation in the prion protein gene.[2])

And your point, Taylor? Well, a lot of the problems I've just listed look like failures of homeostasis, the body's extraordinary maintenance capacity. Ageing builds up damaging factors like oxidative stress and pro-inflammatory cytokines; it reduces healing factors like neurotrophins, growth factors, DNA repair proteins, and chemokines; and it alters delicate balances, for example of blood fats and sugars, and brain neurotransmitters. Genetic variants can alter the rates of change, perhaps by only a small percentage each year; but over a lifetime even small effects can make themselves felt. Young cells recover quickly, but older cells, repeatedly pushed, spring back to homeostasis less easily.

In writing this, I touch on perhaps the two biggest debates in the science of dementia. The first concerns the relationship between familial Alzheimer's, that rare affliction from which we have learned so much, and sporadic Alzheimer's, that common affliction about which we still know so little. Are they similar enough to justify the vast extrapolations that have been made from one to the other? You might think that the answer is obviously 'no', since familial Alzheimer's strikes earlier and is clearly driven by genes, not oxidative stress or infections or any of the other potential causes of the sporadic disease.

But the phrase is misleading, since genes drive nothing by themselves. They express proteins, and that act of creation is driven by changes in the cell's chemistry. Put another way, familial Alzheimer's patients do not live in a timeless vacuum. They too experience stresses, wear and tear, pollution, life. Their genes may simply make them far more vulnerable to these assailants. Those genes have served researchers as a guide to where to look for the processes that cause dementia's damage. They cannot provide certain answers, because the same genes do not seem to be responsible in sporadic Alzheimer's, or in other dementias.

Neurodegenerative processes are fluid, multiple, and interactive. They are also intricately woven into the material life of the cell. We need inflammation, just as we need oxygen, food, and rest; but chronic inflammation and too much oxidative stress, the wrong kind of food and too little activity, can do us great harm. 'All things in moderation', as the saying goes, but we don't yet know where all the tipping points are between moderation and extremity, health and disease. Yet again, the body's complexities preclude any chance of a simple answer.

The second debate, cousin to the first, concerns the relationship between dementia and ageing, and it highlights the problems we have with thinking about diseases. Healthily ageing folk and people with dementia have very different behaviours; their brains look different, and the slide into death is much steeper in dementia. Our instinct, therefore, is to divide the world into 'us' and 'them', 'healthy' and 'sick'. But in a condition with so many small causes, so many stages, and so many synapses and cells to be affected, there may be no clear point at which someone stops being well and starts being ill.

Nothing in the Body is Ever Simple

The vast complexities of our physiology make it remarkably stable for many years. Most gene-reading errors or environmental dangers have little obvious impact on our health. But perfect health is an illusion from day one. Children come into the world marked by their parents' genes and experiences, their time in the womb. Adults accumulate malfunctions throughout life. When we are young, if we're lucky, we possess good health, and it may seem as if we need do little to stay healthy. As we grow older, we learn—sometimes too late—that health requires effort.

The focus of medicine is starting to change accordingly, away from quick fixes and towards using multiple approaches. To quote from the journal *Science*, 'the search for a magic bullet is giving way to combinatorial or convergent solutions. Medications, devices, mobile health apps, social support, education, and team care are all part of the package needed for improving outcomes.'[3] The best ways we will find to treat dementia will involve much more than drugs.

That good health, like illness, is complex is unsurprising. We evolved as wholes, not meat with added spark (whether that spark be thinking power or soul). We descend from organisms that have had four billion years in which to discover what worked. What constraints each system places on other systems, how to get an effective immune response without destroying yourself as well as your attacker, how to manage your waste and find enough fuel: these and many other problems had to be solved. The solutions may not be perfect, but for evolution they don't have to be: they just have to last long enough to give the organism a chance of successful reproduction.

One thing is certain: in creatures made of trillions of cells the solutions were never going to be simple. Nonetheless, over seven billion of us have found a balance by which life can be maintained, sometimes for over a hundred years. Studies have found that although a majority of people aged seventy or older have some chronic disease, only between thirty and forty per cent of people in their nineties or older have dementia. Close on two-thirds of the oldest old are not affected.

Beyond the Science

The complexity of dementia research is a challenge, but it should not be cause for gloom. Our expectations may have been too high in the past, but more realistic hopes will serve us better in the long term. And there is still good reason to be hopeful. We live at a time when there is a wealth of research on the amyloid hypothesis and increasing investigation of other possibilities. We are also seeing astonishingly fast development of new technologies and better understanding of brain mechanisms. Add to that ageing populations in many countries and a change in the political climate, and the conditions are coming together for what could be a golden age for dementia research, bringing a real chance, at last, of finding effective treatments. I hope so.

As I have said, the very complexity of dementia's causes offers a better chance of early intervention and of finding effective treatments, including the 'repurposing' of existing methods such as insulin sprays and ultrasound.

Finally, that same complexity should remind us that there is much we can do beyond sitting back and waiting for science to bring forth a magic pill. Dementia is, after all, an illness suffered by people, not people's brains. There is much we could do to help those people, and ourselves, even if we are not researchers, research funders, or healthcare professionals.

We can help ourselves by adapting our lifestyles, workplaces, and institutions to prioritize not labour and cash, but health and well-being. The social revolution that would be needed to carry that project through can hardly be imagined, it is so far-reaching. Yet it may be forced on us before long by external pressures: shifting demographics; climate change, globalization, and their politics; technologies that alter the kinds of jobs available. And, after all, modern capitalism had a beginning, and not so long ago. We have changed society before, and we can again.

If that is too big a task, then—as noted at the end of Part 2—we can at least take steps to improve our personal health, at whatever age. Acting alone, however, makes failing more likely, and there is much that governments, companies, and regulators could do to make life easier for individuals. Better information would be a good start. Consider the food industry. Hardly anyone has the time—and some don't have the eyesight—to read all the text on the back of every packet of food. We expect what we eat to be harmless unless labelled otherwise, and we rely on our institutions to see that this happens. Yet if those institutions do not insist on good behaviour, corporations will quite rationally aim to maximize profit even if that means heavily promoting unhealthy food.

Insisting that individuals must take responsibility for personal choices is unreasonable if informed choice is unfeasibly difficult. Government could do much to improve this situation, and so could media pressure. If they aren't holding business to account—and particularly big international businesses, whose ethos and constitution factor in profit but don't insist on concern for consumer health—then who else will make them do so, if not us?

We could also consider more inventive approaches to other risk factors. (How about a national drive to collect ideas from the public on how to do this?) One example is the alarming finding that severe stress, especially in early life, increases the risk not just of later dementia but also of many other illnesses, including that underrated disability, major depression. Children can be dreadfully damaged by traumatic experiences, and there is much more that adults could do to protect them.[4]

Some risk factors, like diabetes, are modifiable: they could be reduced by concerted government, media, business, and individual action. Some, like ApoE4, are not at present modifiable. And some look modifiable but in practice don't seem to be. Poverty is one of these. Western governments have struggled with the problem of their poorest citizens for centuries; yet the poor are still with us.

Studies in countries with different ideologies suggest that the solution could be simple: give poor people money, if they adopt better health behaviours. At present, however, that is not politically feasible in many places. Which is a shame, because poverty is so influential on other putative causes—poor diet, stress, environmental pollution, etc.—that it could be described as a 'super-cause' of ill health, and thus of welfare expenditure. Wealth does not spare people from adverse experiences like illness, alcoholism, drug addiction, marital break-up, and unemployment, but it does protect them from the worst consequences, giving them much more resilience under stress. Here again there is much that government and the media could do—and that we as individuals could do—to alter the moral conventions which blame poor people for their poverty. But given the interests vested in this kind of morality, the chances of that happening are small.

Unless you are very wealthy, taking steps towards better health—of body and brain—is often conditional on a decent welfare system and/or an understanding employer. Both are under pressure in the current political climate. This is myopic even by the election-driven standards of democratic societies. To save themselves enormous healthcare costs, governments need to be looking, now, at how to improve life not just for the elderly, but also for working-age people and for children. Health costs—like climate change, biodiversity loss, or job threats from technological advances—often seem to be a future problem, and a vague and abstract one at that. Such problems are the hardest to address politically, because there is no urgent motivation. Until, that is, you notice that the wildlife of your childhood has disappeared, or your work can now be done by a computer...or you, or someone you love, gets a diagnosis of dementia.

As people grow older, dementia and the terror of senility impinge on them more and more. To the young, it may seem impossibly distant, an uninteresting and irrelevant problem compared with all the others they face. To the middle-aged, making grieving and guilt-stricken decisions about how to look after elderly relatives, it is a darkening shadow on their own future as well as that of their loved ones. To older people it is a source of threat and anxiety, as they worry about being a burden, or being left helpless at the mercy of strangers.

In my experience of the medical and care professions, strangers are often remarkably hard-working, kindly, and generous with time, effort, and patience. Having seen good elder care, I am in awe of the people who provide it. But the fear of losing control of one's life is still an issue. And not all the fates awaiting those who need care in later life are benign; far from it. The dread of dependency, like the dread of illness, may sometimes be worse than the thing itself, but illness and old age can leave people extremely vulnerable to abuse.

In the meantime, life is complicated enough even for healthy folk, and there is much that the system could do to help someone with a dementia diagnosis. For starters, how about automatically appointing a named independent financial adviser and healthcare professional, barring and/or heavily penalizing cold callers, notifying local police and health services to treat the person as a priority case, and relieving them of the need to do their tax returns?[5] We could also relieve some of the fears around dementia by making more effort to improve standards of care and to value carers.

We could, in addition, help sufferers of dementia go more gently into that dark night, for example by encouraging people to think of the illness as a gradual withdrawal from life's temptations and stresses, a process which, done well, makes the eventual death less of a shock and less painful for those who are left behind. That withdrawal is, however, uneven. The aspects of life that don't matter so much go first—like knowing what day of the week it is. The important bits, like feeling and loving, linger even in advanced dementia, and people in that state still seem to benefit from kindness and gentle human contact.

Since all life ends in death, the question is not how to dodge the reaper but how to make the living bearable. Dementia is not the kind of death sentence that, like execution, demands that we distance ourselves, morally and physically, from the sufferer; and we as well as they can benefit if we do not. Dementia patients are like us—only us at our most weary, worn, and fragile. Stimuli and emotions that we can easily handle they find overwhelming, because they haven't the energy to deal with them as we would. Knowing this, we can adapt the ways we interact with them. Even small things, like shorter visits and plentiful cups of tea, can help.

We could, moreover, stop seeing dementia patients as nothing more than a burden and a cost. They are people taking on perhaps the worst challenge anyone ever faces: how to handle a terminal disease that not only brings pain, stress, and panic, not only strips away independence and mobility, but will slowly dismember their very identity too. What adventurer's first or sporting triumph comes close to that? Dementia takes courage, and people facing dementia deserve profound respect. We are afraid of dying, and desperately afraid of dementia. They are living with it. If they find that dementia not only makes clear what really matters in life, but also smooths away the fear of dying, then they have achieved a wisdom beyond most of us. In any case, I believe that honour, not avoidance, is the appropriate reaction to dementia.

'If we *are* what we remember, what are they/who don't have memories as we have ours?', asked the poet Tony Harrison. Perhaps we should answer by saying that we are not defined just by what we remember, or our capacity to string sentences together, or our ability to perform the cognitive functions expected of adults by society. Being human involves more than this: a body, a brain, and a history of being loved. (They live in our memories after their own have gone.) Even in the oldest and loneliest dementia patients we should be honouring that recognition by providing kindness and comfort: not as charity to the dying, but as a tribute to heroes.

With proper care, people can live well with neurodegenerative and other brain disorders. Today they live in a better time than ever before to have such conditions, because the strange science of our fragile brains is also an immensely hopeful science. The search for a cure, or some way of delaying neurodegeneration, is accelerating, and recent research has opened up exciting prospects for treatment. Until those prospects bear fruit, we need to make sure patients suffering with age-related brain disorders have the chance to live well and die the kind of death we would like for ourselves and for the people we love.

After all, those patients may one day be us.

Endnotes

Chapter 1

1 Saver, J. L. (2006), 'Time is brain—quantified', *Stroke*, 37, 263–6.
2 UK MS patients have at least benefited from the government's 2010 Equality Act, which for welfare purposes classes them as disabled from the moment of diagnosis, thus sparing them the misery of having to prove their failings to sometimes distant and/or unsympathetic assessors.
3 Taylor, K. (2014), *The Brain Supremacy: Notes from the Frontiers of Neuroscience* (Oxford: Oxford University Press). Actually the language of these sciences is even worse. Acronym soup would at least be easily pronounceable, but many of the abbreviations are initialisms.

Part 1

1 Harrison, T. (1992), *The Gaze of the Gorgon* (Newcastle-upon-Tyne: Bloodaxe Books).

Chapter 2

1 Hughes, T. F. and M. Ganguli (2009), 'Modifiable midlife risk factors for late-life cognitive impairment and dementia', *Current Psychiatry Reviews*, 5, 73–92.
2 I say more about the power of stigma in my book *Cruelty: Human Evil and the Human Brain* (Oxford: Oxford University Press, 2009). The quotation is from the *Atlantic Monthly* in 2000. The original context was an article—'A new way to be mad'—about apotemnophilia (the desire to be an amputee), and the quote is Elliott's summary of an argument made by philosopher of science Ian Hacking. My thanks to Robert Stonjek for drawing my attention to the piece.
3 See, for example (hereafter 'SFE'), a 2015 study which asked participants to rank the importance to them of eight values not directly linked to health ('creativity, friends and family, humor, independence, money, politics, religion, spontaneity') and found that those who affirmed their highest-ranked (versus lowest-ranked) value during the task increased their later activity significantly more. The study is Falk, E. B. *et al.* (2015), 'Self-affirmation alters the brain's response to health messages and subsequent behavior change', *Proceedings of the National Academy of Sciences*, 112, 1977–82.
4 Low socioeconomic status has also been linked to more rapid biological ageing in young people who have done well despite their disadvantaged start. Better-off participants

showed no such effect. See Miller, G. E. *et al.* (2015), 'Self-control forecasts better psychosocial outcomes but faster epigenetic aging in low-SES youth', *Proceedings of the National Academy of Sciences*, 112, 10325–30.

5 Population projections suggest that by mid-century there will be as many older (60 or more years old) as young (up to 15 years old) people on the planet.

Chapter 3

1 Hirtz, D. *et al.* (2007), 'How common are the "common" neurologic disorders?' *Neurology*, 68, 326–37. The US government estimates that in 2010 there were 40 million people over the age of sixty-five in its population.

2 The report, by the Alzheimer's Association, is available from <http://www.alz.org/ downloads/facts_figures_2013.pdf>.

3 The WHO places road injury (1.3 million deaths per year) ninth in its list of top ten causes of death in 2012.

4 Stroke rates are thought to be falling overall, but rising among younger people in Western countries.

5 Mashta, O. (2007), 'Number of people in UK with dementia will more than double by 2050', *British Medical Journal*, 334, 447.

6 See Knapp, M. *et al.* (2007), *Dementia UK: The Full Report* (London, The Personal Social Services Research Unit (PSSRU) at the London School of Economics/The Institute of Psychiatry at King's College London: for the Alzheimer's Society). N.B. re the units used in this book: one billion is a thousand million, 1,000,000,000, 10^9; one trillion is a million million, 1,000,000,000,000, 10^{12}.

7 The Alzheimer's Society's latest report, in September 2014, estimates 850,000 dementia cases by 2015, with costs around £26.3 billion: see Prince, M. *et al.* (2014), *Dementia UK (2nd edn): Overview.* (London: King's College London/London School of Economics: for the Alzheimer's Society). In the United States, the Alzheimer's Association estimates that in 2013 there were 5.2 million people with dementia, of whom 200,000 (4%) had an early-onset form.

8 Hirtz *et al.* (2007) (note 1). Note that if Alzheimer's is rising in the United States, this contradicts findings of potentially falling rates in Europe, e.g. Schrijvers, E. M. *et al.* (2012), 'Is dementia incidence declining? Trends in dementia incidence since 1990 in the Rotterdam Study', *Neurology*, 78, 1456–63. There are, of course, many differences between the two regions.

9 Wu, Y.-T. *et al.* (2016), 'Dementia in western Europe: epidemiological evidence and implications for policy making', *Lancet Neurology*, 15, 116–24.

10 The median length of stay for dementia was twenty-one days, according to United Kingdom government health statistics for 2012–13 (see <http://www.hscic.gov.uk/ catalogue/PUB12566/hosp-epis-stat-admi-summ-rep-2012-13-rep.pdf>). Only hospitalizations for schizophrenia (thirty days), unknown diseases (twenty-four), and antibiotic-resistant infections (forty-six) were longer.

11 The study by the Personal Social Services Research Unit (available from <http://www .pssru.ac.uk/pdf/dp2769.pdf>) was commissioned by the private healthcare provider

BUPA, and considered anonymized data pertaining to 11,565 care home residents who died in BUPA care homes from November 2008 to May 2010. The UK government reports that between 2001 and 2011 the number of care home residents in England and Wales overall (i.e. including private care homes) was fairly stable at around 290,000; for details see <http://www.ons.gov.uk/ons/dcp171776_373040.pdf>.

12 Macdonald, A. and B. Cooper (2007), 'Long-term care and dementia services: an impending crisis', *Age and Ageing*, 36, 16–22.

13 The distribution of care home stay lengths was significantly non-normal, with a long tail at the upper end, so the average given here is the median.

14 The prison population for England and Wales in 2013 was 85,362, including people awaiting deportation, according to UK government figures (available from <https://www.gov.uk/government/publications/prison-population-figures>). Bear in mind that the number of people with dementia is almost certainly an underestimate.

15 The quotation is from a post on the King's Fund blog—'Admission to a nursing home can never become a "never" event' (<http://www.kingsfund.org.uk/blog/2014/08/admission-nursing-home-can-never-become-never-event>)—by visiting fellow David Oliver. It refers to care home residents, most of whom will have dementia.

16 Luengo-Fernandez, R. *et al.* (2015), 'UK research spend in 2008 and 2012: comparing stroke, cancer, coronary heart disease and dementia', *British Medical Journal Open*, 5, e006648.

17 SFE the Alzheimer's Disease International (ADI) 2013 *World Alzheimer's Report*, available from <http://www.alz.co.uk/research/world-report-2013>.

18 Hurd, M. D. *et al.* (2013), 'Monetary costs of dementia in the United States', *New England Journal of Medicine*, 368, 1326–34.

19 ADI states that the figure of $600 billion dollars is 'around 1% of global GDP', which the World Databank estimates (in 2012) to have been $97 trillion. Note that all these figures are guesstimates; no one has gone out and counted the world population of dementia patients, let alone dementia sufferers (given the variation in diagnosis between countries, these are not the same thing). For another, albeit similar, estimate—that the costs of dementia will rise by 85% by 2030—see Banerjee, S. (2012), 'The macroeconomics of dementia—will the world economy get Alzheimer's disease?', *Archives of Medical Research*, 43, 705–9.

20 PwC, 'The World in 2050', available from <http://www.pwc.com/gx/en/issues/the-economy/assets/world-in-2050-february-2015.pdf>.

21 Mullane, K. and M. Williams (2013), 'Alzheimer's therapeutics: continued clinical failures question the validity of the amyloid hypothesis—but what lies beyond?', *Biochemical Pharmacology*, 85, 289–305.

22 Gandy, S. (2014), 'Alzheimer's disease: new data highlight nonneuronal cell types and the necessity for presymptomatic prevention strategies', *Biological Psychiatry*, 75, 553–7.

23 Gandy (2014) (note 22).

24 Scarborough, P. *et al.* (2011), 'The economic burden of ill health due to diet, physical inactivity, smoking, alcohol and obesity in the UK: an update to 2006–07 NHS costs', *Journal of Public Health*, 33, 527–35. For comparison, total government tax receipts for alcohol in 2006–2007 were over £8 billion. This, as is often pointed out by critics of UK tax policy, more than covers the health bill for alcohol. What the critics tend not to add is

that the total costs to society of alcohol are considerably greater, given its role in violent disorder, domestic abuse, unsafe sex, accidents, etc. Of two attempts to estimate overall costs, the lower (in 2003) was £20 billion, the higher (in 2007) £55 billion. Thus, although the health costs for drinking and smoking are similar, and although smoking too has secondary costs, alcohol is a bigger drain on the overall national budget. Data for 2006–7 indicate a net NHS budget of £94.7 billion.

Chapter 4

1 A recent global study estimated the years of life lost through premature death, and the years lived with disability, due to mental illness and substance use. It found 8.6 million years-that-might-have-been: a big number, yet only about half a per cent of the total lost to disease. But look at the years lived with disability: 175 million, almost 23% of the total—according to Whiteford, H. A. *et al.* (2013), 'Global burden of disease attributable to mental and substance use disorders: findings from the Global Burden of Disease Study 2010', *Lancet*, 382, 1575–86. See also Knapp *et al.* (2007) (note 3.6) and the NIH (<http://www.nia.nih.gov/research/publication/longer-lives-and-disability/burden-dementia>).
2 Eustache, M. L. *et al.* (2013), 'Sense of identity in advanced Alzheimer's dementia: a cognitive dissociation between sameness and selfhood?', *Consciousness and Cognition*, 22, 1456–67.

Chapter 5

1 Emil Sioli (1852–1922) is not well known in the English-speaking world; search for him online and most of what you will find is in German. He was known for his compassion and humanity towards patients, encouraging them to work and, where possible, re-enter the community, in an era when institutionalization often meant permanent disappearance from society. The 'agricultural community' he founded in the town of Friedrichsdorf for patients with alcoholism and psychiatric illnesses still exists as the Freundeskreis Waldkrankenhaus Köppern.
2 Devi, G. and W. Quitschke (1999), 'Alois Alzheimer, neuroscientist (1864–1915)', *Alzheimer Disease and Associated Disorders*, 13, 132–7.
3 Various methods of staining body tissues were discovered in the late nineteenth and early twentieth centuries, and they were put to good use in brain research by researchers such as Alzheimer, Nissl, Camillo Golgi (who discovered the Golgi apparatus), and Ramon y Cajal (the latter two shared a Nobel for their work, while Nissl was twice nominated for his). The Nissl stain turns RNA dark blue, making it a useful marker of neural tissue. It particularly highlights the rough endoplasmic reticulum (*aka* 'Nissl body'), where RNA accumulates in ribosomes ('Nissl granules') and is translated into protein.
4 Nissl also later worked with Kraepelin in Munich. The textbook he and Alzheimer produced, *Histologische und histopatologische Arbeiten über die Grosshirnrinde* (*Histologic and Histopathologic Studies of the Cerebral Cortex*), was published between 1907 and 1918.
5 The quotation is from Stelzmann, R. A. *et al.* (1995), 'An English translation of Alzheimer's 1907 paper, "Über eine eigenartige Erkankung [sic: it should be Erkrankung] der Hirnrinde"', *Clinical Anatomy*, 8, 429–31.

6 The title is from Stelzmann *et al.* (1995) (note 5).

7 Katzman, R. (1976), 'The prevalence and malignancy of Alzheimer disease: a major killer', *Archives of Neurology*, 33, 217–18. For more about Katzman, his impact, and legacy see the tribute to him at <http://www.alzforum.org>.

8 See Devi and Quitschke (1999) (note 2) or the biography of Alzheimer: Maurer, K. and U. Maurer (2003), *Alzheimer: The Life of a Physician and the Career of a Disease* (New York, Columbia University Press).

9 More exactly, Alzheimer's 'inaugural dissertation' at the Julius-Maximilian University of Würzburg was on the glands which produce earwax, a topic assigned to him by his tutors. The seventeen-page thesis marks an interest in fatty deposits which is also apparent in his discussion of the 'lipoid saccules' he found in Auguste D.'s brain—perhaps corresponding to abnormally enlarged endosomes (see note 5.26), which are known to be a feature of certain neurodegenerative conditions. His biographers (Maurer and Maurer (2003) (note 8), chapter 3) observe that Alzheimer was in good company; Aristotle commented on earwax. It was first considered a secretion produced by brain activity (perhaps Aristotle suffered from it?) and later seen as a defence against 'various pests that could crawl into the ear during sleep'—like earwigs, presumably, which are accused of this transgression by no less a figure than Pliny (in his *Natural History*). Alzheimer himself refused to speculate on what earwax was for; he was more interested in what it was made of. His answer was: mostly fat.

10 Percentages are from the Alzheimer's Society (see <http://www.alzheimers.org.uk/site/scripts/documents_info.php?documentID=412>).

11 For example, a 2014 review states that 'Alzheimer's disease, vascular dementia, dementia with Lewy body, and fronto-temporal dementia, account for 90% of all cases.' See Abete. P. *et al.* (2014), 'Cognitive impairment and cardiovascular diseases in the elderly. A heart–brain continuum hypothesis', *Ageing Research Reviews*, 18, 41–52.

12 Jellinger, K. A. (2006), 'Clinicopathological analysis of dementia disorders in the elderly—an update', *Journal of Alzheimer's Disease*, 9, 61–70.

13 See the Alzheimer's Association webpage 'What is dementia?' (<http://www.alz.org/what-is-dementia.asp>).

14 SFE Tokuchi, R. *et al.* (2014), 'Clinical and demographic predictors of mild cognitive impairment for converting to Alzheimer's disease and reverting to normal cognition', *Journal of the Neurological Sciences*, 346, 288–92. This publication is a review and meta-analysis of MCI-to-dementia conversion studies. Comparing research using strict and less strict definitions of MCI, in specialist clinics and in community samples, Tokuchi and colleagues found annual conversion rates up to around 10% for the strict definition and specialist setting: specifically, 9.6% for conversion to dementia, 8.1% for Alzheimer's, and 1.9% for vascular dementia. Community samples gave figures of 4.9%, 6.8%, and 1.6%, respectively.

15 H. M. had surgery on his temporal lobes to treat severe epilepsy. The operation left him with profound amnesia, and he became one of the most studied neurological patients in the world. He died in 2008.

16 Multiple processes contribute to tissue loss in healthy ageing. Estimates vary depending on who is measured and when, whether the study is cross-sectional or longitudinal, which corrections are applied (e.g. for head size, as men are generally bigger-headed), and what is analysed (e.g. specific regions, total brain volume, or weight).

17 Svennerholm, L. *et al.* (1997), 'Changes in weight and compositions of major membrane components of human brain during the span of adult human life of Swedes', *Acta Neuropathologica*, 94, 345–52.

18 The percentage change was similar for neurons and glia, though the latter was not statistically significant because that study was on only twelve individuals; see Pakkenberg, B. *et al.* (2003), 'Aging and the human neocortex', *Experimental Gerontology*, 38, 95–9.

19 Azevedo, F. A. *et al.* (2009), 'Equal numbers of neuronal and nonneuronal cells make the human brain an isometrically scaled-up primate brain', *Journal of Comparative Neurology*, 513, 532–41.

20 The area is the mediodorsal thalamus, and the ratios of neurons to glia are 1.06 in newborns and 0.18 in adults. As far as we know the thalamus is not alone in undergoing a shift towards more glia. The study is Abitz, M. *et al.* (2007), 'Excess of neurons in the human newborn mediodorsal thalamus compared with that of the adult', *Cerebral Cortex*, 17, 2573–8.

21 <http://www.Blausen.com> has a short animated video of the ventricles.

22 Psychologist Hermann Rorschach's controversial test involves showing a person complex images (inkblots) and interpreting their reactions.

23 The anterior commissure and corpus callosum link the left and right cortical hemispheres. The fornix arches around the brain's core, bearing information from the hippocampus (star of the memory circuit) to the hypothalamus (important in everything from sex to eating to aggression). The medial forebrain bundle links brain areas involved in reward and emotion processing, such as the medial prefrontal cortex, amygdala, basal ganglia, and hypothalamus. In evolutionary terms, the anterior and hippocampal commissures predate the corpus callosum as ways of linking the brain's left and right halves.

24 Lipid is a term used for fats and oils (it is Greek-derived, whereas 'fat' is from Old English). Dietary fats, the kinds that pile on the poundage, are mostly triglycerides (*aka* triacylglycerols). These have a spine of glycerol (*aka* glycerine) to which three fatty acids are attached like piglets to a sow. Diglycerides and monoglycerides have two fatty acids or one, respectively. Glycerol, formula $C_3H_8O_3$, consists of a three-carbon chain in which each carbon binds to hydrogens and to one hydroxyl (–OH) group. Because the latter tends to be reactive in water, with the hydrogen readily leaving the oxygen, glycerol dissolves quickly. It also easily forms bonds with fatty acids (via their carboxyl groups). The fatty acids do not dissolve quickly: they are hydrophobic.

25 'Soap bubbles have very thin walls. The range can be anywhere from 10 nanometres at the top of a thin-walled bubble to over 1,000 nanometres', according to <http://soapbubble.wikia.com/wiki/Color_and_Film_Thickness>. A cell's membrane is only about four nanometres wide.

26 Vesicles taken in from the cell surface are called endosomes ('inside bodies'). As they are transported within the cell some are recycled, while others are fated for disposal. Enlarged endosomes are found in Alzheimer's brains. Intriguingly, they are also seen in the brains of some people who will go on to develop Alzheimer's—before the appearance of amyloid plaques and tau tangles. In Down's syndrome, which carries a very high risk of midlife dementia, they have been found in third-trimester foetuses. However, they were

not seen in rare cases of Alzheimer's caused by a genetic mutation. This suggests either that familial and sporadic Alzheimer's are two different conditions or that endosomes are a marker of disease but not a cause.

27 The gene for ApoE exists in three common flavours, or alleles. For a review of ApoE4's role in dementia see Michaelson, D. M. (2014), 'APOE ε4: The most prevalent yet understudied risk factor for Alzheimer's disease', *Alzheimer's and Dementia*, 10, 861–8.

28 Clapham, D. E. (2007), 'Calcium signaling', *Cell*, 131, 1047–58.

29 Well over 300 cell surface proteins have been classified in the CD system. The CD proteins are molecules for which we have antibodies; they can therefore be labelled and used to distinguish cell types ('immunophenotyping'). For example, cytotoxic T lymphocytes express CD8 on their surfaces, while T helper cells express CD4. I was taught that CD stands for 'cluster of differentiation', but the organization that decides on these things (<http://www.hcdm.org/>) refers to 'human cell differentiation molecules'.

30 A quiescent neuron maintains a small negative potential (about −70 millivolts) across its membrane, but an activated one opens channels through which sodium ions pour into the cell. This makes the potential much more positive. Other channels then open to let positively charged potassium ions out, bringing the potential swiftly back to rest (with a slight, quickly corrected overshoot). The resulting 'spike' in electrical charge is the action potential.

31 GABA: gamma-amino-butyric acid. It is the main inhibitory neurotransmitter in the adult central nervous system (CNS). During development GABA may have excitatory effects.

32 Whether a cell reacts to a neurotransmitter depends both on whether the substance is released in its vicinity and on the types of receptors for that substance it possesses, because neurotransmitters have more than one kind of receptor. Acetylcholine, for example, has both excitatory and inhibitory types; while some receptors do nothing so simple and obvious as making a neuron more or less likely to fire. Instead they may prompt it to grow in a certain direction, shed a synapse, produce more or less of a certain protein, or do something else that we don't yet understand.

33 Neurotransmitters are not the only molecules capable of opening ion channels; one type has recently been discovered which can be activated by a fatty acid, arachidonic acid, instead of the more usual proteins.

34 In this discussion I have drawn heavily on Clapham (2007) (note 28).

35 Calcium needs careful handling, so many enzymes are involved in its regulation. 'Hundreds of cellular proteins have been adapted to bind Ca^{2+} over a million-fold range of affinities (nM to mM), in some cases simply to buffer or lower Ca^{2+} levels, and in others to trigger cellular processes. The local nature of Ca^{2+} signaling is intimately tied to this large range of affinities', says Clapham (2007) (note 28). Calcium's many regulatory proteins, such as calmodulin and calpain, affect many other cell proteins, including transcription factors, amyloid, and tau.

36 Imaging studies using fluorescent markers show that calcium signals in a healthy cell form intricate patterns of brief spikes or waves moving across the cell's interior. SFE Clapham (2007) (note 28).

37 The endoplasmic reticulum's receptors are activated by internal messenger molecules such as IP_3. The IP_3 receptors are calcium channels.

38 Kang, J.-Q. *et al.* (2015), 'The human epilepsy mutation GABRG2(Q390X) causes chronic subunit accumulation and neurodegeneration', *Nature Neuroscience*, 18, 988–96. The study presents a mouse model of a rare mutation in a type of GABA receptor, which in humans causes epilepsy, abnormal development, misfolding and aggregation of the receptor protein, and neurodegeneration.

39 Functional connectivity measures the correlation between the activity of multiple brain regions, which need not be directly anatomically connected.

40 These subcortical nuclei—cell clusters—are found in the brainstem, basal forebrain (the nucleus basalis of Meynert), and mid-brain. Histamine is used by cells of the tuberomammillary nucleus, noradrenaline (*aka* norepinephrine) in the locus coeruleus, dopamine in the ventral tegmental area and substantia nigra, and serotonin in the raphe. The nucleus basalis uses acetylcholine.

41 The evidence for volume transmission by the acetylcholinergic projections to cortex is unclear.

42 Pissadaki, E. K. and J. P. Bolam (2013), 'The energy cost of action potential propagation in dopamine neurons: clues to susceptibility in Parkinson's disease', *Frontiers in Computational Neuroscience*, 7, 13.

43 SFE Schliebs, R. and T. Arendt (2011), 'The cholinergic system in aging and neuronal degeneration', *Behavioural Brain Research*, 221, 555–63. The authors argue that early severe damage to acetylcholinergic neurons may be one of the main factors distinguishing Alzheimer's from normal ageing. Interestingly, not all such neurons degenerate early in Alzheimer's. The vulnerable ones also express neurotrophin receptors, with which APP is known to interact. A small preliminary trial of neurotrophin-releasing brain implants in Alzheimer patients observed encouraging effects; however, more research is needed on what is, after all, a highly invasive treatment. See Karami, A. *et al.* (2015), 'Changes in CSF cholinergic biomarkers in response to cell therapy with NGF in patients with Alzheimer's disease', *Alzheimer's and Dementia*, 11, 1316–28.

44 The longer form of beta-amyloid, $A\beta_{42}$, appears to be a more potent nicotinic receptor inhibitor (Verdier, Y. and B. Penke (2004), 'Binding sites of amyloid β-peptide in cell plasma membrane and implications for Alzheimer's disease', *Current Protein and Peptide Science*, 5, 19–31).

45 The three anticholinesterase drugs are donepezil (also known as Aricept), galantamine (Reminyl) and rivastigmine (Exelon). The fourth treatment, which targets a type of glutamate receptors (NMDARs), is memantine (Ebixa). Another hypothesis about the causes of Alzheimer's proposes NMDAR over-activation, leading to calcium influx and excitotoxicity, as the core problem. SFE Verdier and Penke (2004) (note 44). (For more on NMDARs see note 13.55.)

46 Quality matters as well as quantity, and acetylcholine's supporters include some of considerable quality, such as the great neuroanatomist M. Marsel Mesulam, whose papers taught me and many others about the brilliance and beauty of brain connections. On acetylcholine, SFE his review 'Cholinergic circuitry of the human nucleus basalis and its fate in Alzheimer's disease' in the esteemed *Journal of Comparative Neurology* (M. M. Mesulam (2013); *JCN*, 521, 4124–44).

47 Biochemical research is also stretching the hypothesis. As I was finishing this book, I received advanced notice, thanks to a colleague at Oxford, of a publication which puts a fascinating twist on the cholinergic idea by proposing that the key molecule is not the neurotransmitter itself but the enzyme which breaks it down: acetylcholinesterase (AChE). The study, since published, reports that AChE is found in cells (including cells not using acetylcholine as a transmitter) that are selectively vulnerable to early damage in Alzheimer's. Like APP, it can be cleaved to produce a smaller, neurotoxic peptide. This is structurally similar to Aβ and can stimulate production of both amyloid and tau (via effects on calcium and on an enzyme called glycogen synthase kinase, both of which have been linked to Alzheimer's). The AChE-peptide acts as a neurotrophin during development but becomes toxic later in life. (Recall the preponderance of acetylcholinesterase inhibitors among successful Alzheimer drugs.) Excitingly, a modified version of the peptide not only blocks its damaging effects but those of Aβ also. See Garcia-Ratés, S. *et al.* (2016), '(I) Pharmacological profiling of a novel modulator of the alpha7 nicotinic receptor: blockade of a toxic acetylcholinesterase-derived peptide increased in Alzheimer brains', *Neuropharmacology*, 105, 487–99.

48 Carrière, I. *et al.* (2009), 'Drugs with anticholinergic properties, cognitive decline, and dementia in an elderly general population: the 3-city study', *Archives of Internal Medicine*, 169, 1317–24; Gray, S. L. *et al.* (2015), 'Cumulative use of strong anticholinergics and incident dementia: a prospective cohort study', *Journal of the American Medical Association Internal Medicine*, 175, 401–7.

49 'The circuitry of the nucleus basalis allows it to influence rapidly every part of the cerebral cortex in response to afferents not only from the brainstem but also from the cerebral cortex' (Mesulam 2013) (note 46).

50 Acetylcholine also inhibits activity in the cortex's input layer (Layer IV). This makes stronger signals more distinct, 'modulating the impact and memorability of incoming sensory information'. SFE Mesulam (2013) (note 46).

51 Meynert's nucleus may thus help 'to modulate the neural impact of ambient events and mental experiences in accordance with their motivational and motional significance' (Mesulam 2013) (note 46).

52 Cortex and subcortical nuclei are grey matter—clusters of cell bodies comprising about half the brain's volume—while the rest is white matter.

53 The ligand that activates a receptor does so via an 'active site' on the receptor, but that may not be the only place where chemical bonds can form. Other molecules may be attracted to other sites, and they too may affect the receptor's function. This is called allosteric binding (from the Greek word for 'other', and 'steros', a term used to refer to objects' position in space; a stereotaxic frame, for instance, is an essential tool for determining the precise locations of parts of the brain before surgery). Allosteric binding may increase, decrease, or demolish the usual effects of the receptor's activation. An example involves calcium signalling in cells, triggered when inositol trisphosphate (IP_3) binds to its receptor, IP3R. It has recently been discovered that another protein can bind allosterically to the IP3R molecules and lock them into an unhelpful shape, thereby disrupting calcium signalling. This protein, transglutaminase type 2, has been linked to inflammation and to Alzheimer's disease.

54 The study, on a small sample of male brains, is mentioned in Pakkenberg *et al.* (2003) (note 18); but no specific citation is given.

55 I simplify. Not all neurons have this shape, and they vary in size, number of dendrites, how much their axons branch, how many synapses they form with other cells, etc.

56 One nanometre (nm) is one billionth, 0.000000001, 10^{-9}, of a metre (m).

57 Data are from Washington University, available from <https://faculty.washington.edu/chudler/facts.html - neuron>. Synapses are 20–40 nm wide, while dendrites may extend up to 2 mm, according to figures from the Dana Foundation, available from <http://www.dana.org/News/Details.aspx?id=43512> and, for macaque brain, from the University of Texas, available from <http://www.synapses.clm.utexas.edu/pubs/dendrites.pdf>.

58 Studies of 'functional connectivity'—i.e. which brain regions talk to each other during a given task—are a hot topic in current brain research. The neuroscience has been boosted by the development of neuroimaging techniques for measuring structural connectivity, such as DTI (diffusion tensor imaging). See Taylor (2014) (note 1.3), chapter on fMRI for more details.

59 The comparison overlooks a big difference: in electrical cables electrons flow along the wire, whereas in white matter cabling, ions flow in and out of the cable. Robert Stonjek, whom I thank for reminding me of this point, notes that the comparison is more apt for undersea electrical cables (Robert Stonjek, 2014, personal communication); see also his 'Essay: are axons like electrical wires?' on the psychiatry-research group, available from <https://groups.yahoo.com/neo/groups/psychiatry-research/conversations/messages/42067>.

60 SFE de Groot, M. *et al.* (2014), 'Tract-specific white matter degeneration in aging: the Rotterdam Study', *Alzheimer's and Dementia*, 11, 321–30; Lebel, C. *et al.* (2012), 'Diffusion tensor imaging of white matter tract evolution over the lifespan', *NeuroImage*, 60, 340–52. Both studies use diffusion tensor imaging, a form of MRI, to investigate brain white matter tracts.

61 Two signature white matter brain disorders are multiple sclerosis and a set of genetic diseases called leucodystrophies. The former was brought to public notice by the great classical cellist Jacqueline du Pré, the latter by the 1992 film *Lorenzo's Oil*. A recent estimate puts the prevalence of leucodystrophy at around 13 per 100,000 live births (Bonkowsky, J. L. *et al.* (2010), 'The burden of inherited leukodystrophies in children', *Neurology*, 75, 718–25).

62 Larger axons are those with diameters greater than a fifth of a micron. For a guide to myelin, see *Nature's SciTable* website (<http://www.nature.com/scitable/topicpage/myelin-a-specialized-membrane-for-cell-communication-14367205>). NB: one micrometre or micron (μm) is one millionth, 0.000001, 10^{-6}, of a metre.

63 Neural activity appears to be an important signal in myelination and may not require synapses between oligodendrocytes and neurons.

64 The calculation assumes a step length of one-third of a metre per person. Data are from Caminiti, R. *et al.* (2013), 'Diameter, length, speed, and conduction delay of callosal axons in macaque monkeys and humans: comparing data from histology and magnetic resonance imaging diffusion tractography', *Journal of Neuroscience*, 33, 14501–11.

65 The quotation is from *Nature's SciTable* website (note 62).

66 This is a simplification of how so-called saltatory conduction works. A more in-depth, physics-oriented take on the topic would note that the cell membrane, which is made up of pairs of phospholipid molecules placed tail-to-tail, can be modelled as an insulator (the lipid tails) between two conductors (the phosphate head groups). This allows nodes of Ranvier—exposed areas of membrane at which ion channels tend to gather—to be modelled as resistor–capacitor circuits, set in parallel along the axon's length.

67 One of the pioneers of brain research, Stenson is probably better known as Nikolaus di Steno or Nicolai Steno. 'Deus et natura nihil faciunt frustra' is taken from p. 61 of his 1671 dissertation *De Cerebri Anatome*, Steno (1671). The 'finest work' quotation is translated from p. 4: 'de exquissitissimo naturae opere'. It is available online (in image form, complete with large pink thumb) from the Bayerische Staatsbibliothek Munich (<http://reader .digitale-sammlungen.de/resolve/display/bsb10842494.html>).

68 A caveat: our perception of brain space is heavily inflected by the methods we use to study it. Different methods of fixing brains after death, for example, have different effects on the gaps between cells. Since those gaps are full of busy molecules, however, they are far from frivolously excessive, whatever their size.

69 Estimates of cognitive dysfunction in MS vary; SFE Langdon, D. W. (2011), 'Cognition in multiple sclerosis', *Current Opinion in Neurology*, 24, 244–9.

70 In brief, in most animal models, such as the EAE (experimental autoimmune encephalomyelitis) rodent, researchers administer some kind of toxin or antigen—a substance to which the immune system reacts—in order to set off an inflammatory reaction in the animal's brain tissue, mimicking the as-yet-undetermined triggers of disease in people.

71 About 80% of patients with MS may have the relapsing-remitting form initially, according to *Nature's SciTable* website (note 62).

72 Kingwell, E. *et al.* (2013), 'Incidence and prevalence of multiple sclerosis in Europe: a systematic review', *BMC Neurology*, 13, 128.

73 Braak, H. and E. Braak (1997), 'Frequency of stages of Alzheimer-related lesions in different age categories', *Neurobiology of Aging*, 18, 351–7.

74 Bartzokis, G. (2011), 'Alzheimer's disease as homeostatic responses to age-related myelin breakdown', *Neurobiology of Aging*, 32, 1341–71.

75 My short story 'Freedom' (available on my website <https://neurotaylor.com/2013/08/22/ freedom-from-a-neurons-point-of-view/>) can be read as a gentle satire of this metaphor.

76 The use of 'association' to describe areas of cortex outside the primary sensory and motor areas can be traced back to three great figures in the history of brain research: Theodor Meynert (1833–1892), who proposed that when ideas associate a physical linkage is happening in the brain (he also did foundational work on the structure of the brain); William James, who popularized the idea of association and its neural basis; and Korbinian Brodmann, whose maps of human cortex helped define modern neuroanatomy.

77 Douaud, G. *et al.* (2014), 'A common brain network links development, aging, and vulnerability to disease', *Proceedings of the National Academy of Sciences*, 111, 17648–53.

78 Memory comes in several varieties, which appear to involve different brain networks. For example, after an unpleasant social interaction with a work colleague you may remember

every painful detail for a while (short-term or working memory). In the longer term, you may recall some of what was said (semantic memory) and the situation where it happened (episodic memory). Or the details may fade until you have no memory of the encounter, but retain an awareness that you don't much like that colleague (emotional memory). Scientists also distinguish procedural memory, which allows you to remember how to do things—the things you might want to do to your colleague, for instance. The theory of fluid and crystallized intelligence is set out in Horn, J. L. and R. B. Cattell (1966), 'Refinement and test of the theory of fluid and crystallized general intelligences', *Journal of Educational Psychology*, 57, 253–70. They summarize it as follows: 'primary abilities which can be said to involve intelligence to any considerable degree are organized at a general level into two principal classes or dimensions. One of these, referred to as fluid intelligence (abbreviated Gf) is said to be the major measurable outcome of the influence of biological factors on intellectual development—that is, heredity, injury to the central nervous system (CNS) or to basic sensory structures, etc. The other broad dimension, designated crystallized intelligence (abbreviated Gc), is said to be the principal manifestation of a unitariness in the influence of experiential-educative-acculturation influences.' That is, fluid intelligence has to do with capacity and plasticity, crystallized intelligence with knowledge and life history.

79 Regions included: 'lateral prefrontal cortex, frontal eye field, intraparietal sulcus, superior temporal sulcus, posterior cingulate cortex, and medial temporal lobe' as well as 'the parietal operculum (especially OP1), crus of the cerebellum, fusiform and lingual gyrus, supplementary motor area (SMA), and a focal, lateral portion of the primary motor cortex (M1)', say Douaud et al. (2014) (note 77).

80 Bartzokis (2011) (note 74). See the tribute to George Bartzokis by his institution, the University of California, Los Angeles, available from <http://newsroom.ucla.edu/stories/in-memoriam:-dr-george-bartzokis-neuroscientist-who-developed-the-myelin-model-of-brain-disease>. See also Lebel et al. (2012) (note 60), which found similar lifespan trends in white matter function.

81 Douaud et al. (2014) (note 77). Older people may also use both halves of the brain more, whereas younger people's brain function tends to be less symmetrical and makes more use of different networks for different tasks. Interestingly, carriers of a major genetic risk factor for Alzheimer's, ApoE4, show 'more diffuse neural activity', as if their brains were ageing faster (Evans, S. et al. (2014). 'Cognitive and neural signatures of the APOE E4 allele in mid-aged adults', *Neurobiology of Aging*, 35, 1615–23).

82 A 2009 meta-analysis reported that 'early Alzheimer's disease affects structurally the (trans)entorhinal and hippocampal regions, functionally the inferior parietal lobules and precuneus'. See Schroeter, M. L. et al. (2009), 'Neural correlates of Alzheimer's disease and mild cognitive impairment: a systematic and quantitative meta-analysis involving 1351 patients', *NeuroImage*, 47, 1196–206.

83 Technically, the overlying cortex is neocortex; some researchers see the hippocampus as an evolutionarily older form of cortex.

84 Gomez-Isla, T. et al. (1997), 'Neuronal loss correlates with but exceeds neurofibrillary tangles in Alzheimer's disease', *Annals of Neurology*, 41, 17–24.

85 Davies, C. A. et al. (1987). 'A quantitative morphometric analysis of the neuronal and synaptic content of the frontal and temporal cortex in patients with Alzheimer's disease',

Journal of the Neurological Sciences, 78, 151–64, cited in Selkoe, D. J. (2002), 'Alzheimer's disease is a synaptic failure', *Science*, 298, 789–91. Selkoe glosses the findings as follows: 'This revealed a ~25 to 35% decrease in the numerical density of synapses (painstakingly counted in electron micrographs) in biopsied AD cortex, and a ~15 to 35% decrease in the number of synapses per cortical neuron.'

86 Selkoe (2002) (note 85).

87 For example, a study of 58 post-mortem brains found correlations between a measure of brain structural integrity in dorsolateral prefrontal cortex and IQ (van Veluw, S. J. *et al.* (2012), 'Prefrontal cortex cytoarchitecture in normal aging and Alzheimer's disease: a relationship with IQ', *Brain Structure and Function*, 217, 797–808).

88 The degree of correlation is measured statistically by the correlation coefficient r, which puts a number on the extent to which one variable changes when another one does. For example, in patients with mild cognitive impairment, levels of gene expression for certain genes involved in synaptic plasticity are highly correlated with the patients' cognitive performance on a standard test, the MMSE (Berchtold, N. C. *et al.* (2014), 'Brain gene expression patterns differentiate mild cognitive Impairment from normal aged and Alzheimer's disease', *Neurobiology of Aging*, 35, 1961–72). The correlation coefficients were greater than 0.8. (In principle, r can range from magnitude 0 if there is no correlation to 1, perfect correlation, usually only obtained in real life by correlating a variable with itself.) Correlations can be positive (r from 0 to +1) or negative (0 to −1). For the Berchtold *et al.* study, to its authors' surprise, they were negative. 'Unexpectedly, we found that gene expression changes that facilitate synaptic excitability and plasticity were overwhelmingly associated with poorer MMSE, and conversely that gene expression changes that inhibit plasticity were positively associated with MMSE.'

89 The clock-drawing test may be useful in diagnosing moderate to severe dementia, but is not recommended for diagnosing mild dementia or moderate cognitive impairment. It has also been used in other neurological syndromes, most notably hemispatial neglect. Often a consequence of damage to right parietal cortex, neglect causes patients to act as if one side (usually the left) of their world is unavailable to them. They may apply make-up to one half of their face only, eat half the food on their plate, and when drawing a clock, squash all its numbers into one half of its area.

90 Boyle, P. A. *et al.* (2013), 'Much of late life cognitive decline is not due to common neurodegenerative pathologies', *Annals of Neurology*, 74, 478–89.

91 Note that synapse numbers are usually measured in one of two ways: by counting them on electron microscopes (for simple organisms like flies and worms) or by estimating them using levels of a synaptic protein, synaptophysin, as a proxy (SFE Selkoe 2002) (note 85). Synaptophysin levels reflect the number of vesicles in the synapse, so the connection with synapse function and/or loss is somewhat indirect.

92 Many statistical methods assess how variables change across a sample, and whether variation in the quantity of interest (the dependent variable, e.g. brain volume loss per year) correlates with variation in other, independent variables (e.g. levels of certain proteins in the CSF). A full explanation of what causes brain volume loss would be achieved by a model in which variation in the independent variables accounted for 100% of the variance in the dependent variable. In practice, each independent variable

may account for a proportion of the variance, but some remains unaccounted for even when all of them are considered. If there is a strong relationship—such that, say, protein X is always low when brain volume loss is high and *vice versa*—then protein X may be worth exploring further. Unfortunately, proteins Y and Z may show the same relationship, necessitating more complex statistics—and it is an informal rule in brain research that the more complicated the statistics required to show a result, the less trustworthy that result.

93 This is not strictly accurate; senile plaques had been observed by earlier researchers. Alzheimer's work, however, was foundational in defining the disease.

94 Cell loss is variable between patients and between brain regions. For example, among cholinergic neurons in the nucleus basalis of Meynert 'the number of large neurons decreases while that of small neurons increases', according to Swaab, D. F. and A. M. Bao (2011), '(Re)activation of neurons in aging and dementia: lessons from the hypothalamus', *Experimental Gerontology*, 46, 178–84.

95 SFE Ellison, D. *et al.* (2012), *Neuropathology: A Reference Text of CNS Pathology* (London: Elsevier Health Sciences UK). This textbook has useful pictures of tau and amyloid pathologies, and much else of interest. I recall an image of atherosclerosis that would have put me right off a junk food diet if other deterrents hadn't already done so. My thanks to John Stein for recommending the book.

96 According to a 2016 review, 'aggregation of tau into paired helical filaments (PHFs; initially observed by Kidd) and neurofibrillary tangles (NFTs) characterizes a wide range of neurodegenerative diseases known as tauopathies, including Alzheimer disease (AD; initially described by Alzheimer), progressive supranuclear palsy (PSP), corticobasal degeneration (CBD), agyrophilic grain disease (AGD), Pick disease (PiD), Huntington disease (HD) and frontotemporal dementia with parkinsonism-17 (FTDP-17)' (Wang, Y. and Mandelkow, E. (2016), 'Tau in physiology and pathology', *Nature Reviews Neuroscience*, 17, 22–35). The early papers referred to are Alzheimer, A. (1907), 'Über eine eigenartige Erkrankung der Hirnrinde', *Allgemeine Zeitschrift für Psychiatrie und Psychisch-gerichtliche Medizin*, 64, 146–8; Kidd, M. (1963), 'Paired helical filaments in electron microscopy of Alzheimer's disease', *Nature*, 197, 192–3.

97 I simplify. There are various stages of plaque development and the dense amyloid core is only present in some of them.

Chapter 6

1 Glenner, G. G. and C. W. Wong (1984), 'Alzheimer's disease: initial report of the purification and characterization of a novel cerebrovascular amyloid protein', *Biochemical and Biophysical Research Communications*, 120, 885–90.

2 An analysis of amyloid plaques found them to be relatively rich in twenty-six proteins (Liao, L. *et al.* (2004), 'Proteomic characterization of postmortem amyloid plaques isolated by laser capture microdissection', *Journal of Biological Chemistry*, 279, 37061–8). As well as Aβ, they include molecules involved in cell adhesion (collagen, fibrinogen), a chaperone (heat shock) protein, a calcium channel ATPase, cytoskeletal proteins including tau, the enzyme phosphofructokinase, which has an important role in glucose

metabolism, inflammation-related molecules (glial fibrillary acidic protein (GFAP) and vimentin), proteins involved in membrane trafficking (clathrin, dynamin, dynein), regulatory proteins (kinases, phosphatases), and proteins with roles in waste disposal (antitrypsin, lysosomal ATPases, cathepsin D, cystatin B and C, ubiquitin-activating enzyme E1).

3 PET (positron emission tomography) imaging detects radioactive emissions from marker compounds injected into the body. It requires radioactive labelling of a compound with the desired biological function—i.e. one that marks the process of interest. Developing compounds to bind amyloid is technically challenging, but one such compound is carbon 11–labelled Pittsburgh Compound B (^{11}C-PiB). This is a compound derived from thioflavin T—long used to stain amyloid plaques post-mortem—which has been made with a radioactive form of carbon, ^{11}C.

4 An example is the protein amylin, which is released by pancreatic cells. In type two diabetes it can form damaging amyloid deposits in the pancreas and elsewhere—perhaps including the brain.

5 See Glenner's obituary in the New York Times, 14 July 1995. For more about the clinical symptoms of amyloidosis, see its NHS webpage (<http://www.nhs.uk/Conditions/ amyloidosis/Pages/Introduction.aspx>).

6 Kyle, R. A. (2001), 'Amyloidosis: a convoluted story', British Journal of Haematology, 114, 529–38.

7 Glenner, G. G. and C. W. Wong (1984), 'Alzheimer's disease and Down's syndrome: sharing of a unique cerebrovascular amyloid fibril protein', Biochemical and Biophysical Research Communications, 122, 1131–5.

8 SFE Prasher, V. P. et al. (1998), 'Molecular mapping of Alzheimer-type dementia in Down's syndrome', Annals of Neurology, 43, 380–3. The study reports a rare case of Down's in which the extra copy of chromosome 21 was only partial and did not include the region encoding the APP gene. The patient lived into her seventies and did not develop dementia.

9 Amyloid plaques are sometimes called 'senile' or 'neuritic' plaques. Technically a neuritic plaque is one that contains identifiable bits of damaged neuronal processes (neurites), plus evidence of disrupted tau processing. Not all amyloid deposits have such evidence of neuron damage. Neuritic plaques correlate better with cell loss than either amyloid plaques or tau tangles.

10 Data are from Braak and Braak (1997) (note 5.73). Amyloid was found in around 10% of individuals aged sixty or under and around 5% of those aged fifty or under.

11 The study analysed thirty-five pollution-exposed frontal cortices, of which half showed diffuse Aβ plaques, and eight controls, none of which had plaques (Calderón-Garcidueñas, L. et al. (2012), 'White matter hyperintensities, systemic inflammation, brain growth, and cognitive functions in children exposed to air pollution', Journal of Alzheimer's Disease, 31, 183–91). The finding should be regarded as provisional until repeatedly replicated, bearing in mind that it is much easier to get hold of elderly brains than young ones.

12 Hardy, J. A. and G. A. Higgins (1992), 'Alzheimer's disease: the amyloid cascade hypothesis', Science, 256, 184–5.

13 Goldgaber, D. et al. (1987), 'Characterization and chromosomal localization of a cDNA encoding brain amyloid of Alzheimer's disease', Science, 235, 877–80; Tanzi, R. E. et al.

(1987), 'Amyloid beta protein gene: cDNA, mRNA distribution, and genetic linkage near the Alzheimer locus', *Science*, 235, 880–4.

14 Studies in mice confirm the importance of APP. There are three known members of the APP family: APP itself, and APP-like proteins 1 and 2. The latter two seem to be less relevant for Alzheimer's, but it also seems that they can substitute to some extent for an artificially absent APP gene (as in APP knockout mice). Thus APP-lacking mice survive with minor problems—they are a bit smaller and weaker—but about 80% of those missing both APP and APLP-2 die soon after birth (von Koch, C. S. *et al.* (1997), 'Generation of APLP2 KO mice and early postnatal lethality in APLP2/APP double KO mice', *Neurobiology of Aging*, 18, 661–9).

15 These processes include phosphorylation, which adds a phosphate group, acetylation, which adds an acetyl group ($-COCH_3$), and glycosylation, which adds glycans (sugar molecules made from carbohydrates). These chemical transactions are an essential part of cells' internal control and communication, and are widely used. For example, acetylation is key to gene control, while phosphorylation of the insulin receptor inactivates it and can be used as a marker of insulin resistance (see Chapter 14 for more details).

16 Recent research suggest that changes in cell lipids, as well as proteins, can trigger the endoplasmic reticulum's stress responses. ER stress can also stimulate NFκB, linking cellular protein problems to inflammation.

17 Tau has also been linked to effects on chromatin (Frost, B. *et al.* (2014), 'Tau promotes neurodegeneration through global chromatin relaxation', *Nature Neuroscience*, 17, 357–66) and to impaired dendrite function before synapses are lost (Hoover, B. *et al.* (2010), 'Tau mislocalization to dendritic spines mediates synaptic dysfunction independently of neurodegeneration', *Neuron*, 68, 1067–81).

18 Tau is important for holding microtubules in place, and it seems that the part of tau that binds to the microtubules is also essential for its abnormal aggregation (Kadavath, H. *et al.* (2015), 'Tau stabilizes microtubules by binding at the interface between tubulin heterodimers', *Proceedings of the National Academy of Sciences*, 112, 7501–6).

19 SFE Selkoe (2002) (note 5.85). One way in which tau tangles have been proposed to do their damage is by blocking the passage of mitochondria along axons, thereby starving the latter of energy. Tau also seems to be necessary for amyloid to exert its damaging effects, since reducing tau levels in mice engineered to have high levels of Aβ prevents the usual behaviour deficits (e.g. in water maze learning; for details see Roberson, E. *et al.* (2007), 'Reducing endogenous tau ameliorates amyloid beta-induced deficits in an Alzheimer's disease mouse model', *Science*, 316, 750–4). Interestingly, Aβ levels were still high; and tau reduction in non-transgenic animals was protective against glutamate excitotoxicity.

20 Since 1988, Barbara Pearse has been one of a very rare kind: a lady Fellow of the Royal Society. A gene associated with clathrin processing, PICALM (phosphatidylinositol binding clathrin assembly protein), is one of the better-validated risk genes for Alzheimer's. For more about PICALM, search online for its page on NCBI *Gene*.

21 BDNF, which ever since I wrote *Cruelty* has unfortunately reminded me of BDSM, regulates synapse growth and plasticity, and is also implicated in schizophrenia and bipolar disorder (Gatt, J. M. *et al.* (2015), 'Specific and common genes implicated across

major mental disorders: a review of meta-analysis studies', *Journal of Psychiatric Research*, 60, 1–13). For more about the roles of BDNF and NGF in neurodegeneration, see Allen, S. J. *et al.* (2013), 'GDNF, NGF and BDNF as therapeutic options for neurodegeneration', *Pharmacology and Therapeutics*, 138, 155–75. GDNF is glial-derived neurotrophic factor, another neurotrophin.

22 A study in animals found that altering certain histone-related genes could boost BDNF production and synaptic plasticity (Zeng, Y. *et al.* (2011), 'Epigenetic enhancement of BDNF signaling rescues synaptic plasticity in aging', *Journal of Neuroscience*, 31, 17800–10).

23 APP can also bind to collagen and to the anticoagulant heparin, which is thought to inhibit the toxic effects of Aβ. Heparin is best known as an anticoagulant, but it also forms part of the extracellular matrix, and thus plays important roles in the interactions of many brain proteins. Heparan sulphate inhibits cleavage of APP by β- but not α-secretase, and heparin treatment has been proposed for dementia (Scholefield, Z. *et al.* (2003), 'Heparan sulfate regulates amyloid precursor protein processing by BACE1, the Alzheimer's β-secretase', *Journal of Cell Biology*, 163, 97–107).

24 I simplify, as there is more than one length of Aβ protein. The two most important species identified to date are both made intracellularly, and differ by very little, structurally: one has forty amino acids, the other forty-two. $A\beta_{42}$ is made in the endoplasmic reticulum, while $A\beta_{40}$ is made in the Golgi apparatus.

25 The so-called 'non-amyloidogenic' pathway can still produce shortened versions of the Aβ protein, again released by γ-secretase. Their function is unclear, but they may be able to form amyloid.

26 I simplify: β-secretase has two very similar forms, commonly known as BACE1 and BACE2 (beta-site amyloid precursor protein cleaving enzymes 1 and 2). The former cleaves APP as described; the latter is a potent destroyer of Aβ proteins.

27 For aggregates of the same kind of molecule researchers use Greek prefixes: 'mono' for one, 'oligo' for a few, and 'poly' for a lot. (Polysaccharides contain more sugar molecules than do oligosaccharides or monosaccharides.) Proteins often form aggregates with one of two characteristic patterns: a long, twisted strand (the alpha-helix) or a flat, spreading structure (the beta-sheet). Amyloid fibrils, cross-linked by hydrogen bonds, form beta-sheets; hence the name amyloid-beta. For more details of the physics see <http://www.proteinstructures.com/Structure/Structure/secondary-sructure.html>.

28 I simplify: two presenilins, PSEN1 and PSEN2, are involved, and in both rare mutations have been linked to familial Alzheimer's.

29 This assumption has been challenged, as will be made clear later in the book.

30 Jonsson, T. *et al.* (2012), 'A mutation in APP protects against Alzheimer's disease and age-related cognitive decline', *Nature*, 488, 96–9.

31 Drugs could also target β-secretase, but that enzyme 'is critical in myelin formation, so some possibility of central nervous system toxicity is present' (Gandy 2014) (note 3.22). If an enzyme does more than one thing, however, it may still be possible to block only one of its effects—*if* it does its different things in different places. For a recent use of this logic—targeting only β-secretase's APP-cleaving activity by restricting the arena to endosomes—see Ben Halima, S. *et al.* (2016), 'Specific inhibition of β-secretase processing of the Alzheimer disease amyloid precursor protein', *Cell Reports*, 14, 2127–41.

32 Tests for amyloid protein found a drop in blood, but not in CSF levels (Doody, R. S. *et al.* (2013), 'A Phase 3 trial of semagacestat for treatment of Alzheimer's disease', *New England Journal of Medicine*, 369, 341–50).

33 One other protein cleaved by γ-secretase is Notch, whose signalling pathways are involved in angiogenesis (blood vessel growth) as well as in 'embryonic development, hematopoiesis, cell adhesion, and other cell–cell contacts' (Doody *et al.* 2013) (note 32). Haematopoiesis is the creation of blood cells.

34 SFE Nordberg, A. (2004), 'PET imaging of amyloid in Alzheimer's disease', *Lancet Neurology*, 3, 519–27.

35 The search was done on *Web of Science* on 6 May 2015, selecting for English-language articles and reviews.

36 Monomers have also been found to act as transcription factors—proteins that directly regulate gene expression by binding to DNA.

37 Aβ oligomers have not yet definitively been shown to damage living human brains, but in primates, where it is ethically acceptable (to scientists at least) to administer Aβ oligomers and observe the results, damage has been shown. 'Cardinal features of AD pathology, including synapse loss, tau hyperphosphorylation, astrocyte and microglial activation, were observed in regions of the macaque brain where Aβ oligomers were abundantly detected. Most importantly, oligomer injections induced AD-type neurofibrillary tangle formation in the macaque brain' (Forny-Germano, L. *et al.* (2014), 'Alzheimer's disease-like pathology induced by amyloid-β oligomers in nonhuman primates', *Journal of Neuroscience*, 34, 13629–43).

38 A study of the mechanics finds that the forces generated by amyloid aggregation are 'comparable to that observed for actin and tubulin, systems that have evolved to generate force during their native functions'. Actin helps muscles work, and both actin and tubulin are crucial for the cytoskeleton and intracellular transport. See Herling, T. W. *et al.* (2015), 'Force generation by the growth of amyloid aggregates', *Proceedings of the National Academy of Sciences*, 112, 9524–9.

39 In humans, APP exists in three varieties, or isoforms, created at the RNA stage by alternative splicing. Post-translational modifications also occur, providing cells with even more variations on the APP theme. The isoforms—APP_{695}, APP_{751}, and APP_{770}—are found throughout the body. The amounts of each isoform differ by location. In healthy neurons, APP_{695} is the dominant variety. However, some researchers have found that levels of the longer isoforms are increased in the brains of Alzheimer patients. Among other differences, this may make APP and its protein products more resistant to cellular recycling. Longer APP isoforms contain a section that acts to inhibit proteases, the enzymes which break up proteins for recycling. Levels of this inhibitor seem to rise in Alzheimer's—as if slowing down protein recycling is part of the disease. Or perhaps keeping APP around for longer is part of the brain's attempt to resolve its problems. In technical language, the APP gene contains a Kunitz protease inhibitor (KPI) domain, and isoforms of APP mRNA/protein containing the KPI—APP_{770} and APP_{751}—seem to be over-produced in Alzheimer's relative to healthy brains. The shorter APP_{695}, characteristic of normal neurons, lacks the KPI.

Chapter 7

1 Atoms have no overall electrical charge because they have the same number of protons (+) as electrons (-). However, each atomic electron shell can accommodate a specific number of electrons, and the outermost shell is generally not full; if it is, the atom is chemically inert. Atoms tend to seek out arrangements with each other—to form molecules—whereby the gaps can be filled, or else their outermost electrons given away; a quiet life, for an atom, is one with either no shells or full shells. For example, a hydrogen atom, H, readily donates its one electron to become a hydrogen ion, H^+, a single proton.

2 As an example, both kinds of chemical bond can be formed from that deceptively simple everyday molecule, water. H_2O tends to split into hydroxide ions, $-OH^-$, and protons, H^+. (Water's supply of free-floating protons affects the behaviour of many cellular proteins and is also essential for powering cells.) As well as hydroxide ions, however, oxygen bonded to a single hydrogen can also be found in the covalent form of a hydroxyl group, $-OH$. More details are available at Colorado State University's website, <http://www.vivo .colostate.edu/hbooks/pathphys/misc_topics/radicals.html>.

3 Carbon (C) can form up to four single chemical bonds, and frequently forms hydrocarbon chains: strings of linked carbon atoms bonded to each other by single (C–C) or double (C=C) bonds. The 'spare' carbon bonds are with hydrogen. Hydrocarbon bonds are especially tough, which is why hydrocarbons like petrol and many fats don't dissolve in water.

4 When a particular molecule's presence as part of a larger compound determines how that compound behaves—its characteristic function—the molecule is called a functional group. Hydroxyl groups are one of the most common types.

5 Saturated fats also tend to keep better, because unsaturated fats, with more double bonds, are more likely to react with other molecules and go rancid.

6 EPA: eicosapentaenoic acid; DHA: docosahexaenoic acid.

7 Clapham (2007) (note 5.28). The heading, 'Protein function...', is a quotation from this work.

8 SFE a study modelling the molecular dynamics for beta-amyloid which finds that electrostatic interactions between nearby charges affect the functional properties of various parts of the molecules (Yun, S. et al. (2007), 'Role of electrostatic interactions in amyloid β-protein (Aβ) oligomer formation: a discrete molecular dynamics study', *Biophysical Journal*, 92, 4064–77).

9 The bases are adenosine (A), thymine (T), guanine (G), and cytosine (C); and for RNA, uracil (U).

10 The twenty standard amino acids required by the human body (which can be converted into many others) are: alanine, arginine, asparagine, aspartic acid, cysteine, glutamic acid, glutamine, glycine, histidine, isoleucine, leucine, lysine, methionine, phenylalanine, proline, serine, threonine, tryptophan, tyrosine, and valine. All amino acids contain an amino group ($-NH_2$). In body fluids this tends to bind to a passing proton (H^+) and become positively charged.

11 I discuss epigenetics in more detail in Taylor 2014 (note 1.3).

12 To make a histone more negative, specialized enzymes bolt on certain functional groups, such as acetyl groups. This pushes the histone away from the DNA, prising open the

chromatin and rendering the DNA more accessible by other enzymes. Acetylation, which is done by enzymes called histone acetyl transferases, attaches an acetyl group ($-COCH_3$) to a positively charged amino acid (lysine) in the histone, and in doing so changes it to an electrically neutral molecule, thereby making the histone overall less positive (i.e. more negative). An acetylated histone is more likely to repel nearby DNA, which loosens the chromatin coils and makes the DNA more accessible to other enzymes, including those responsible for transcribing DNA into RNA. Thus acetylation tends to increase gene expression. It can be reversed by sets of enzymes known as histone deacetylases (HDACs); and other enzymes can attach a methyl group ($-CH_3$) to one of the DNA bases, cytosine. Methylation tends to silence a gene. Modifications like phosphorylation (attaching a phosphate group), which is done by enzymes called kinases, can likewise alter gene expression.

13 One way in which histones may influence brain health is by regulating the production of neurotrophins such as BDNF. One of the enzymes regulating histone acetylation, HDAC2, also modulates production of this neurotrophin (Zeng *et al.* 2011) (note 6.22).

14 These receptors include the liver X receptors, which detect oxysterols (metabolites of cholesterol), vitamin D receptors, retinoic acid and retinoid X receptors, which detect metabolites of vitamin A, and PPAR-γ, which among other things binds to unsaturated fatty acids like arachidonic acid and also regulates glucose metabolism. PPAR-γ is the target of a major class of drugs (e.g. Avandia) for type two diabetes. 'PPAR' stands for 'peroxisome proliferator-activated receptor'.

15 Pahl, H. L. (1999). 'Activators and target genes of Rel/NF-kappaB transcription factors', *Oncogene*, 18, 6853–66.

16 NFκB is not the only link between stress and inflammation. For example, the danger-associated molecular pattern HMGB1 (short for high mobility group box-1), which can stimulate inflammatory responses, appears to be inducible by glucocorticoids.

17 Histone acetylation is boosted by neural activity. The proteins are from the Tet family, one of which I discuss in more detail in Taylor (2014) (note 1.3). They oxidize one of the methylated DNA bases, cytosine, and this triggers DNA repair mechanisms which demethylate the DNA, altering expression of the GluR1 glutamate receptor. Similar mechanisms may regulate other neurotransmitter systems. Interestingly, one of the Tet proteins has recently been found to be an important contributor to the processes that resolve inflammation—and it does so by way of histone deacetylation (Zhang, Q. *et al.* (2015), 'Tet2 is required to resolve inflammation by recruiting Hdac2 to specifically repress IL-6', *Nature*, 525, 389–93).

18 I describe the remarkable methods of optogenetics and genetic modification in Taylor (2014) (note 1.3).

19 Matsui, T. *et al.* (2007), 'Expression of APP pathway mRNAs and proteins in Alzheimer's disease', *Brain Research*, 1161, 116–23.

20 Mawuenyega, K. G. *et al.* (2010), 'Decreased clearance of CNS β-amyloid in Alzheimer's disease', *Science*, 330, 1774.

Chapter 8

1 The pH scale measures how acid—pH lower than 7—or alkaline—pH higher than 7—a liquid is. The pH of a watery solution, such as blood or brain fluids, reflects the number of positive electrical charges (free hydrogen ions, H^+, *aka* protons) available for transfer between atoms. Some compounds, when added to water, hoover up passing protons, leaving a surfeit of negative charges; these are alkalis, also called bases. Other compounds have protons that can float free in water, boosting the level of H^+; these are acids. The pH scale is inverse, so solutions with high levels of H^+—i.e. acidic—have a pH below 7.0; alkalis have a pH above 7.0. Bleach (pH 13) and baking soda (pH 9) are alkalis, while lemon juice (pH 2) and stomach acid (pH 1) are acids. See *ChemWiki*'s treatment of the topic, available from <http://chemwiki.ucdavis.edu/Core/Physical_Chemistry/Acids_and_Bases/Acid>.

2 The phrase is immunologist Richard Ransohoff's (Ransohoff, R. M. (2014), 'Good barriers make good neighbors', *Science*, 346, 36–7).

3 'A typical human cell might be one-tenth of the diameter of your hair (10 microns)', according to <http://science.howstuffworks.com/life/cellular-microscopic/cell1.htm>. The words 'endothelium' and 'endothelial', which refer to cells lining certain body cavities including blood vessels, are derived from the Greek words for 'within' and 'nipple', presumably because that was the first cavity where they were identified.

4 For this description of the blood–brain barrier I have leaned heavily on a review by William Pardridge (Pardridge, W. M. (2005), 'The blood–brain barrier: bottleneck in brain drug development', *NeuroRx*, 2, 3–14). Note that he does not give a source for many of his figures. They are widely cited in the literature, but tracing them back to their origin, or obtaining independent corroboration, is not easy. They should therefore be consumed with caution.

5 Pardridge (2005) (note 4).

6 Skin measures a little under 2 square metres in adult humans—a sizeable if irregularly shaped rug—according to <http://hypertextbook.com/facts/2001/IgorFridman.shtml>.

7 Assuming an average total brain volume for female adults of 1250 ml, the percentage would be 0.4%.

8 Human red blood cells also average about 8 µm across, so it is as well that they are shape changers, able to squeeze through tiny blood vessels.

9 Radiolabelling builds a normally non-radioactive compound using a radioactive form of certain elements, such as hydrogen or carbon, so that the compound can be tracked inside an organism. For example, my chapter on positron emission tomography (PET) in Taylor (2014) (note 1.3) describes how radiolabelling is used in brain scanning.

10 Ehrlich used dyes rather than radiolabelling because for the latter he'd have needed time-travel. In 1885, when his work was published—around the time when Alzheimer started his doctorate—there was still another decade to go before Röntgen, Becquerel, and the Curies opened up the science of radioactivity. Wilhelm Röntgen, discoverer of X-rays, won the first Nobel Physics Prize in 1901. Henri Becquerel found that uranium salts are spontaneously radioactive. Pierre and Marie Curie shared the 1903 Nobel Prize

for Physics with Becquerel for their work on radioactivity. Radiolabelling only came into use after World War II.

11 Large-molecule drugs are often produced in living systems like genetically modified yeast or algae.

12 Pardridge (2005) (note 4). The italics are my addition.

13 Levels of amyloid-beta were reduced in the study (Leinenga, G. and J. Götz (2015), 'Scanning ultrasound removes amyloid-β and restores memory in an Alzheimer's disease mouse model', *Science Translational Medicine*, 7, 278ra233).

14 Endothelial cells are not entirely forbidding, thanks to a structure called the glycocalyx. This is a sugar-and-protein mesh on their inner surface, between them and the blood rushing through the vessel's inner space, or lumen. The glycocalyx is similar to the extracellular matrix and is made up of cross-linked molecules of various kinds: proteoglycans, glycoproteins, and glycosaminoglycans (for definitions see note 9.16). These molecules don't just help to structure the space between cells. They assist cells in forming physical connections, and also hold molecules such as the neurotrophin BDNF on the cell surface until they are released by enzymes, e.g. in response to inflammation. The glycocalyx is constantly changing as molecules dissolve in and out of it, but is more solid closer to the vessel wall. Like a climbing net spread across a smooth cliff face, it allows molecules and cells to get a better grip on endothelial cells—the first step to passing through them. Many contenders get no further.

15 Pathogens such as *Streptococcus pneumoniae*, which causes meningitis, can penetrate the blood–brain barrier by binding to receptors on endothelial cells; these receptors are then endocytosed. Candidate receptors include PAFR, the receptor for platelet-activating factor; however, a 2013 review finds uncertainty over whether the interaction is direct or whether *S. pneumoniae* is activating inflammatory pathways involving PAF, which then activates its receptor (Iovino, F. *et al.* (2013), 'Signalling or binding: the role of the platelet-activating factor receptor in invasive pneumococcal disease', *Cellular Microbiology*, 15, 870–81). Clarification is essential if effective treatments are to be developed, and for understanding why *Strep*, which normally lives in us without doing great harm, can occasionally turn so nasty.

16 Restrictions on lipid-soluble trans-blood–brain barrier transport include molecules with rotatable bonds, a large polar surface, or a predilection for forming hydrogen bonds.

17 For example, Aβ has been shown to depress occludin levels.

18 In children with Down's syndrome—from toddlers to teenagers—both blood and brain Aβ levels are higher than in healthy controls; and this is seen before amyloid plaques are observed in their brains, which is consistent with blood being a source of Aβ (Mehta, P. D., *et al.* (2007), 'Increased amyloid beta protein levels in children and adolescents with Down syndrome', *Journal of the Neurological Sciences*, 254, 22–7).

19 RAGE abbreviates 'receptor for advanced glycation end products'. The latter are sugar-protein compounds produced by high-temperature cooking. Among its other effects, RAGE alters the function of MAPKs (mitogen-associated protein kinases), which have fingers in too many cellular pies to list here.

20 Proteins expressed by activated platelets include fibrinogen, which binds cells together in sealing clots, and specialized 'cell adhesion' molecules which act like grappling hooks,

allowing the platelets to latch on to damaged tissue instead of getting swept away by the bloodstream. For more details see the European Bioinformatics Institute description at <http://www.ebi.ac.uk/interpro/potm/2006_11/Page2.htm>.

21 The omega-6 fatty acid arachidonic acid, found in red meat and grain products (e.g. hamburgers), is able to activate platelets, one of numerous pro-inflammatory pathways in which AA is thought to be involved.

Chapter 9

1 Takeda, S. *et al.* (2013), 'Brain interstitial oligomeric amyloid beta increases with age and is resistant to clearance from brain in a mouse model of Alzheimer's disease', *FASEB Journal*, 27, 3239–48. Aβ oligomers were also found in control 'wild-type' mice, but did not increase with age.

2 Mawuenyega *et al.* (2010) (note 7.20).

3 Taylor, K. (2006), *Brainwashing: The Science of Thought Control* (Oxford: Oxford University Press).

4 Magistretti , P. J. *et al.* (2000), 'Brain energy metabolism: an integrated cellular perspective', in *Psychopharmacology: The Fourth Generation of Progress*, eds F. E. Bloom and D. J. Kupfer (Brentwood, TN: American College of Neuropsychopharmacology).

5 Hypoglycaemia is acutely damaging. 'If blood glucose falls below 2 mmol/l for as little as 5 minutes, it can cause lethal brain damage', according to Cantley, J. and F. M. Ashcroft (2015), 'Q&A: insulin secretion and type 2 diabetes: why do β-cells fail?', *BMC Biology*, 13, 33. The authors suggest that this is why there are multiple hormones which raise blood sugar (e.g. glucagon, glucagon-like peptide 1, growth hormone, etc.) and only one hormone that lowers it (insulin).

6 Reduced glucose supply would be expected to affect cellular energy production. It could also have other effects, since glucose levels regulate functionally important post-translational modifications of many cellular proteins, including some implicated in Alzheimer's.

7 'Patients with Alzheimer's disease (AD) show prominent reduction in ^{18}F-FDG uptake [a marker of glucose uptake] in the precuneus/posterior cingulate (PP), parietotemporal, and frontal regions' (Ishibashi, K. *et al.* (2015), 'Reduced uptake of ^{18}F-FDG and ^{15}O-H$_2$O in Alzheimer's disease-related regions after glucose loading', *Journal of Cerebral Blood Flow and Metabolism*, 35, 1380–5).

8 Correia, S. C. *et al.* (2011), 'Insulin-resistant brain state: the culprit in sporadic Alzheimer's disease?', *Ageing Research Reviews*, 10, 264–73.

9 Ishibashi *et al.* (2015) (note 7).

10 A common form of arteriosclerosis involves the build-up of plaques containing calcium and cholesterol on blood vessel walls: atherosclerosis. The 'athero' derives from the prolific Greek doctor Galen, whose 'atheroma' (ἀθήρωμα) is translated—by the great Greek dictionarians Liddell and Scott—as 'tumour full of gruel-like matter'. Gruel-like plaques in the carotid arteries, which feed the brain, have been found to be risk factors for vascular dementia, independent of other known risk factors like stroke.

11 The superficial veins contain blood from the cortex and nearby white matter; other structures are drained by the deep venous system. Unlike veins in other parts of the body, brain veins lack the valves that prevent blood from reversing flow; they also dilate less.

12 The external jugulars deal more with blood from the face. For images of the brain's venous system, see Salamon's Neuroanatomy and Neurovasculature Web-Atlas Resource, available at <http://www.radnet.ucla.edu/sections/DINR/Part 16/Part16A1.htm>.

13 IMCOTT (it's more complicated than that): CSF may be produced by brain tissue—such as the ependymal cells that line the ventricles—as well as by the choroid plexus. The blood–brain barrier may also actively produce interstitial fluid; but both suggestions remain to be confirmed.

14 The term 'sloshing' covers patterns of flow which are complex and not yet fully understood, but which include a bulk flow through the ventricles, a pulsing, 'to-and-fro' flow throughout the brain, and many small-scale, local flows across the borders between blood, CSF, and interstitial fluid. In humans, the flow appears to be propelled mostly by the rhythm of our breathing, though heartbeats also affect it a little.

15 See the press release by the Spine Health Institute, available from <http://www .thespinehealthinstitute.com/news-room/health-blog/george-clooney-back-on-track>.

16 A note on terminology. Components of the extracellular matrix include proteoglycans, glycoproteins, and glycosaminoglycans. Glycans are polysaccharides: strings of sugar molecules. Glycosaminoglycans (GAGs) such as heparin and chondroitin sulphate are a subset of glycans: long, unbranched sugars often containing nitrogen and sulphur. GAGs are sometimes called mucopolysaccharides because they are found in mucus; being highly charged, they form sticky substances in water. They are also important molecules in the nervous system, e.g. because of their roles in the extracellular matrix and the formation of neural connections. GAGs are found in the amyloid plaques characteristic of Alzheimer's disease and may be important contributors to plaque formation and stability. Proteoglycans are proteins to which at least one GAG is attached. They are also thought to be central to the formation of atherosclerosis, as they can bind low-density lipoprotein. Glycoproteins are also protein/sugar mixes; they have glycan chains with side chains of polypeptides (small proteins).

17 For example, a study of 1,818 participants selected to exclude dementia found status cribrosum (= 'état criblé') in 1.3% (Zhu, Y. C. et al. (2011), 'Frequency and location of dilated Virchow-Robin spaces in elderly people: a population-based 3D MR imaging study', American Journal of Neuroradiology, 32, 709–13).

18 Durand-Fardel's 'Traduction libre' of Dante's great work is still available, libre, from <http://www.archive.org>.

19 The amount of fluid in the body is of vital importance. Blood loss can kill, and the effects of the acute stress response include attempts to minimise blood loss. Fluid balance in the body is maintained by the renin-angiotensin system, problems with which have been linked to Alzheimer's. Angiotensinogen made in the liver is converted by the kidney enzyme renin into inactive angiotensin I; this in turn is converted to active angiotensin II by the enzyme angiotensin-converting enzyme (ACE), which is found in kidney and lung tissue. Angiotensin regulates not just water content and blood pressure, but the amount of salts such as sodium in the water. (Too high

a sodium content—hypernatremia—is rare and can be lethal.) Under stress, sympathetic nervous system activation triggers the production of angiotensin II—which is a potent constrictor of blood vessels—and of other molecules such as aldosterone and noradrenaline.

20 The idea of interstitial spaces becoming blocked should not be confused with the far more controversial hypothesis of chronic cerebrospinal venous insufficiency, which proposes that reduced flow in the major cerebral veins is a cause of multiple sclerosis; for a vigorous refutation see Valdueza, J. M. et al. (2013), 'What went wrong? The flawed concept of cerebrospinal venous insufficiency', Journal of Cerebral Blood Flow and Metabolism, 33, 657–68.

21 Louveau, A. et al. (2015). 'Structural and functional features of central nervous system lymphatic vessels', Nature, 523, 337–41. The publication attracted criticism for not citing previous findings, and a corrigendum was published online.

22 Note that glymphatics postulates a flow of CSF into the brain along arteries, whereas other research suggests an outward flow along these vessels.

23 The perivascular space also contains pericytes and smooth muscle cells, which help to control blood flow by wrapping around blood vessels and actively relaxing or tautening. They can thus regulate the delivery of blood to the brain in response to neural activity—varying supply in response to demand. (I simplify: capillaries, the smallest blood vessels, are wrapped in pericytes, which may not be contractile. Larger arterioles and arteries are surrounded by the tunica media, a wall of smooth muscle cells, which can contract and thereby regulate blood flow.) Like microglia, pericytes are thought to help defend the brain against immune attack, and the brain's blood vessels also have their own resident perivascular macrophages, as do the meninges. Pericytes can regulate vascular permeability—how easy blood vessels are to penetrate—by changing the production of proteins involved in tight junctions. And although they can last a lifetime, their numbers shrink as people age, as does the production of major tight junction proteins like occludin. In addition, pericytes share with people the phenomenon of rigor mortis after death. When a harmful event like an ischaemic stroke kills cells, dead pericytes may contract around their blood vessels, reducing the blood supply still further and worsening the damage.

24 This pathway along the sides of blood vessels, by which CSF can circulate through the brain, also involves glial cells called astrocytes. Their position between the arterial and venous systems, and their ability to transport water actively via special channels called aquaporins, is thought to allow them to couple the inflow and outflow.

25 I am simplifying by referring to astrocytes as if they are all the same; they are not. Most, for example, express a protein called GFAP (glial fibrillary acidic protein), but not all. SFE <http://www.networkglia.eu/en/astrocytes> for more details on astrocyte subtypes, from Bergmann cells (in the cerebellum) to radial glia (which help neurons find their way during brain development). The same website also offers useful introductory guides to microglia and oligodendrocytes.

26 Pakkenberg et al. (2003) (note 5.18).

27 Jensen, C. J. et al. (2013), 'Immune players in the CNS: the astrocyte', Journal of Neuroimmune Pharmacology, 8, 824–39.

28 Astrocytes make and release lactate (the chemical commonly associated with muscle cramps during exercise, though cramps' exact causes remain unclear). Lactate stimulates neurons to produce more proteins associated with synaptic plasticity, i.e. with the mechanics of memory.

29 Song, Y. *et al.* (2013), 'Evolutionary etiology of high-grade astrocytomas', *Proceedings of the National Academy of Sciences*, 110, 17933–8.

30 The perivascular spaces are too small for APCs to squeeze through, suggesting that these immune sentinels have a lesser role in monitoring grey matter compared with white. Interestingly, the brain's native population of immune cells, microglia, tend to be more prevalent in white matter—in humans at least. This is one of numerous differences between human and mouse brains, a besetting problem in dementia and immunology research.

31 The study is preliminary in that it is in mice: Xie, L. *et al.* (2013), 'Sleep drives metabolite clearance from the adult brain', *Science*, 342, 373–7.

32 Lee, H. *et al.* (2015), 'The effect of body posture on brain glymphatic transport', *Journal of Neuroscience*, 35, 11034–44. The authors argue—again extrapolating from rodents—that the best position for effective flushing of brain waste is to sleep on your side.

33 Other substances can also cause harm. One example in the scientific literature is a thirty-six-year-old man who suffered repeated strokes. He appeared to have healthy blood vessels, but a brain biopsy revealed the build-up of collagen, the key component of connective tissue. Collagen is the body's most plentiful protein, but too much in the wrong place can still be a problem. See McKinney, J. S. *et al.* (2012), 'Noninflammatory cerebral vasculopathy associated with recurrent ischemic strokes', *Journal of Stroke and Cerebrovascular Diseases*, 21, 417–21.

34 Conventional methods of assessing brain blood flow include fMRI and cerebral angiography, which injects an X-ray-blocking substance and then X-rays the brain. The prefix 'angio' has to do with blood vessels, and its etymology is intriguing: it derives from the Greek word used by the Gospel writer Matthew (25:4)—in the parable of the wise and foolish virgins—for the containers in which the smart girls carried the oil for their lamps. (In the interests of damping down the mutual abuse between some areas of science and religion I like to cite the Bible now and then.)

35 Orexin, also called hypocretin, is released by a specific set of neurons in the hypothalamus. The cells 'are activated during waking, stress, exposure to novel environments, and undernutrition', say Grossberg, A. *et al.* (2011), 'Inflammation-induced lethargy is mediated by suppression of orexin neuron activity', *Journal of Neuroscience*, 31, 11376–86. They keep the brain wakeful, monitor the body's energy levels, and prompt food seeking when these drop. Grossberg *et al.* also note that orexin neurons 'are linked to other motivated behaviors as well, including drug-seeking and sexual behavior'. During infections, however, eating well is less important than fighting pathogens, so the activity of orexin neurons is suppressed. You're more likely to fall asleep when you're battling flu.

36 Liguori, C. *et al.* (2014), 'Orexinergic system dysregulation, sleep impairment, and cognitive decline in Alzheimer disease', *Journal of the American Medical Association Neurology*, 71, 1498–505.

37 The Aβ–ApoE complex binds with a cell surface lipoprotein receptor which takes it inside the cell. The brain has numerous kinds of lipoprotein receptors, expressed by neurons,

glia, and endothelial cells, with different preferences for Aβ and other molecules (e.g. they also bind APP). Aβ taken into endothelial cells can then be ejected into the bloodstream.

38 Receptors implicated in microglial processing of Aβ include complement receptors, TLRs, CD33, and RAGE. For example, CD33 activation is thought to inhibit microglia from taking up Aβ, whereas complement receptors seem to facilitate uptake.

39 The king is Erysichthon, and his story is told in Book VIII of Ovid's *Metamorphoses*. Ovid does not say at what point the auto-consumption process stopped.

40 Two cathepsins, B and D, may have important roles in Alzheimer's, but the story is not a simple one. Cathepsin B can act as a β-secretase to cleave APP, producing Aβ, and both CatB and CatD also seem able to degrade Aβ. A 2014 meta-analysis of cathepsin gene associations found no link with Alzheimer's (Mo, C. *et al.* (2014), 'Lack of association between cathepsin D C224T polymorphism and Alzheimer's disease risk: an update meta-analysis', *BMC Neurology*, 14, 13), though they have been linked to a raised risk of cancer as well as to atherosclerosis and osteoporosis. On the other hand, a mutation in the gene for the neuroprotective protein cystatin C, which inhibits cathepsins, has been linked to Alzheimer's in Caucasians. Cystatin levels seem to drop in the disease, and drug trials of cathepsin inhibitors have shown promise in animal models. For a condition like Alzheimer's, which takes decades to cast its shadow, having a deficit in a regulatory protein, rather than in the lysosomal system itself, makes sense. In a major cellular system, direct disruption of one enzyme would likely have more noticeable effects than 'second-level' disruption to one of that enzyme's regulators. Furthermore, one small failure could be worked around, but as failures accumulated the brain's resilience would gradually weaken. Except in rare cases, this is what the genetics of dementia suggests: many genes, each with a small effect.

41 The acidity of lysosomes is around pH 4.5–5.0 (Mindell, J.A. (2012), 'Lysosomal acidification mechanisms', *Annual Review of Physiology*, 74, 69–86).

42 There are also 'cold shock proteins'. Useful for hibernation, these encourage synapses that die off during the animal's torpor to reform when it resumes normal existence. Genetically tampering with one such protein worsens the effects of prion infection and amyloid in transgenic animals, whereas enhancing it is beneficial, so cold shock proteins are currently being investigated for their potential therapeutic value in dementia.

43 The quotation is from Snoeckx, L. H. *et al.* (2001). 'Heat shock proteins and cardiovascular pathophysiology', *Physiological Reviews*, 81, 1461–97.

44 One heat shock protein has been identified as being among relatively few proteins (twenty-six) which are selectively enhanced in amyloid plaques; see note 6.2.

45 Josephin is the cellular equivalent of a last-minute presidential pardon; it reverses ubiquitination and so spares proteins from being crunched up by the proteasome. I simplify: there is a family of Josephin proteins, and they form part of a bigger protein called ataxin. Furthermore, Josephin is one regulator among many: according to a recent review, 'nearly a hundred enzymes' have been found which take off ubiquitin chains. This is further testament to the critical role of UPS processes. See Eletr, Z. M. and K. D. Wilkinson (2014), 'Regulation of proteolysis by human deubiquitinating enzymes', *Biochimica et Biophysica Acta*, 1843, 114–28.

46 SFE Jones, L. *et al.* (2015), 'Convergent genetic and expression data implicate immunity in Alzheimer's disease', *Alzheimer's and Dementia*, 11, 658–71. This analysis of genetic data

looked for biochemical pathways associated with disease. Ubiquitination activity was one of four areas identified as relevant to Alzheimer's: the others were immune function, cholesterol transport (e.g. ApoE), and the regulation of endocytosis (by which cells take in molecules including spent surface receptors and APP).

Part 2

1 Taylor, J. (1649/1990), *Holy Living and Holy Dying. Selected* Works, ed. T. K. Carroll (New York: Paulist Press), Classics of Western Spirituality, 75, 428–71.

Chapter 10

1 See the Washington Post's WONKBLOG post by Christopher Ingraham, 12 November, 2014. The piece is an instance of the html address <http://www.washingtonpost.com/blogs/wonkblog/wp/2014/11/12/study-having-just-one-drink-doubles-your-risk-of-going-to-the-e-r/> being more accurate than the headline.

2 A 2014 analysis of media health reporting looked at exaggerated claims and found that many originated not with the media but with the press releases issued by institutions and journals, which often provide substantial content for media reports (Sumner, P. *et al.* (2014), 'The association between exaggeration in health related science news and academic press releases: retrospective observational study', *British Medical Journal*, 349, g7015). The authors blame the increased pressures in academia, which demand ever more self-promotion and competition—more, it seems, on ideological grounds than on the basis of evidence that this ferocious individualism is the best way to run a university. Pressures on the media—e.g. fewer specialist science journalists—may also play a part.

3 You are, after all, physiologically as well as socially unique. Science relates to masses. This is one reason why it struggles with issues like free will and consciousness, which are so utterly individual. It also makes accurately predicting one person's health an insuperable challenge in all but a very few cases.

4 For example, socioeconomic status (SES) is usually approximated by recording educational achievement. There is a strong correlation between them; children from rich families do better academically in many countries. But the relationship isn't perfect, or social mobility would be even lower than it is in the well-educated West. Some children who do well at school will have low adult SES, and some working-class children will drop out of school and go on to achieve enormous wealth.

5 Cataldo, J. K. *et al.* (2010), 'Cigarette smoking is a risk factor for Alzheimer's disease: an analysis controlling for tobacco industry affiliation', *Journal of Alzheimer's Disease*, 19, 465–80.

6 Chen, R. (2012). 'Association of environmental tobacco smoke with dementia and Alzheimer's disease among never smokers', *Alzheimer's and Dementia*, 8, 590–5.

7 Anstey, K. J. *et al.* (2007), 'Smoking as a risk factor for dementia and cognitive decline: a meta-analysis of prospective studies', *American Journal of Epidemiology*, 166, 367–78.

8 The critique is of nutrition research, but is relevant elsewhere. See Ioannidis, J. (2013), 'Implausible results in human nutrition research', *British Medical Journal*, 347, f6698.

9 Cherpitel, C. J. *et al.* (2014), 'Relative risk of injury from acute alcohol consumption: modeling the dose–response relationship in emergency department data from 18 countries', *Addiction*, 110, 279–88.

10 As well as odds ratios (ORs) there are three other widely used measures of risk: the relative risk, the hazard ratio, and the effect size (*d*). Relative risks and hazard ratios are not strictly comparable with ORs, but for relatively rare events such as getting Alzheimer's they can be treated as working the same way. Effect sizes are slightly different. One is familiar: *r*, the correlation coefficient (see note 5.88). The statistician Jacob Cohen, who did much to popularize effect sizes, thought that *r* = 0.5 signalled a large effect and *r* = 0.3 a medium one (Cohen, J. (1988), *Statistical Power Analysis for the Behavioral Sciences*, New York, NY, Routledge Academic; cited in Lakens, D. (2013), 'Calculating and reporting effect sizes to facilitate cumulative science: a practical primer for t-tests and ANOVAs', *Frontiers in Psychology*, 4, 863).

Cohen also gave his name to another measure of effect size, Cohen's *d*. This measures the difference *d* between the average values (means) of two groups, taking their variability (the average of their standard deviations) into account. When *d* = 1, the groups' means differ by 1 standard deviation; when d = 0 there is taken to be no difference between the groups. Here 0.8 is considered a large effect and 0.5 a medium one. For more about effect sizes, see Bath University's statistics site, <http://staff.bath.ac.uk/pssiw/stats2/page2/page14/page14.html>.

NB: to obtain the mean of a set of X numbers, add them all up and divide by X.

The standard deviation (SD) is a way of assessing the variability of a sample. Imagine taking the entire population of your country, weighing each person, and drawing a graph which shows, for each weight, how many people weighed that much. The graph would show a characteristic bell-shaped curve called a 'normal' distribution, whose mid-point is the population mean. About two-thirds of the population (68%) will have weights within one SD of the mean value (half will be lighter, half heavier). A further quarter (27%) will fall between one and two SDs of the mean, and almost all of the rest (totalling more than 99%) will fall within three SDs of the mean. So you are very unlikely to measure a weight that is more than three SDs different from the mean. To obtain the standard deviation, for each number in your sample, subtract the mean from it and square the result (this gets rid of any minus signs and gives a measure of how the number differs from the average value). Add up all the squares and divide by X-1, then take the square root of the result.

11 For clarity's sake I will only be citing odds ratios, but if you are starting to read epidemiology research there are two more measures you need to know about: the *p* value and the confidence interval. Epidemiology papers, especially more recent ones, often include statements like the following: 'Midlife diabetes was associated with subcortical infarctions (odds ratio, 1.85 [95% confidence interval, 1.09–3.15]; p = 0.02)' (Roberts, R. O. *et al.* (2014), 'Association of type 2 diabetes with brain atrophy and cognitive impairment', *Neurology*, 82, 1132–41). In this example an odds ratio of 1.85 gives us the authors' conclusion that midlife diabetes raises the risk of a subcortical stroke by 85%.

The *p* value shows that the researchers did a significance test to see how likely it was that their result—an apparent link between stroke and diabetes—came about by chance.

In its traditional misinterpretation, a value of p less than 0.05 is considered a 'pass': that is, significant. It implies that there is a less than one in twenty chance of the result being a fluke. In our example the p value is less than 0.05, but not a great deal less.

The confidence interval, which ranges from 1.09 to 3.15, also shows that the estimate is not very precise; narrower confidence intervals are more encouraging than broader ones. To interpret it, the question to ask is whether the range—here, 1.09–3.15—includes the null value at which risk is unchanged, i.e. odds ratio = 1.00. If it does, then the 'null hypothesis' that there is no real effect cannot be excluded. In our example it doesn't, but 1.09 is not far off 1.00, so again, the study should be treated with a certain amount of caution.

Chapter 11

1 For more about the risk factors for dementia, see the *AlzRisk* epidemiology database. I have been unable to find research addressing the question of whether sexuality—as opposed to gender—influences dementia risk, or whether sex reassignment surgery could alter the risk. However, if this is not being studied yet, I trust it will be soon.

2 The quotation is from Kawas, C. H. and M. M. Corrada (2006). 'Alzheimer's and dementia in the oldest-old: a century of challenges', *Current Alzheimer Research*, 3, 411–19.

3 Data are from the Alzheimer's Society's 2014 report (Prince *et al.* 2014) (note 3.7). See also its previous report (Knapp *et al.* 2007) (note 3.6).

4 'A newborn baby boy could expect to live 79.1 years and a newborn baby girl 82.8 years if mortality rates remain the same as they were in the United Kingdom in 2012–2014 throughout their lives', according to data from the Office for National Statistics, available from <http://www.ons.gov.uk/peoplepopulationandcommunity/ birthsdeathsandmarriages/lifeexpectancies/bulletins/ nationallifetablesunitedkingdom/2015-09-23>.

5 Data are from the World Bank's Aid Effectiveness indicators, available from <http://data. worldbank.org/indicator?display=default>.

6 Madabhushi, R. *et al.* (2014), 'DNA damage and its links to neurodegeneration', *Neuron*, 83, 266–82. See also Isaiah 40:6 ('All flesh is grass'), John Dryden's *Mac Flecknoe* ('All human things are subject to decay'), etc.

7 Iyama, T. and D. M. Wilson (2013), 'DNA repair mechanisms in dividing and non-dividing cells', *DNA Repair*, 12, 620–36; Madabhushi *et al.* (2014) (note 6).

8 Hewitt, G. *et al.* (2012), 'Telomeres are favoured targets of a persistent DNA damage response in ageing and stress-induced senescence', *Nature Communications*, 3, 708.

9 SFE Price, L. H. *et al.* (2013), 'Telomeres and early-life stress: an overview', *Biological Psychiatry*, 73, 15–23.

10 Belsky, D. W. *et al.* (2015), 'Quantification of biological aging in young adults', *Proceedings of the National Academy of Sciences*, 112, E4104–10.

11 Ramunas, J. *et al.* (2015), 'Transient delivery of modified mRNA encoding TERT rapidly extends telomeres in human cells', *FASEB Journal*, 29, 1930–9.

12 SFE Madabhushi *et al.* (2014) (note 6); Iyama and Wilson (2013) (note 7).

13 To divide, a cell must first make a copy of its DNA (replication, done during a 'synthesis' or S phase). This needs preparatory work—chromosomes must be untangled, histones

pushed apart—which takes place immediately before replication during the first gap phase, G1. After replication and before division the cell takes another breather, G2. Then it undergoes the physical division into two daughters (the mitosis or M phase). Finally, there is G0, the resting phase. Cells in G0 are post-mitotic: they have finished their growing and are no longer playing the division game, at least for now. Cells in any other phase (G1, S, G2, or M) are mitotic: they are still dividing.

14 A cancer cell takes on average two to four days to complete a cell cycle.

15 Inflammatory responses involve many interacting molecules, including cytokines, chemokines, adhesion molecules, and bioactive lipids such as free fatty acids. By referring only to the first of these I am simplifying, not excluding.

16 Pakkenberg *et al.* (2003) (note 5.18). The increase in the average size of the cell nucleus was significant, which is consistent with cell cycle problems such as duplicated DNA.

17 The free energy obtained by breaking one of ATP's phosphate bonds has been calculated as 7.3 kcal/mol (Lodish, H. *et al.* (2000), 'Section 2.4, Biochemical Energetics', in *Molecular Cell Biology*, eds H. Lodish *et al.*, New York, W. H. Freeman). Moles count amounts of stuff. Large amounts: $6 * 10^{23}$ atoms or molecules per mole, a value known to generations of schoolchildren as Avogadro's number. One mole (mol) of a substance is the amount of that substance containing the same number of atoms as are found in 12 grams of pure carbon, i.e. $6.02 * 10^{23}$ atoms. Physiological amounts—of substances in blood, for instance—tend to range from millimoles per litre (mmol/l) down to picomoles (pmol, 10^{-12}) per litre.

18 In the liver, the process of gluconeogenesis can convert pyruvate back into glucose. Pyruvate can be used to make lactate, used by astrocytes as a messenger molecule. (Researchers have proposed that astrocytes may in addition offer lactate as fuel for needy neurons, like a sports coach standing by with energy drinks as athletes train. Recent work, however, suggests that neurons can take up glucose directly, their uptake rising when they are more active.) Pyruvate can also be turned into ketones, molecules that can serve as an alternative fuel source for the brain when glucose supplies are limited. (Ketones contain a carbon atom double-bonded to an oxygen atom; the carbon's other two bonds are both with some type of hydrocarbon.) Ketones are exploited in high-fat, low-carbohydrate 'ketogenic' diets, which are used to treat some cases of epilepsy and brain cancer. They have also been tried in mild cognitive impairment and dementia, with encouraging, if preliminary, results. Ketones can be converted back to acetyl-CoA and used in the Krebs cycle, providing an alternative fuel source for neurons.

19 I have simplified considerably. For one thing, glucose can also be produced from fat, in the form of triglycerides. These can be broken down by lipolysis, 'fat-splitting', into glycerol and free fatty acids. (The liver and fat cells reverse this process to build triglycerides and create fat stores: lipogenesis. Too much of this can lead to obesity and to dangerous conditions like fatty liver disease, as fat—adipose tissue—builds up around the viscera.) Glycerol can then be converted into either glucose or pyruvate. Free fatty acids can also be used in the Krebs cycle by breaking them down into acetyl-CoA (acetyl-Coenzyme A, a key player in cellular energy production). They produce much more energy than glucose, so cells need less fat than sugar to generate energy. This is why losing fat is difficult, and especially difficult if you eat lots of sugary foods. Glucose can, conversely, be used to make

fat. Some of the molecules produced during glycolysis can be used to produce triglycerides; and pyruvate, converted to acetyl-CoA, can be used to produce fatty acids.

In addition, proteins can be used for energy if necessary. Proteins are broken down by digestion into two types of amino acids. Glucogenic amino acids can be converted into pyruvate, and hence used by the Krebs cycle to produce energy. They can be used to make glucose, glycogen, or fatty acids. Ketogenic amino acids can be converted into acetyl-CoA, and hence used in the Krebs cycle; or they can be converted to ketones or fatty acids.

20 The Krebs cycle is also known as the TCA (tricarboxylic acid) cycle or the citrate cycle. Plants use photosynthesis to turn carbon dioxide and water into glucose and oxygen. Animals use the Krebs cycle to do the reverse. It begins with acetyl-CoA being turned into citrate and ends by producing citrate, thus completing the cycle.

21 Nicotinamide adenine dinucleotide has many names, and a chemical structure too daunting to repeat here (for details see its *PubChem* entry). As well as its role in energy production, NADH is a useful measure of the cell's metabolism: its energy efficiency. This is because it is formed from NAD^+ during glycolysis and the Krebs cycle, so levels of NADH indicate how effectively these processes are using glucose. The electron transport chain turns NADH back into NAD^+, so if there is plenty of NAD^+ the mitochondria are making good use of oxygen. A recent neuroimaging study has found that in human brains NAD^+ levels drop with age and NADH levels increase. (The study used a form of MRI modified to detect NAD; see for details Zhu, X.-H. *et al.* (2015), 'In vivo NAD assay reveals the intracellular NAD contents and redox state in healthy human brain and their age dependences', *Proceedings of the National Academy of Sciences*, 112, 2876–81.) This suggests that failing mitochondria, more than lack of glucose, may be affecting older neurons.

22 The charge builds up because, as each protein shifts the electrons along, protons (H^+) are pumped across the inner membrane into the space between the inner and the outer membrane. This builds up an energy gradient between the positively charged space and the inner mitochondrion.

23 The term 'three-parent' embryo was coined to describe foetuses containing DNA from a mother, a father, and mitochondrial DNA from another source. Given that a mitochondrial genome contains all of thirty-seven genes and is thought to have minimal impact on the offspring, and given that parenting is about a great deal more than mere DNA donation, the phrase is not particularly helpful; it is, however, more familiar, and shorter, than 'meiotic nuclear transplantation techniques'.

24 Oxygen's outer electron shell needs two electrons to fill it.

25 ROS are prone to engaging in redox reactions. These chemical exchanges were first identified as oxygen transfers between molecules, though they are now often described in terms of electron transfer. When oxygen is moved from molecule A to molecule B, A is said to be reduced (it loses oxygen) by a reduction reaction, while B is oxidized (it gains oxygen) by an oxidation reaction. Every reduction is balanced by an oxidation: hence 'redox'. In terms of electrons, reduced A gains electrons while oxidized B loses them (because the oxygen which binds to B avidly accepts them into its outer shell).

26 Technically not all reactive species are free radicals because the latter are defined as having an unpaired electron in the outermost shell of an atom (this makes them particularly reactive).

27 As well as reactive oxygen species, other highly reactive molecules have been implicated in biochemical wear and tear. One example is reactive nitrogen species like nitric oxide (NO); the term used for their effects is nitrosative stress. I will refer to 'oxidative stress' throughout, but in doing so I am not excluding other radicals.

28 According to a 2015 study, this is because having better anti-oxidants would interfere with neurons' specialized development. Anti-oxidant gene expression is regulated by a transcription factor called Nrf2, but in maturing neurons its gene expression is reduced. Experiments that switch Nrf2 back on have found that the neurons fail to develop normal synapses and neurites. See Bell, K. F. *et al.* (2015), 'Neuronal development is promoted by weakened intrinsic antioxidant defences due to epigenetic repression of Nrf2', *Nature Communications*, 6, 7066.

29 Tarczyluk, M. A. *et al.* (2015), 'Amyloid β 1–42 induces hypometabolism in human stem cell-derived neuron and astrocyte networks', *Journal of Cerebral Blood Flow and Metabolism*, 35, 1348–57.

30 This is why the differences in percentage terms between men and women are smaller than the raw numbers of affected individuals would suggest; the total population is bigger for women.

31 Except when cultural factors have changed the balance, as in China, India, and Iran, the countries that contribute most to dementia research—the United States, the United Kingdom, other Western nations, Australia, and Japan—thus contain more females than males.

32 Ferreira, L. *et al.* (2014), 'Rate of cognitive decline in relation to sex after 60 years-of-age: a systematic review', *Geriatrics and Gerontology International*, 14, 23–31.

33 SFE Jorm, A. F. and D. Jolley (1998). 'The incidence of dementia: a meta-analysis', *Neurology*, 51, 728–33.

34 For more about the relationship between oestrogen and cognition, see the special issue of the journal *Hormones and Behaviour* of August 2015, volume 74.

35 Prince *et al.* (2014) (note 3.7).

36 I simplify: for the two major neuropathological markers of Alzheimer's, amyloid and tau proteins, research found that the three familial Alzheimer's genes linked to amyloid processing (APP, PSEN1, PSEN2) were probably not doing much in late-onset Alzheimer's, but there might have been something going on with tau. SFE Gerrish, A. *et al.* (2012), 'The role of variation at AβPP, PSEN1, PSEN2, and MAPT in late onset Alzheimer's disease', *Journal of Alzheimer's Disease*, 28, 377–87.

37 CRISPR (clustered, regularly interspaced, short palindromic repeat) technology is a method of gene editing which adapts a system used by bacteria to rid themselves of invasive genetic material such as viruses. For more about CRISPR, see Ledford, H. (2015), 'CRISPR, the disruptor', *Nature*, 522, 20–4; or *Nature*'s online special feature on CRISPR. For more (highly technical) detail, try Sander, J. D. and Joung, J. K. (2014), 'CRISPR-Cas systems for editing, regulating and targeting genomes', *Nature Biotechnology*, 32, 347–55.

38 There are numerous kinds of apolipoproteins, and some may transport certain proteins as well as lipids.

39 Fats are transferred from the liver to the bile ducts, concentrated in the gall bladder, and then passed into the intestine. During this transit they are chemically modified to make

them more soluble in water, allowing better digestion. Some are excreted, especially if excess dietary cholesterol has been consumed, and some are reabsorbed for re-use by the liver.

40 Phospholipids are another major component of cell membranes. They are diglycerides: a glycerol spine with two fatty acids attached. In the third position is a phosphate group. Like the –OH group, this prefers water, so phospholipids are also amphipathic. As with cholesterol, this makes them useful in cell membranes and also in the transport of fat through the body, since they can interact both with fat and water. For more on the structures, functions, and synthesis of phospholipids, and indeed other lipids, the online database *LipidLibrary* (see the Further Reading section for details) has a lot of information.

41 Cholesterol, $C_{27}H_{46}O$, is produced from acetyl-CoA. Sterols, cholesterol included, are steroid alcohols. They are built, like steroids, of linked carbon rings with a hydrocarbon tail at one end; being alcohols, they also have an –OH group at the other end. This format makes cholesterol amphipathic, and that enables it to do its job.

42 A Cochrane review (McGuinness, B. *et al.* (2014), 'Statins for the treatment of dementia', *Cochrane Database of Systematic Reviews*, 7, CD007514), found insufficient evidence to recommend statin use in patients with dementia. Although some epidemiological studies have suggested they may have a slight preventative effect if taken earlier in life, not all agree.

43 There are three main female sex hormones: estradiol, estriol, and estrone. I have followed the convention of using the collective noun oestrogen.

44 Chylomicrons by weight are roughly four-fifths triglyceride, the rest being cholesterol, phospholipid, and protein. They may be up to 600 nm across, though the sizes given here are ballpark indications only. Next in size are very low-density lipoprotein particles (VLDL, around 60 nm), which are about half triglyceride. Low-density lipoprotein (LDL, around 25 nm) contains about one-tenth triglyceride, and high-density lipoprotein (HDL, up to 12 nm) about one-twentieth. VLDL and LDL are often lumped together as LDL. Data are taken from *LipidLibrary* (<http://lipidlibrary.aocs.org/Lipids/lipoprot/index.htm>). The site gives size data in angstroms; to convert to nanometres, divide by ten.

45 Oxidized LDL is a variable and complex mess of damaged and disrupted lipids and proteins with, overall, a net negative charge. Many of its contents trigger immune responses (possibly including antibody reactions).

46 LDL associates with proteoglycans on the arterial inner wall.

47 Stimulated macrophages increase their production of pro-inflammatory cytokines and may also present bits of digested oxLDL as antigen to passing T cells.

48 Animal studies suggest that some neurons may also produce ApoE as part of the response to damage: SFE Mahley, R. W. and Y. Huang (2012), 'Apolipoprotein E sets the stage: response to injury triggers neuropathology', *Neuron*, 76, 871–85.

49 Global frequency estimates of 6.4% for allele ε2, 78.3% for ε3, and 14.5% for ε4—based on (highly variable) samples from 225 populations—are from Eisenberg, D. T. *et al.* (2010), 'Worldwide allele frequencies of the human apolipoprotein E gene: climate, local adaptations, and evolutionary history', *American Journal of Physical Anthropology*, 143, 100–11.

50 ApoE2 and ApoE3 have a cysteine at position 112, while ApoE4 has an arginine instead. ApoE2 has a cysteine at position 158, while ApoE3 and ApoE4 have an arginine instead. The amino

acid sequence of human ApoE was identified by Rall, S.C. *et al.* (1982). 'Human apolipoprotein E. The complete amino acid sequence', *Journal of Biological Chemistry*, 257, 4171–8.

51 The cytoskeleton and mitochondria seem particularly affected (Huang, Y. and Mahley, R.W. (2014), 'Apolipoprotein E: structure and function in lipid metabolism, neurobiology, and Alzheimer's diseases', *Neurobiology of Disease*, 72, 3–12).

52 SFE the Alzheimer's Society (<http://www.alzheimers.org.uk/site/scripts/documents_info.php?documentID=168>). Other estimates put the fraction of Alzheimer's patients with ApoE4 at up to four-fifths; SFE Mahley, R. W. *et al.* (2006), 'Apolipoprotein E4: a causative factor and therapeutic target in neuropathology, including Alzheimer's disease', *Proceedings of the National Academy of Sciences*, 103, 5644–51.

53 Various studies have found that, relative to $\varepsilon3/\varepsilon3$ genotypes, the risk of Alzheimer's ranges from less than double to more than thirty times higher in $\varepsilon4/\varepsilon4$ genotypes. A 2013 meta-analysis finds an increased risk of conversion from MCI to Alzheimer's in ApoE4 carriers (Fei, M. and W. Jianhua (2013), 'Apolipoprotein $\varepsilon4$-allele as a significant risk factor for conversion from mild cognitive impairment to Alzheimer's disease: a meta-analysis of prospective studies', *Journal of Molecular Neuroscience*, 50, 257–63).

54 Mayeda, E.R. *et al.* (2016), 'Inequalities in dementia incidence between six racial and ethnic groups over 14 years', *Alzheimer's and Dementia*, 12, 216–24. The study's authors comment that 'the patterns we report defy simple explanations', because the sample they used was population-based and had equal healthcare access; comorbidity (e.g. vascular disease) and education didn't seem to explain the results, and they were consistent across age. There were gender differences: the gap between African-American and Asian-American males was greater than for females. 'In most racial/ethnic groups, dementia incidence rates were similar for women and men until ages 90+ years.'

55 Just because ApoE2 protects against Alzheimer's in some populations, however, does not make it altogether benign. There may be, for example, a greater risk of fracture and low bone mass in $\varepsilon2/\varepsilon2$ individuals, and of severe diarrhoea in children.

56 Kulminski, A. M. *et al.* (2014), 'Age, gender, and cancer but not neurodegenerative and cardiovascular diseases strongly modulate systemic effect of the Apolipoprotein E4 allele on lifespan', *PLoS Genetics*, 10, e1004141.

57 'Of 7.6 million children who died in the first five years of their life in 2010, 64.0% (4.879 million) died of infectious causes'. The main culprits were pneumonia (1.40 million), diarrhoea (0.80 million), and malaria (0.56 million). Other major causes of death included birth complications (1.79 million), sepsis and meningitis (0.39 million), injury (0.35 million), and congenital abnormalities (0.27 million). Data were gathered from the WHO, UNICEF, and individual countries. For the methods and uncertainties associated with these figures, see the publication Liu, L. *et al.* (2012), 'Global, regional, and national causes of child mortality: an updated systematic analysis for 2010 with time trends since 2000', *Lancet*, 379, 2151–61.

58 Vitamin D status by country is reviewed by Hilger, J. *et al.* (2014), 'A systematic review of vitamin D status in populations worldwide', *British Journal of Nutrition*, 111, 23–45. To explain the differences between nations the authors suggest a mixture of cultural factors (e.g. traditions relating to clothing, working and leisure habits, and diet) and environmental factors (e.g. amounts of sunlight).

59 See the WHO report on global health risks, available from <http://www.who.int/healthinfo/global_burden_disease/GlobalHealthRisks_report_full.pdf>.

60 Oriá, R. B. *et al.* (2010). 'ApoE polymorphisms and diarrheal outcomes in Brazilian shanty town children', *Brazilian Journal of Medical and Biological Research*, 43, 249–56.

61 Genes repeatedly linked to Alzheimer's include: PICALM and BIN1, which are involved in clathrin-mediated endocytosis; CD33, which helps immune cells interact and is involved in clathrin-independent endocytosis; ABCA7 and CLU (the apolipoprotein clusterin, *aka* APOJ), which are involved with ApoE; and TREM2, which has to do with microglial clearance. See the *AlzGene* website.

62 In captive chimpanzees, for example, 'although mild to moderate atherosclerosis was observed in the aorta and other major blood vessels in some of the chimpanzee necropsies, no major blockages of the coronary arteries were observed in any case', and 'a search of the extant literature revealed only rare instances of acute coronary thrombosis in chimpanzees and gorillas, typically under dietary or blood lipid circumstances that would have been expected to maximize the risk of severe atherosclerosis in humans', according to Varki, N. *et al.* (2009), 'Heart disease is common in humans and chimpanzees, but is caused by different pathological processes', *Evolutionary Applications*, 2, 101–12.

Chapter 12

1 The quotation is from Chauhan, N. B. (2014), 'Chronic neurodegenerative consequences of traumatic brain injury', *Restorative Neurology and Neuroscience*, 32, 337–65. Compare the CDC (<http://www.cdc.gov/traumaticbraininjury/get_the_facts.html>), which states that in the United States in 2010, 'TBI was a diagnosis in more than 280,000 hospitalizations and 2.2 million ED [emergency department] visits' and a factor in more than 50,000 deaths.

2 DeKosky, S. T. *et al.* (2013), 'Acute and chronic traumatic encephalopathies: pathogenesis and biomarkers', *Nature Reviews Neurology*, 9, 192–200.

3 Meaney, D. F. *et al.* (2014). 'The mechanics of traumatic brain injury: a review of what we know and what we need to know for reducing its societal burden', *Journal of Biomechanical Engineering*, 136, 021008.

4 Cole, J. H. *et al.* (2015), 'Prediction of brain age suggests accelerated atrophy after traumatic brain injury', *Annals of Neurology*, 77, 571–81.

5 'People sustaining TBI are ~4 times more likely to develop dementia at a later stage than people without TBI' (Chauhan 2014) (note 1).

6 The singular form of meninges, meninx, is vanishingly rare today; the term, also used for the scum on milk, was first applied to brain membranes by Hippocrates (he of the oath). The work in question is *On the Sacred Disease*, thought to have been written around 400 BC. The sacred disease is epilepsy, and this text, which may or may not be by Hippocrates, contains one of its earliest descriptions. See also Part 3, note 1.

7 Someone has worked out how much force you need to get a surgical needle through the dura mater (of corpses). The answer is around five to seven Newtons, apparently, depending on the angle. For comparison, ten Newtons is roughly the weight of (the force

exerted by gravity on) a 1kg bag of sugar. See Lewis, M. C. *et al.* (2000), 'How much work is required to puncture dura with Tuohy needles?' *British Journal of Anaesthesia*, 85, 238–41.

8 Buoyancy results from the displacement of fluid. The apparent weight of an object immersed in fluid will depend on the object's weight, and the object's and fluid's specific gravities (i.e. their densities, relative to a reference substance which for liquids is usually water). The specific gravity of brain tissue is around 1.04 and that of CSF around 1.007, according to Johanson, C. E. (2008), 'Choroid plexus–cerebrospinal fluid circulatory dynamics: impact on brain growth, metabolism, and repair', in *Neuroscience in Medicine*, ed. P. M. Conn (Totowa, NJ: Humana Press), 173–200.

9 Holland, J. N. and Schmidt, A. T. (2015), 'Static and dynamic factors promoting resilience following traumatic brain injury: a brief review', *Neural Plasticity*, 2015, 902802.

10 For example, the mechanical stretching of epithelial cells has been shown to trigger cell cycle re-entry (Benham-Pyle, B. W. *et al.* (2015), 'Mechanical strain induces E-cadherin–dependent Yap1 and β-catenin activation to drive cell cycle entry', *Science*, 348, 1024–7). Could this also happen in neurons? We don't know yet.

11 Fakhran, S. *et al.* (2013), 'Symptomatic white matter changes in mild traumatic brain injury resemble pathologic features of early Alzheimer dementia', *Radiology*, 269, 249–57.

12 A 2014 study of 646 US Marines which attempted to study both emotional distress and cognitive dysfunction found that both were increased in soldiers who had been concussed multiple times, but that a single or recent concussion was linked only to emotional distress. See Spira, J. L. *et al.* (2014), 'The impact of multiple concussions on emotional distress, post-concussive symptoms, and neurocognitive functioning in active duty United States marines independent of combat exposure or emotional distress', *Journal of Neurotrauma*, 31, 1823–34.

13 Chen, C.-W. *et al.* (2014). 'Increased risk of dementia in people with previous exposure to general anesthesia: a nationwide population-based case–control study', *Alzheimer's and Dementia*, 10, 196–204.

14 Scott, D. A. *et al.* (2014). 'Cardiac surgery, the brain, and inflammation', *Journal of Extra-Corporeal Technology*, 46, 15–22.

Chapter 13

1 Heppner, F. L. *et al.* (2015), 'Immune attack: the role of inflammation in Alzheimer disease', *Nature Reviews Neuroscience*, 16, 358–72.

2 SFE Tate, J. A. *et al.* (2014), 'Infection hospitalization increases risk of dementia in the elderly', *Critical Care Medicine*, 42, 1037–46.

3 I am determined to make it through this book without once using the phrase 'arms race'.

4 The microbiome itself is one tiny part of a global 'unseen majority' of single-celled organisms, totalling about five nonillion, quintillion, or decillion cells, depending on what you prefer to call a one followed by thirty zeros. These are classed as prokaryotes or eukaryotes; only the latter have their genetic material membrane-wrapped in a nuclear package. The former—bacteria and archaea, the 'unseen majority' of life on Earth—have been estimated to store up to as much carbon as the world's plants, to number up to 6×10^{30} cells, and to renew themselves at a rate of 1.7×10^{30} cells per year (Whitman, W. B. *et al.*

(1998). 'Prokaryotes: the unseen majority', *Proceedings of the National Academy of Sciences*, 95, 6578–83). The number of bacterial cells in an adult human body is said to outnumber the human cells by about ten to one (Turnbaugh, P. J. *et al.* (2007), 'The human microbiome project', *Nature*, 449, 804–10). That this has only recently been established is because the required gene-sequencing technology is still quite new. Researchers have been able to 'read' DNA for years (I used the already-standard technique, PCR, as an undergraduate). Only lately, however, have they been able to read it fast enough to get through all those extra genomes—smaller than the human genome, but far more numerous—before their universities began complaining about their publication rate.

5 The microbiome may be necessary for normal immune development. It has been suggested, for example, that lack of these bacteria, or changes in their composition, may have contributed to the rise in allergies in Western countries over recent decades.

6 Ian Fleming's novel *You Only Live Twice* was published in 1964; the movie, starring Sean Connery, appeared three years later.

7 The result, some researchers argue, is an 'inflammatory bias'—the immune system's tendency to react, and sometimes over-react, as if it is better safe than sorry. SFE Raison, C. L. and A. H. Miller (2013), 'Malaise, melancholia and madness: the evolutionary legacy of an inflammatory bias', *Brain, Behavior, and Immunity*, 31, 1–8.

8 The most recent study I could find was Granerod, J. *et al.* (2013), 'New estimates of incidence of encephalitis in England', *Emerging Infectious Diseases*, 19, 130064. The authors assessed encephalitis incidence in England between 2005 and 2009. Using two methods, they estimated it as 4.32 per 100,000 per year (from hospital data) or 5.23 (from modelling data), with a potential range between 2.75 and 8.66. All the figures are significantly higher than the only previous estimate of 1.5 (Davison, K. L. *et al.* (2003), 'Viral encephalitis in England, 1989–1998: what did we miss?' *Emerging Infectious Diseases*, 9, 234–40). Using population data from the ONS and assuming no major change in incidence between 2009 and 2012, when my relative was infected, gives an estimate of the incidence for that year as between 1,450 and 4,633.

9 The data are average values based on laboratory-confirmed cases. The statistic is from the NHS (<http://www.nhs.uk/conditions/Meningitis/Pages/Introduction.aspx>).

10 Meningitis—inflammation of the membranes wrapping the brain—can be caused by multiple pathogens. Viral cases are considered less severe than bacterial infections. Data, based on the ten years from 2000, are from the Meningitis Research Foundation (<http://www.meningitis.org/facts>). I have lumped various forms of the disease together.

11 The lower figure is for lab-confirmed infections (<http://www.food.gov.uk/science/ microbiology/campylobacterevidenceprogramme>), the higher is the UK government's estimate of the total number (<https://www.gov.uk/government/publications/ campylobacter-cases-2000-to-2012>).

12 Bacteria are often classified as either Gram-positive or Gram-negative. This depends on whether they turn purple or pink when washed with the staining procedure named after nineteenth-century Danish researcher Hans Christian Gram. The different colours reflect different structures. Bacteria have three wrappings: an inner and an outer cell membrane separated by a cell wall made of peptidoglycan, a combination of sugars and amino acids

that forms a lattice-like structure. The cell wall is thinner in Gram-negative bacteria, and tends to wash away during Gram staining; these cells are stained by another chemical added to the solution. Gram-positive cells retain their thicker cell wall and the initial violet stain. Gram-negative bacteria include *V. cholerae* and *E. coli*, syphilitic spirochaetes, *H. pylori* (linked to stomach ulcers, inflammation, and cancer), and the *Neisseria* species *N. gonorrhoeae* and *N. meningitidis*. Gram-positive bacteria include the well-known *Listeria* and its similarly troublesome fellows *Staphylococcus* and *Streptococcus*.

13 Francis, D. (1973), *Bonecrack* (London: Pan Books).

14 Miklossy, J. (2011), 'Alzheimer's disease—a neurospirochetosis. Analysis of the evidence following Koch's and Hill's criteria', *Journal of Neuroinflammation*, 8, 90.

15 The rabies virus is an especially useful example of a neural tracer. Some pathogens enter the brain by hitching a ride across the blood–brain barrier; rabies does likewise but by way of nerves. It gets into a nerve ending, which may be far distant from the brain, and co-opts the nerve's internal transport mechanisms, used to move proteins from their production site in the cell body to the synapses. The virus travels up inside the nerves, remarkably fast, to reach the brain, and when tagged with a suitable marker it can thus blaze a speedy trail for researchers to follow. In its wild form it attacks the grey matter, especially in the cranial nerves, brainstem, thalamus, and basal ganglia. The changes caused, however, are subtle. Rabies, though almost always fatal, seems to use a strategy of not destroying too much tissue too fast. Post-mortem there may not be much cell loss or inflammation, and the blood–brain barrier appears intact until late on, when the sufferer sinks into a coma.

16 Herpes simplex virus is found in two forms, HSV1 and HSV2. HSV1 has been linked to coldsores and to Alzheimer's: SFE Urosevic, N. and R. N. Martins (2008), 'Infection and Alzheimer's disease: the APOE ε4 connection and lipid metabolism', *Journal of Alzheimer's Disease*, 13, 421–35. HSV2 is more associated with genital effects.

17 The website is <http://www.life-worldwide.org/>. The infections are cryptococcal meningitis, invasive and chronic pulmonary aspergillosis, *Pneumocystis* pneumonia, and infection of the bloodstream by *Candida* yeast species. One of these fungi, the mould *Aspergillus*, kills more than half a million victims per year. In the West, however, we usually only hear of it when some unfortunate gardener breathes it in and expires; *Aspergillus* likes compost.

18 The CDC (<http://www.cdc.gov/fungal/diseases/candidiasis/index.html>) says that candidiasis affects up to ten in 100,000 people in the United States.

19 *P. falciparum* and *T. gondii* are protozoa (single-celled organisms). *Taenia* is a helminth, a worm.

20 I exaggerate, but *T. gondii* does exert a disconcerting degree of behaviour control over its victims. As with the cordyceps 'zombie ant' fungus, the outcome for the target is not good. *T. gondii*-infected animals lose their fear of cats—it has even been suggested that they may find them sexually arousing—raising the chance that they will be killed and eaten. (Or, if your cat is like the ones that kill my garden birds, nibbled and then left somewhere unhelpful.) It is thought that *T. gondii* may operate by altering brain levels of the neurotransmitter dopamine. Once back in the cat, *T. gondii* reproduces sexually, producing oocysts that the cat then excretes, contaminating the food of so wide a variety

of animals—including humans—that *T. gondii* has been described as 'the world's most successful parasite' (<http://web.utk.edu/~xzha09/research/Tgondii/Tgondii.html>). When consumed, the oocysts reproduce asexually, clustering in muscles and the viscera—and also in nerves and brain. *T. gondii* is a worldwide problem and is thought to infect about 30% of humans, though studies have found widely varying rates, from minimal to around 40% in the United Kingdom and the United States, with variation between and within countries, and by gender, background, and age.

21 For more details of neurocysticercosis, including MRI images of the cysts, see DeGiorgio, C. M. *et al.* (2004), 'Neurocysticercosis', *Epilepsy Currents*, 4, 107–11. *Taenia* infection is said to be 'the leading cause of secondary epilepsy in Central and South America, East and South Asia, and sub-Saharan Africa'. It is also found elsewhere, including Western countries, and has been labelled an emerging public-health problem in Europe and the United States, especially in poor areas.

22 Note that the distinction between innate and adaptive immune systems is a convenient tradition, but not absolute. T cells, for instance, have immune memory, but they also respond to innate signals. Monocytes, which are cells of the innate immune system, have also recently been found to show memory. The phenomenon, which has yet to be fully understood, is called 'trained immunity'.

23 Infections vary in their effects on the brain. For example, cerebral malaria may not involve brain tissue penetration by cells of the adaptive immune system, and sleeping sickness may do so only late in the disease, according to Bentivoglio, M. *et al.* (2011), 'Neuroinflammation and brain infections: historical context and current perspectives', *Brain Research Reviews*, 66, 152–73.

24 Other PAMPs include the bacterial component peptidoglycan, zymosan, found on fungi, protozoan mucins, glycans from worms, double-stranded RNA from certain viruses, and glycoproteins from viral capsids, the protein coats in which viruses do their travelling. Viruses are segments of either DNA or RNA, sheathed in a protein coat which they shed before inveigling their way into cellular DNA. Some are single-stranded, some double.

25 The best-known pattern recognition receptors are a family of molecules called TLRs. The abbreviation stands for toll-like receptor, and the name arose because the receptor proteins look similar to a protein in fruit flies, *Drosophila melanogaster*, whose discovery so startled the German scientists involved—notably Nobel prize winner Christiane Nüsslein-Volhard—that they are said to have reacted by exclaiming 'Toll!'—a word whose meanings include 'Great!', 'Weird!' and 'Amazing!'

26 TLR2 recognizes peptidoglycan, found on bacteria, but it can also react to zymosan, mucins, and glycoproteins—from fungi, parasites, and viruses, respectively. TLR3 specializes in viral RNA, while TLR4 responds to bacterial LPS. (You see how the abbreviations accumulate.) TLR5 is also stimulated by bacteria and TLR11 is especially good at detecting *T. gondii*—at least in mice; the mechanism in humans remains unclear. Not all TLRs result in the stimulation of immune responses: TLR10 appears to be mainly inhibitory.

27 Humoral immunity is named after an ancient Greek theory of medicine, in which blood was one of the four humours, bodily fluids identified by Hippocrates. The other humours are black bile, yellow bile, and phlegm.

28 Sebum is just one of the substances we shed from skin (and elsewhere), as a stomach-turning analysis of swimming-pool water makes clear (Keuten, M. G. *et al.* (2014), 'Quantification of continual anthropogenic pollutants released in swimming pools', *Water Research*, 53, 259–70).

29 If you do your housework energetically, you will find that sweat is a product of household cleaning.

30 Another set of immune proteins that has become very interesting to neuroscientists is MHC (see also note 13.59). This classic immune system component, the holder in which T cells present antigen on their surfaces, also has a neural function: it regulates how neurons connect to one another, both during development and thereafter. MHC molecules are involved with the developmental processes that turn a baby's brain, with its chaotic mass of potential neural circuits, into a system refined by experience of the world. Having shaped brain pathways, they then help to maintain synaptic plasticity. (MHC stands for major histocompatibility complex. In humans it is also called HLA: human leucocyte antigen. Looking at the DNA, there are three main MHC regions, labelled I, II, and III. Perhaps someone was fed up with Greek and fancied a change to Latin.)

31 Astrocytes also help prune synapses.

32 CD33 and similar molecules are linked to ageing, as they interact with a family of cell surface molecules called 'siglecs' which when activated damp down both inflammation and oxidative stress. Siglecs are thought to have evolved to help cells control ROS levels. Mammal species with more genes coding for siglecs seem to live longer.

33 The other part of Mac-1 is integrin β2, *aka* CD18.

34 For example, variation in the gene coding for CD11b has been strongly linked to the autoimmune disease lupus, while CD18 deficit leads to a rare immunodeficiency syndrome called leucocyte adhesion deficiency, featuring repeated and dangerous bacterial infections.

35 CR3 also detects beta-glucan, a protein made by yeasts. As per note 13.33, Mac-1 (macrophage-1 antigen) is also known as the receptor integrin αMβ2, and/or CD11b/CD18.

36 The 'cascade' contains several complement pathways, e.g. 'classical' and 'alternative'.

37 Most children will have learned about exponential growth from reading Harry Potter. (I daresay complement ought to remind me of something with more cultural heft, like James Joyce's *Ulysses*, but I never finished *Ulysses*, precisely because of its habit of expanding minor observations into vast screeds.) In the last book of J. K. Rowling's series about the schoolboy wizard, he and his friends are trying to rob a bank when they encounter treasure bewitched with a Geminius charm. It causes objects to multiply, and within seconds the thieves are nearly drowned by the expanding mass of metal. (Joyce's way with words can have a similarly smothering effect.)

38 Many complement proteins bind near to where they are formed, or else are rapidly inactivated. Some must bind to other members of the complement family in order to exert their amplifying effects, which also restricts them. In addition, regulatory proteins also dampen the cascade.

39 Regulatory proteins include the complement receptor CR1 and Factor H, both of which have been linked to Alzheimer's. Factor H is also associated with the eye condition age-related macular degeneration—which can cause blindness—as well as with certain

rare kidney problems. Haemolytic uraemia, in which kidneys become blocked by protein (including complement) deposits, is thought to involve a genetic defect that results in complement overactivation, together with an environmental trigger such as *E. coli* infection.

40 B cells and T cells emerge from the bone marrow and thymus, respectively.

41 I simplify: stem cells mature into a variety of immune cells, including megakaryocytes, 'big-bodied' cells which produce platelets, and granulocytes. These latter, short-lived cells are so called because they contain distinctive granules that can be stained different colours: pink for the majority neutrophils, red for eosinophils, and purple for the rarest type, the basophils. The stain used is a combination of hematoxylin, which is basic and stains purple-blue, and eosin, which is acidic and stains red-orange. (Granulocytes are sometimes called polymorphonuclear cells. Confusingly, the name is also sometimes used for neutrophils, a subset of granulocytes.) Mast cells, which cluster around blood vessels, also contain granules, but opinions differ on whether they are granulocytes or not, as they live longer (for weeks rather than days). Unlike granulocytes they are not usually found in blood in their mature form, but in connective tissues. The granules are chemical weapons, containing substances like histamine, which are deleterious to pathogens and stimulatory to other immune cells. Eosinophils, basophils, and mast cells are key players in the development of allergic reactions such as eczema and asthma.

42 A quick rummage in Google's cornucopia (other search engines are available) makes the point about the relative obscurity of immune organs. When I looked for 'What does the [X] do?', results for 'brain' (22,300) and 'heart' (35,400) greatly outnumbered those for 'thymus' (1,300), or even for 'bone marrow' (1,970). This is probably not because most people know all about their thymus but have no idea what their heart does.

43 The thymus, where T cells mature, has a growth rate far faster than that of a cancer cell. It is thought to contain between one and two hundred million thymocytes (junior T cells), which proliferate at a rate of 50 million a day; meanwhile 2 million T cells leave each day. That we do not all die young, our heart and lungs crushed by a ballooning thymus, is because 96–98% of T cells are rejected and then commit suicide, their carcasses quickly cleared by macrophages. This is a higher rejection rate than the United Kingdom's famous military elite the SAS. Besides, soldiers who don't make it into the SAS can usually resume their duties elsewhere. About thirty of 200 pre-selected candidates are accepted into the most selective of the three SAS regiments (the 22nd), according to <http://www .sasregiment.org.uk/>. Estimates of T cell numbers are from young adult mouse thymus; see the chapter 'Generation of lymphocytes in bone marrow and thymus' in Janeway, C. A. *et al.* (2001), *Immunobiology: The Immune System in Health and Disease* (New York: Garland Science). I have cited the fifth edition of Janeway's *Immunobiology* because it can be accessed freely from *PubMed* (<http://www.ncbi.nlm.nih.gov/books/NBK27140/>); there are later editions.

44 Neutrophils have long been considered the frontline cannon fodder of the immune army. When, for example, cells in the brain's choroid plexus detect an invading bacterium—such as *E. coli*, which can cause fatal meningitis in babies—they chemically scream for help. This calls neutrophils, which are constantly patrolling the bloodstream, to flood the scene, crossing the blood–brain barrier to seek and destroy the invader. Neutropenia, a lack of

neutrophils, is one of the problems oncologists look out for when giving chemotherapy, because it renders cancer patients extremely vulnerable to infection, with potentially severe or lethal consequences. Neutrophils live for days only and readily sacrifice themselves to kill the body's enemies; the white pus in wounds and spots is mostly the corpses of heroic neutrophils. Even cannon fodder may be highly skilled, and neutrophils are now known to engage in complex interactions with other immune cells. They are involved in acute and also in chronic inflammation. They also become more common with age, whereas other leucocytes tend to decrease in number. In animal models of Alzheimer's they have been found to enter the brain and migrate towards amyloid plaques. Stem cells can also turn into natural killer cells. These are lymphocytes, a type of white blood cell often found in lymph nodes which is capable of engulfing and digesting pathogens and infected cells.

45 The technical terms for cell eating are phagocytosis if the cell is wholly consumed and trogocytosis if bits of it are nibbled off. Trogocytosis is used by the immune system as a quick way of transferring information from antigen-presenting cells to lymphocytes. It also seems to be a way of killing cells.

46 Other immune cells such as dendritic cells have similar APC functions. Dendritic cells, for example, are found in the borderlands of the body—tissues such as skin and gut—where they detect and process antigen before moving to the lymph nodes. They also contribute to the regulation of other immune cells' reactions, and hence to immune tolerance.

47 A Phase III clinical trial of solanezumab was initially thought to have failed (Doody, R. S. *et al.* (2014), 'Phase 3 trials of solanezumab for mild-to-moderate Alzheimer's disease', *New England Journal of Medicine*, 370, 311–21), but re-analysis suggested that patients with the mildest stages of dementia might have better-preserved cognitive function, and that the drug might be altering brain amyloid (see the comment by the Alzheimer's Association at <http://www.alz.org/aaic/releases_2015/wed-7amET.asp>). If so, this would make it the first truly disease-modifying treatment for Alzheimer's. It also provides encouragement for proponents of the amyloid hypothesis (see Part 3).

48 Antibodies are a type of immunoglobulin (Ig), a group of proteins found in blood plasma. Humans have five kinds of Ig, denoted A, D, E, G, M, with different structures and roles. IgE, for example, is particularly associated with allergic reactions, while IgA predominates in the various sticky oozes we humans produce to defend ourselves. IgD is mainly found on cell surfaces. IgM's domain is the bloodstream, where it facilitates humoral immune processes. IgG is a general-purpose molecule. It is also the only type to cross the placenta. There is some evidence that antibodies from the mother can in some cases—e.g. in autoimmune disorders like lupus—harm the foetal brain, causing learning disorders such as autism.

49 Trying to estimate vocabulary size is like trying to classify mental illnesses: it has been done but the attempt was inevitably flawed. For English, estimates vary hugely but generally range up to about 100,000 words.

50 In brief, antibodies are Y-shaped proteins made up of four subunits: two 'heavy chain' and two 'light chain' proteins. The chains are made by splicing together segments of DNA of three types, called V, D, and J. For the human heavy-chain protein, it is thought there are about thirty-nine V, twenty-seven D and six J segments. See for details 'The generation of diversity in immunoglobulins' in Janeway (2001) (note 43).

51 See the Nobel Prize website (<http://www.nobelprize.org/nobel_prizes/medicine/laureates/1987/tonegawa-bio.html>). Tonegawa's sole award is an honour rare in the post-war period: from 1946–2010 only a fifth of medicine/physiology prizes were singletons. For the physics and chemistry prizes the figures are 28% and 48%, respectively. Perhaps biology is more of a team sport?

52 'Thus, the immunological evolution of antibodies recapitulates on a much shorter timescale the natural evolution of enzymes' (Wang, F. *et al.* (2013), 'Somatic hypermutation maintains antibody thermodynamic stability during affinity maturation', *Proceedings of the National Academy of Sciences*, 110, 4261–6). Whether the B cells' tendency to replicate if they make better matches is analogous to the human situation is surprisingly hard to discover, as there has been much more research on what having babies does to relationship satisfaction than on whether more satisfied partners tend to have more babies. One study suggests that they may be more likely to have babies, as long as they are not so delighted with the status quo that another child appears as a threat rather than a promise (Rijken, A. and A. Liefbroer (2009), 'The influence of partner relationship quality on fertility', *European Journal of Population*, 25, 27–44).

53 For vaccines to provide lasting protection, the body must remember previous immune experiences. This capacity, immune memory, involves B cells. They detect antigens via receptors that are simply membrane-bound antibodies, and once activated, those receptors prompt B cells to mature into antibody-spewing plasma cells. They also replicate, producing clones with identical antibody specificities that can spread through the bloodstream, multiplying the defence force available to tackle the identified threat. As well as making antibodies, activated B cells may also proliferate, acquire immune tolerance, commit suicide, alter the numbers of BCRs (B cell receptors) on their surface—thereby adjusting their sensitivity to immune stimuli—and so on.

54 Doody *et al.* (2013) (note 6.32).

55 Anti-NMDAR encephalitis is more common in women and may be linked to undiagnosed ovarian cancer. The Encephalitis Society offers a useful factsheet for patients, available from <http://www.encephalitis.info/files/9813/4012/7830/FS057V1.pdf>. (Another rare autoimmune disease, Rasmussen's encephalitis, also involves autoantibodies to glutamate receptors.) In laboratory studies the glutamate receptors in question were found to be activated by a glutamate analogue called n-methyl-d-aspartate, hence the name NMDA receptors (NMDARs). They are of particular interest to dementia researchers because they have great influence on calcium signalling and are involved in triggering excitotoxicity. They are also central players in learning, memory, and stress responses because their unusual structure allows them to associate stimuli together. NMDARs are calcium channels, but in the resting state the channel is usually blocked by a magnesium ion. To be activated, the receptor must not only bind to glutamate emitted from another cell, but the magnesium block must also be lifted. This happens when the cell membrane is depolarized in response to signals from a second cell. When coincidental firing occurs among cells connected to it, the receiving cell's NMDARs allow it to adjust its synaptic strength so as to boost the neural network linking senders and receiver.

56 Note that immunization can be either active or passive. Active immunization, which takes longer but lasts longer, stimulates the immune system with antigen so that it forms antibodies. Passive immunization provides the antibodies ready-made.

57 See, from the drug company, Schenk, D. (2002), 'Amyloid-β immunotherapy for Alzheimer's disease: the end of the beginning', *Nature Reviews Neuroscience*, 3, 824–8.

58 The poem referred to is Lewis Carroll's 'The Walrus and the Carpenter'.

59 T cell receptors recognize antigen fragments—proteins from munched pathogens presented on the surfaces of APCs. The trophies are not displayed naked, but in a specialized chemical holder: an MHC protein (see also note 13.30). These are of great interest to immunologists because they help phagocytes to tell self from nonself—and to kill accordingly. Which MHC proteins you have affects your immune function, including your chances of getting an autoimmune disease. MHC gene variants are also among the list of risk genes identified for Alzheimer's. When microglia and other APCs around brain blood vessels detect and consume Aβ, they are thought to release proteins that prompt the cells of the blood–brain barrier to express more MHC. That in turn attracts T cells to cross the barrier. They are found in the brains of advanced Alzheimer's patients only late in the disease, whereas other inflammatory processes seem to happen at an earlier stage. How and when in the disease the blood–brain barrier is breached, and the extent to which the brain is then flooded with white blood cells, is unclear, not least because it has until recently been hard to distinguish microglia, especially when retracted, from peripheral macrophages.

60 C5a is thought to stimulate prostaglandin E2, which binds to receptors on the vagus nerve, which connects with the brain's ventromedial preoptic area, which regulates body temperature. PGE2, which like other prostaglandins is produced within the body from the omega-6 fatty acid arachidonic acid, is an interesting molecule: among its effects is an increase in tissue regeneration in multiple organs. Needless to say, the enzyme which degrades PGE2 is being investigated as a potential therapeutic target, given that inhibiting it in mice was found to speed up their recovery after injury (Zhang, Y. *et al.* (2015), 'Inhibition of the prostaglandin-degrading enzyme 15-PGDH potentiates tissue regeneration', *Science*, 348, aaa2340).

61 The verb is luo (λύω). I remember it because it was the first verb my textbook used to try to teach me biblical Greek—most of which I have forgotten except for the science-relevant bits. This shows the importance of relating what you learn to what you know already.

62 Obviously one cannot give Aβ oligomers to people to see if their brains shrink, so claims of Aβ toxicity rely heavily on animal and cell culture work.

63 As well as ROS, complement, CRP, and cytokines, humoral (blood-borne) chemical signals used by the innate immune system include chemokines (which control many aspects of cells' movement and behaviour) and adhesion molecules (which help cells form physical connections). Operating alongside the various protein messengers are bioactive lipids (fats with signalling capacities which can active immune reactions). These include fatty acids such as arachidonic acid, platelet-activating factor, prostaglandins, and leukotrienes. Their many roles extend beyond immune function: one of the leukotrienes

(C4), for example, has recently been identified as key to the triggering of oxidative stress (Dvash, E. *et al.* (2015), 'Leukotriene C4 is the major trigger of stress-induced oxidative DNA damage', *Nature Communications*, 6, 10112). This is potentially of great clinical interest for neurodegeneration, because drugs inhibiting LTC4 already exist and are used to treat asthma. One has already been shown to slow disease progression in an Alzheimer's mouse model (Tang, S. S. *et al.* (2014), 'Protective effect of pranlukast on Aβ1-42-induced cognitive deficits associated with downregulation of cysteinyl leukotriene receptor 1', *International Journal of Neuropsychopharmacology*, 17, 581–92).

64 There are also interferons and growth factors, which may be lumped in with cytokines or treated separately. Growth factors play many roles in development, maintenance, and repair. Interferons were identified in the context of viral infection: infected cells produce interferons to 'warn' other cells and stimulate immune reactions. They have been instrumental in research into the link between the immune system and depression following the observation that some cancer patients given interferon therapy became severely depressed. Interferons are not the only immune mediators linked to depression, however. A review observes that 'Depression as an inflammatory disorder is mediated by pro-inflammatory cytokines, interleukin-1, interleukin-6, TNFα, soluble interleukin-2 receptors, interferon-α, interleukin 8, interleukin-10, hs-CRP, acute phase proteins, haptoglobin, toll like receptor 4, interleukin-1beta, mammalian target of rapamycin pathway, substance P, cyclooxygenase-2, prostaglandin-E2, lipid peroxidation levels and acid sphingomyelinase' (Lang, U. E. and S. Borgwardt (2013), 'Molecular mechanisms of depression: perspectives on new treatment strategies', *Cellular Physiology and Biochemistry*, 31, 761–77). Is that all? Probably not.

65 Cytokines can be classified by their structure, by their function (e.g. pro-inflammatory or anti-inflammatory), or by their source (the Th1/Th2 division). The latter refers to cytokines produced by two types of helper T cell. Th1 cells are more focused on intracellular threats; they regulate the macrophages that can eat affected cells. Th2 cells target mainly extracellular threats and regulate B cells, the makers of antibodies.

T cell biology is an enormous topic. Mature T cells come in several flavours, distinguished by their behaviours and by the markers on their surfaces. The primary distinction is between killers and helpers. Killer T cells specialize in devouring cells with internal problems, like viral infection or the beginnings of cancer. Helpers secrete a range of molecules into the bloodstream to regulate the immune response. Killer T cells, also known as cytotoxic T lymphocytes, express a molecule called CD8 on their surfaces which is a co-receptor: it participates in the cell's activation by binding to the APC alongside the T cell receptor (which recognizes fragments of antigen presented by the APC). Helper T cells express CD4. These are the cells notably attacked by HIV, and they have been suggested to contribute to neurodegeneration. Which type predominates in an immune response affects the character of that response. (A clear guide to T cells can be found at Cardiff University's T Cell Modulation Group, <http://www.tcells.org/>.)

There are also memory T cells (as with B cells) and T regulatory cells (Tregs) whose complex functions are not yet fully understood. That last statement should not encourage you to infer that the rest of T cell biology is done and dusted. As elsewhere, I have simplified greatly.

66 We owe the four cardinal signs of inflammation to the Roman writer Celsus (not to be confused with the eighteenth-century Swedish astronomer Celsius, he of the temperature scale). Celsus recorded that 'Notae vero inflammationis sunt quattuor: rubor et tumor cum calore et dolore': 'The signs of inflammation are four: redness and swelling with heat and pain.' The quotation is from his *De Medicina*, Liber III, Section 10. A fifth sign— 'functio laesa', the loss or disturbance of function—has also been proposed. SFE Graeber, M. B. *et al.* (2011), 'Role of microglia in CNS inflammation', *FEBS Letters*, 585, 3798–805.

67 The 'other factors' include growth factors like transforming growth factor β (TGFβ) and enzymes such as the matrix metalloproteinases. MMPs break up the extracellular matrix to assist with damage clearance and repair, so that remodelling can take place. They also help with other aspects of healing like blood vessel regrowth and the gradual disappearance of scar tissue. MMPs and TGFβ, like some cytokines, promote the growth of new neurons as well. Excess MMP function has been linked to inflammatory disorders like arthritis and to the neurodegenerative condition amyotrophic lateral sclerosis (ALS), a form of motor neuron disease also called Lou Gehrig's disease. For a clinical guide to motor neuron disease see <http://www.patient.co.uk/health/Motor-Neurone-Disease.htm>.

68 TNFα, for instance, is expressed by macrophages that encounter bacteria. It contributes to pain, e.g. in arthritis, and can interact with neurons in the hypothalamus to trigger fever. It also makes endothelial cells in blood vessels stickier, so that leucocytes can more easily attach to them. I have referred to TNFα as if it were a single thing, but immunologists more precisely refer to the TNF superfamily. Like Aβ, pro-inflammatory cytokines such as TNFα can activate the transcription factor NFκB, stimulating microglia to ramp up cytokine production.

69 These cytokines are involved in allergic reactions (e.g. IL-4, IL-13) and also in wound healing (e.g. IL-10).

70 Mizwicki, M. T. *et al.* (2013), '1alpha,25-dihydroxyvitamin D3 and resolvin D1 retune the balance between amyloid-β phagocytosis and inflammation in Alzheimer's disease patients', *Journal of Alzheimer's Disease*, 34, 155–70.

71 SFE Murta, V. *et al.* (2015), 'Chronic systemic IL-1β exacerbates central neuroinflammation independently of the blood–brain barrier integrity', *Journal of Neuroimmunology*, 278, 30–43. This study models the effects of inflammation using the cytokine IL-1β and shows that its administration peripherally aggravates pre-existing damage in the brain whether the blood–brain barrier is healthy or not.

72 Krstic, D. *et al.* (2012), 'Systemic immune challenges trigger and drive Alzheimer-like neuropathology in mice', *Journal of Neuroinflammation*, 9, 151.

73 Some researchers have even linked genetic variation in cytokine production to personality traits such as harm avoidance (MacMurray, J. *et al.* (2014), 'The gene-immune-behavioral pathway: gamma-interferon (IFN-γ) simultaneously coordinates susceptibility to infectious disease and harm avoidance behaviors', *Brain, Behavior, and Immunity*, 35, 169–75).

74 Psychoneuroimmunology is a young, controversial, and fascinating science. The standard textbook is Schedlowski, M. and U. Tewes (1999), *Psychoneuroimmunology: An Interdisciplinary Introduction* (New York: Kluwer Academic/Plenum).

75 A 2005 meta-analysis, for example, concluded that bias might be responsible for the apparent association between NSAID use and lower dementia risk, because the strength

of the association was greatest in studies of dementia patients, less in studies where some patients developed dementia during the study, and least in studies where cognitive decline, rather than a diagnosis, was being assessed (De Craen, A. J. et al. (2005), 'Meta-analysis of nonsteroidal antiinflammatory drug use and risk of dementia', *American Journal of Epidemiology*, 161, 114–20). Other drugs used to treat inflammation, such as glucocorticoids, have different problems.

76 Beeri, M. S. et al. (2012), 'Corticosteroids, but not NSAIDs, are associated with less Alzheimer neuropathology', *Neurobiology of Aging*, 33, 1258–64.

77 Harry, G. J. (2013), 'Microglia during development and aging', *Pharmacology and Therapeutics*, 139, 313–26.

78 Hortega learned his craft from a master: Ramon y Cajal, to whom we owe the idea that neurons communicate by way of synapses. He also worked with the neurosurgeon Wilder Penfield, better known for his experiments with electrical stimulation of human brains.

79 A search of the literature for studies with 'neuroinflammation' in the title brings up over 6,000 results. For both publications and citations (how often papers are referred to, a measure of influence) the growth is exponential since 1996. For comparison, a search on 'Alzheimer' over the same period gives almost 170,000 results.

80 SFE Graeber et al. (2011) (note 66).

81 For example, markers for MHC-II, expressed by microglia and upregulated during their activation, are a common tool for identifying them post-mortem.

82 For instance, many more neutrophils enter the injured spine, and the inflammatory response there is much greater.

83 The condition is due to a mutation in sodium ion channels. A personal communication from Oxford expert David Bennett via Angela Vincent and John Stein says 'he is not aware of the sodium channel mutations having a direct effect on the inflammatory response'.

84 Cribbs, D. H. et al. (2012), 'Extensive innate immune gene activation accompanies brain aging, increasing vulnerability to cognitive decline and neurodegeneration: a microarray study', *Journal of Neuroinflammation*, 9, 179.

85 Filiou, M. D. et al. (2014), '"Neuroinflammation" differs categorically from inflammation: transcriptomes of Alzheimer's disease, Parkinson's disease, schizophrenia and inflammatory diseases compared', *Neurogenetics*, 15, 201–12.

86 Graeber et al. (2011) (note 66).

87 Neumann, H. et al. (2009), 'Debris clearance by microglia: an essential link between degeneration and regeneration', *Brain*, 132, 288–95.

88 TREM2 abbreviates 'triggering receptor expressed on myeloid cells-2'.

89 Ludvigsson, J. F. et al. (2013), 'Influenza H1N1 vaccination and adverse pregnancy outcome', *European Journal of Epidemiology*, 28, 579–88.

90 Basha, M. R. et al. (2005), 'The fetal basis of amyloidogenesis: exposure to lead and latent overexpression of amyloid precursor protein and beta-amyloid in the aging brain', *Journal of Neuroscience*, 25, 823–9.

91 The proverb says that cleanliness is next to godliness. Perhaps surprisingly, it resonates with modern science in two ways. The first is that studies of religion suggest that purity is

a major pillar and obsession driving both traditional conservative and more extremist forms of belief in religion, and also in politics. The second is that research into the psychology of disgust shows that cleansing activities make people feel more virtuous, even though they may actually then behave less morally and judge others more harshly. See my book *Cruelty* for further details (note 2.2).

92 If the hygiene hypothesis is correct, many modern ailments may be at least in part a consequence of modern living arrangements. That is encouraging, since arrangements can be changed. Indeed, attempts to reintroduce urban children to the natural world, in the hope of boosting their physical and mental health, are already underway. The hygiene hypothesis was proposed by David Strachan in 1989 (Strachan, D. P. (1989). 'Hay fever, hygiene, and household size', *British Medical Journal*, 299, 1259–60). Since then it has developed numerous variants and embellishments. One such is the 'old friends' hypothesis (Rook, G. A. (2012), 'Hygiene hypothesis and autoimmune diseases', *Clinical Reviews in Allergy and Immunology*, 42, 5–15). It states that in the past, humans had to put up with a certain level of infestation and co-evolved with certain invaders (like worms or *T. gondii*) to tolerate their presence; only recently have we been able to remove these organisms, and their loss may have disrupted immune development. These ideas have generated considerable debate, for example over which infectious agents might be involved.

Chapter 14

1 The estimate of chronic illness is from a 2012 UK government report on long-term conditions (available from <https://www.gov.uk/government/publications/long-term-conditions-compendium-of-information-third-edition>). Estimates from the United States are even higher. Some diseases raise the risk of acquiring others; for example, patients with Alzheimer's are more likely to get Parkinson's.

2 SFE the CDC (<http://www.cdc.gov/nchs/fastats/deaths.htm>), which lists the top ten causes of death as 1) heart disease; 2) cancer; 3) chronic lower respiratory diseases; 4) accidents; 5) stroke (cerebrovascular diseases); 6) Alzheimer's disease; 7) diabetes; 8) influenza and pneumonia; 9) nephritis, nephrotic syndrome, and nephrosis; and 10) intentional self-harm (suicide).

3 Statistics are from a British Heart Foundation report on trends in coronary heart disease, available from <https://www.bhf.org.uk/~/media/files/research/heart-statistics/bhf-trends-in-coronary-heart-disease01.pdf>.

4 Listed by the number of deaths they caused in the United Kingdom in 2013, the top five illnesses killing men were ischaemic heart diseases (15.4% of all deaths), cancer of the windpipe and lungs (6.8%), dementia (6.2%), chronic lower respiratory diseases (6.1%), and cerebrovascular diseases (5.7%). For women, dementia topped the list (12.2%), followed by ischaemic heart diseases (10.0%), cerebrovascular diseases (7.9%), influenza and pneumonia (5.9%), and chronic lower respiratory diseases (5.7%).

5 The WHO factsheet on stroke deaths (<http://www.who.int/mediacentre/factsheets/fs317/en/>) refers to data from 2008.

6 The term 'ischaemic' comes from a Greek combination: a verb meaning 'to hold back' or 'restrain', and the noun meaning 'blood'; and in an ischaemic stroke a vessel becomes

blocked by a lump of material (a thrombus), such as a piece of an atherosclerotic plaque; this cuts off the supply to part of the brain. It has been estimated that ischaemic thromboses account for 85% of all strokes (Orlowski, P. *et al.* (2011), 'Modelling of pH dynamics in brain cells after stroke', *Interface Focus*, 1, 408–16).

7 SFE Sabayan, B. *et al.* (2012), 'Cerebrovascular hemodynamics in Alzheimer's disease and vascular dementia: a meta-analysis of transcranial Doppler studies', *Ageing Research Reviews*, 11, 271–7.

8 Amin-Hanjani, S. *et al.* (2015), 'Effect of age and vascular anatomy on blood flow in major cerebral vessels', *Journal of Cerebral Blood Flow and Metabolism*, 35, 312–18.

9 Definitions of high blood pressure vary, but typically a reading of 140 over 90, or higher, would be cause for further investigation. The first number is the systolic pressure—the actual heartbeat, in which blood is ejected into the aorta—and the second the diastolic pressure, when the heart is gathering its energies for the next beat.

10 High salt intake appears to alter blood pressure via effects on pituitary neurons, and can also affect kidney function. A recent review suggests that most of us are now aware that salt is bad for our blood pressure, if somewhat confused about how to reduce our intake (Sarmugam, R. and A. Worsley (2014), 'Current levels of salt knowledge: a review of the literature', *Nutrients*, 6, 5534–59).

11 Deckers, K. *et al.* (2014), 'Target risk factors for dementia prevention: a systematic review and Delphi consensus study on the evidence from observational studies', *International Journal of Geriatric Psychiatry*, 30, 234–46. The risk change percentage is from Barnes, D. E. and K. Yaffe (2011), 'The projected effect of risk factor reduction on Alzheimer's disease prevalence', *Lancet Neurology*, 10, 819–28.

12 Angiotensin also increases sympathetic nervous system activity.

13 Diabetes was first named by a Greek gentleman called Aretaeus of Cappadocia, according to <http://www.diabetes.co.uk/diabetes-history.html>.

14 Blood sugar—glucose—levels are usually measured either directly, when fasting, or by the HbA1c test. This assesses longer-term levels: usually three months or thereabouts, the average lifespan of a red blood cell. The A1c test uses the fact that haemoglobin (Hb) binds to blood glucose, forming glycated haemoglobin. Diabetes is typically diagnosed when HbA1c levels reach 48 mmol/mol, or 6.5% (depending on the test used). For fasting glucose, the diagnosis requires multiple tests and values of ≥ 7.0 mmol/l (from blood plasma) or ≥ 6.1 mmol/l (from whole blood). Note that glucose, not insulin, is used; the former is much easier and cheaper to measure. Note also the different units; conversion charts are available online. Prediabetes is typically indicated by HbA1c levels between 42 and 47 mmol/mol (6.0–6.4%) or glucose between 5.5 and 6.9 mmol/l.

15 Protein consumption also stimulates the liver to produce insulin-like growth factor IGF-1, which, as the name suggests, is similar to insulin and can bind to its receptor (although see note 14.29). IGF-1 is an important regulator of growth, metabolism, longevity, and ageing.

16 The estimates are from Perreault, L. and K. Faerch (2014), 'Approaching pre-diabetes', *Journal of Diabetes and its Complications*, 28, 226–33.

17 'In 2009–2012, based on fasting glucose or A1C levels, 37% of U.S. adults aged 20 years or older had prediabetes (51% of those aged 65 years or older). Applying this percentage

to the entire U.S. population in 2012 yields an estimated 86 million Americans aged 20 years or older with prediabetes.' The quotation is from the CDC, available from <http:// www.cdc.gov/diabetes/pubs/statsreport14/national-diabetes-report-web.pdf>.

18 Mainous, A. G. *et al.* (2014), 'Prevalence of prediabetes in England from 2003 to 2011: population-based, cross-sectional study', *British Medical Journal Open*, 4, e005002. The diabetes statistic is the UK average of 4.6%, according to Diabetes UK (<http://www .diabetes.org.uk/prevalence-2012>).

19 Mainous *et al.* (2014) (note 18).

20 Estimates based on data from the American Diabetes Association (available from <http:// www.diabetes.org/diabetes-basics/statistics/>) suggest that around 1% of diagnosed US diabetics are on dialysis or have had a kidney transplant, and around one-third of a percent suffer 'non-traumatic lower-limb amputations'.

21 Data are for 2010 from the American Diabetes Association (note 20).

22 Janson, J. *et al.* (2004), 'Increased risk of type 2 diabetes in Alzheimer disease', *Diabetes*, 53, 474–81.

23 A 2006 cohort study (not among the nineteen) found no link overall, but in participants without known risk factors like an ApoE4 genotype, there was a statistically significant association (Akomolafe, A. *et al.* (2006), 'Diabetes mellitus and risk of developing Alzheimer disease: results from the Framingham Study', *Archives of Neurology*, 63, 1551–5). The study excluded participants with ApoE risk alleles and/or high homocysteine levels. It found that 'relative risk for AD comparing diabetic patients with nondiabetic patients was 2.98 (95% confidence interval, 1.06–8.39; P = .03)', or higher in patients over seventy-five years of age.

24 Buzsaki, G. *et al.* (2007). 'Inhibition and brain work', *Neuron*, 56, 771–83. Other studies suggest a narrower range of 60–70%. Data are from animal research.

25 Data are from neuroimaging studies (as reported in Shulman, R. G. *et al.* (2009), 'Baseline brain energy supports the state of consciousness', *Proceedings of the National Academy of Sciences*, 106, 11096–101). One mole of glucose weighs just over 180g (see also note 14.14). In physiology, milli-, micro-, or nanomoles (mmol, μmol, or nmol) are more common units.

26 XKCD (<http://xkcd.com/1035/>), source of the soda comparison, also observes that one Cadbury's crème egg contains 20–25g sugar, so 120g is equivalent to 5 or 6 crème eggs a day. This is not an encouragement to eat crème eggs, but an illustration of brains' metabolic rapacity: if your brain were a person, he or she would be eating nearly 10% of his or her body weight in sugar daily, while gradually losing weight (as noted earlier, brains tend to shrink with age). Real persons eat far less, proportionately—UK adults, who weigh on average about 76 kg, consume somewhat over 2 kg of food and drink (less than 4% of their bodyweight) per day—and many are gaining weight.

27 No overall change also allows for the possibility of glucose within the brain moving from one compartment to another (e.g. from astrocytes to neurons). For a review of insulin function in the brain see Ghasemi, R. *et al.* (2013), 'Insulin in the brain: sources, localization and functions', *Molecular Neurobiology*, 47, 145–71.

28 SFE de la Monte, S. M. and J. R. Wands (2008), 'Alzheimer's disease is Type 3 diabetes— evidence reviewed', *Journal of Diabetes Science and Technology*, 2, 1101–13.

ENDNOTES

29 Talbot, K. *et al.* (2012), 'Demonstrated brain insulin resistance in Alzheimer's disease patients is associated with IGF-1 resistance, IRS-1 dysregulation, and cognitive decline', *Journal of Clinical Investigation*, 122, 1316–38. Bear in mind that although the authors refer to their cases being without diabetes, it is not clear from the article whether the brains tested came from people with peripheral insulin resistance, since their pre-death glucose levels are not reported. Furthermore, a clinical diagnosis is typically based on a continuous scale (see note 14.14), on which above a certain point is taken to 'mean' prediabetes, and above a higher point diabetes. A person might therefore be very nearly diabetic without actually having the diagnosis.

30 Talbot *et al.* (2012) also found evidence of brain resistance to IGF-1, which seems to use a different insulin receptor subtype and signalling pathway from insulin, at least in the human brain. Insulin itself seemed to be at normal levels and to be activating the usual intracellular pathways via its receptors.

31 'Controlling for age, education, diabetes duration, fasting blood glucose, vascular and non-vascular risk factors, metformin use showed a significant inverse association with cognitive impairment in longitudinal analysis (OR = 0.49, 95% CI 0.25–0.95)' (Ng, T. P. *et al.* (2014), 'Long-term metformin usage and cognitive function among older adults with diabetes', *Journal of Alzheimer's Disease*, 41, 61–8). OR: odds ratio; CI: confidence interval.

32 SFE Claxton, A. *et al.* (2014), 'Long-acting intranasal insulin detemir improves cognition for adults with mild cognitive impairment or early-stage Alzheimer's disease dementia', *Journal of Alzheimer's Disease*, 44, 897–906.

33 In theory. Because insulin is thought to be involved in regulating the hypothalamus, however, delivering insulin to the brain via intranasal spray could affect metabolism centrally, by altering hypothalamic functions like the control of food and water intake (SFE Ghasemi *et al.* 2013) (note 27). Clinical trials will no doubt be looking out for such side effects.

34 Calling Alzheimer's 'Type 3 diabetes' implies that insulin acts as an energy gatekeeper in the brain—as it does in the body—but more research is needed to determine whether this is the case. The reason is that although insulin encourages cells to import glucose, its role is supervisory. The molecules that do the actual sugar-shifting work are called glucose transporters; and there are various kinds of these, some of which are insulin-sensitive and some of which work very well on their own. Neurons, and their axons, possess both kinds; and astrocytes, microglia, and oligodendrocytes need feeding too; they also have both kinds of glucose transporters. Recent research has confirmed that most neurons, and also the endothelial cells of the blood–brain barrier, get their sugar rush using a type of glucose transporter which is not controlled by insulin (see Gray, S. M. *et al.* (2014), 'Insulin regulates brain function, but how does it get there?' *Diabetes*, 63, 3992–7). Much is yet to be clarified about these molecules and their interactions with insulin in brain tissues, though it is known that they vary from region to region. I would not be surprised if this science changed considerably over the next few years; early conclusions are often rewritten.

35 Winkler, E. A. *et al.* (2015), 'GLUT1 reductions exacerbate Alzheimer's disease vasculo-neuronal dysfunction and degeneration', *Nature Neuroscience*, 18, 521–30. The particular

type of glucose transporter investigated by Winkler *et al.* has also been found to be reduced in Alzheimer's patients.

36 Another problem for the hypothesis is sourcing its insulin. Recall that in type two diabetes insulin resistance is due to high levels of the hormone pulsing repeatedly into the bloodstream. But in the healthy brain insulin is low, so how is it getting enough to bring on insulin resistance? The hormone can be transported across the choroid plexus into the CSF—and hence to brain tissue by way of the Virchow-Robin spaces discussed in Chapter 9. It can also cross the blood–brain barrier; but high blood sugar is thought to reduce this latter capacity rather than increasing it, though the science is not conclusive (Gray *et al.* 2014) (note 34). Research suggests that the first pathway (via the choroid plexus) would be very slow, so the second (via the blood–brain barrier) may be the preferred route. High blood sugar also uses up more peripheral insulin, at least to start with, and this would also reduce the quantities reaching the brain.

37 Talbot *et al.* (2012) (note 30), for example, prefer 'insulin-resistant brain state': a lack of functioning insulin receptors without, as far as we know, the driving sugar surges found in the body. It is not yet clear whether, in a brain somewhat protected by its ability to get glucose through other means, brain insulin resistance could be enough by itself to cause all the symptoms of Alzheimer's, or whether other mechanisms such as mitochondrial dysfunction must also be involved.

38 The nucleus basalis of Meynert, also known as Meynert's nucleus, was named after the nineteenth-century neuroanatomist—and respected poet—Theodor Meynert.

39 Other brain disorders, such as Down's syndrome, are associated with increased risk of certain cancers, like leukaemia, and a lower risk of others, e.g. solid tumours. SFE Tabares-Seisdedos, R. and J. L. Rubenstein (2013), 'Inverse cancer comorbidity: a serendipitous opportunity to gain insight into CNS disorders', *Nature Reviews Neuroscience*, 14, 293–304; and for the numbers, Catala-Lopez, F. *et al.* (2014), 'Inverse and direct cancer comorbidity in people with central nervous system disorders: a meta-analysis of cancer incidence in 577,013 participants of 50 observational studies', *Psychotherapy and Psychosomatics*, 83, 89–105. This meta-analysis found significant effects for Alzheimer's, Parkinson's, MS, and Huntington's, but not amyotrophic lateral sclerosis.

40 As a review in the high-impact journal *Nature Reviews Neuroscience* puts it, 'patients with neurodegenerative disorders (AD, HD, PD, multiple sclerosis and ALS) have a substantially lower overall risk of developing cancer' (Tabares-Seisdedos and Rubenstein 2013) (note 39). AD: Alzheimer's; HD: Huntington's; PD: Parkinson's; ALS: amyotrophic lateral sclerosis.

41 Another candidate is the important regulatory protein PIN1 (peptidyl-prolyl *cis-trans* isomerase NIMA-interacting 1). PIN1 is a prolyl isomerase: it operates on the amino acid proline, which exists in two distinct, differently shaped forms (isomers). PIN1 switches proline from one form to the other, altering its function.

42 Aubry, S. *et al.* (2015), 'Assembly and interrogation of Alzheimer's disease genetic networks reveal novel regulators of progression', *PLoS One*, 10, e0120352.

43 Neural stem cells initially divide repeatedly in two. Later they start dividing asymmetrically, producing one mature neuron and one neural stem cell. Eventually the neurons stop dividing (becoming 'post-mitotic').

44 Microglia are often described as 'myeloid', a term used to describe immune cells originating from stem cells in bone marrow (as opposed to 'lymphoid' cells like T lymphocytes which are born in lymphatic tissues like the thymus). However, recent research suggests that microglia may derive from stem cells in the embryonic yolk sac—which exists in humans as well as birds, and provides early access to nutrients while the placenta develops.

45 Origins matter: astrocytes born from neural stem cells behave differently from astrocytes derived from oligodendrocyte precursors.

46 I am grateful to the organizers of the second Oxford Dementia Research Day, held on 16 July 2015 at St John's College Oxford, for allowing me to attend and sample researchers' immense enthusiasm about stem cell research.

47 Scientists' enthusiasm about new methods can sometimes distract them from the need to stay focused on patients: cells, after all, are much easier to deal with and understand. Good criticism—a pearl beyond price, though it may not feel like it to the recipient—is essential to keep that focus and find the quickest, most efficient route to successful treatments for neurodegeneration. For example, one stem cell critic at the Oxford Dementia Research Day in June 2015 noted doubts about how well stem cells model mature neurons and their environment, and over the techniques used to derive them. (These were developed in mice, which are not necessarily the same in all relevant cellular respects.)

48 The quotation is from Gold, P. W. (2015), 'The organization of the stress system and its dysregulation in depressive illness', *Molecular Psychiatry*, 20, 32–47.

49 The estimate of global depression prevalence is from the WHO, available from <http://www.who.int/mediacentre/factsheets/fs369/en/>.

50 Deckers *et al.* (2014) cite the relative risk for dementia/depression as 1.85, following Diniz, B. S. *et al.* (2013), 'Late-life depression and risk of vascular dementia and Alzheimer's disease: systematic review and meta-analysis of community-based cohort studies', *British Journal of Psychiatry*, 202, 329–35.

51 The odds ratios were 1.85 and 1.66 for dementia, 2.52 and 1.89 for vascular dementia, in the two meta-analyses (Diniz *et al.* (2013) (note 50) and Gao, Y. *et al.* (2013), 'Depression as a risk factor for dementia and mild cognitive impairment: a meta-analysis of longitudinal studies', *International Journal of Geriatric Psychiatry*, 28, 441–9).

52 For an impression of some of the biochemical and physiological mechanisms thought to be at play in depression, see the abstract of Lang and Borgwardt (2013) (note 13.64), which is basically a list of them.

53 A study of extreme stress, however, found that survivors of the Holocaust and concentration camps were not at increased risk of dementia (Ravona-Springer, R. *et al.* (2011), 'Exposure to the Holocaust and World War II concentration camps during late adolescence and adulthood is not associated with increased risk for dementia at old age', *Journal of Alzheimer's Disease*, 23, 709–16). Survivor bias may be relevant here. As the authors comment, 'Individuals who survived concentration camps and then lived into old age may carry survival advantages that are associated with protection from dementia and mortality.'

54 The SNS uses the neurotransmitters acetylcholine and noradrenaline.

55 The HPA axis is regulated by brain areas including the prefrontal cortex, amygdala, and hippocampus. It is activated when the hypothalamus releases corticotropin-releasing hormone (CRH). This stimulates the pituitary to release ACTH into the bloodstream. When ACTH reaches the adrenal glands, which sit above the kidneys, it triggers the release of glucocorticoids—cortisol in humans, corticosterone in rodents—into the bloodstream. I have simplified: other substances such as vasopressin (from the hypothalamus) and aldosterone (from the adrenal glands) are also released. They are needed to mediate the numerous effects of the stress response, such as changes in blood pressure. The two branches of the stress response interact. Adrenaline boosts the production of CRH and ACTH, enhancing HPA axis activity. Cortisol, however, reduces CRH production, damping it down.

56 Gerstein, M. B. *et al.* (2014), 'Comparative analysis of the transcriptome across distant species', *Nature*, 512, 445–8.

57 Less flexible neurotransmission due to poorer synaptic plasticity, reduced neurogenesis, and dying dendrites have been observed in animal brains chronically exposed to glucocorticoids, and some people with depression have high blood cortisol levels.

58 This is poetic licence and entirely inappropriate for a science book. In reality, the Greek verb from which we get 'hormesis' means 'to stimulate' or 'urge on'.

59 The physiology of young children is in some ways more flexible than that of adults, but also more vulnerable to abnormal environmental factors. In particular, there seem to be 'critical periods' of development for certain brain and body systems, such as vision and language. Problems during this time can have a lifelong impact. It has recently been suggested, following a study of orphaned children either fostered or raised institutionally, that the stress response also has a particularly sensitive period (before age two), with autonomic and HPA axis reactivity being significantly blunted in the institutionally raised children (McLaughlin, K.A. *et al.* (2015), 'Causal effects of the early caregiving environment on development of stress response systems in children', *Proceedings of the National Academy of Sciences*, 112, 5637–42).

Chapter 15

1 Since Karl Marx's famous critique in *Das Kapital* (1867), many authors have commented on the problems with consumerism. It is environmentally destructive. It depends on feelings, both pleasurable and aversive—lust and envy, contempt and anxiety, the sense of belonging and the sense of control—and these may lead us to act against our own rational self-interest. You might expect experience to have an impact on our ability to be rational, but in one respect at least that appears not to be the case. A study of people who have spent years bargaining over policy—and who might therefore be expected to have honed their rational capacities to excellence—found that if anything they are more likely to act against self-interest (LeVeck, B. L. *et al.* (2014), 'The role of self-interest in elite bargaining', *Proceedings of the National Academy of Sciences*, 111, 18536–41).

Consumerism also favours youth over age and short-term desires over long-term ones, as indeed our brains evolved to do. And it is biased against reasoning, because when people think about products they all too often decide they don't really need them. This is why so much marketing is focused on making the time between desire-creation and purchase as short as possible; or on distracting the buyer while they buy; or on presenting them with so much choice that to avoid sensory overload they grab the nearest or nicest-looking package—without doing detailed checks on value and—for food—nutritional content.

2 One estimate by the *Grocer* magazine (reported by the BBC at <http://www.bbc.co.uk/news/business-16450526>) reckoned that in 1852 UK citizens spent about one-third of their income on food, while today they spend about one-tenth.

3 Bilton, R. (2013), 'Averting comfortable lifestyle crises', *Science Progress*, 96, 319–68.

4 It has also been suggested that the human taste for spices evolved because they have anti-microbial properties, and are hence protective in areas with a high pathogen load.

5 Hidaka, B. H. (2012), 'Depression as a disease of modernity: explanations for increasing prevalence', *Journal of Affective Disorders*, 140, 205–14.

6 Chan, K. Y. *et al.* (2013), 'Epidemiology of Alzheimer's disease and other forms of dementia in China, 1990–2010: a systematic review and analysis', *Lancet*, 381, 2016–23. The researchers found that the prevalence of dementia also rose: 'in 1990 [it] ranged from 0.5% in people aged 55–59 years to 42.1% in people aged 95–99 years'. In 2010, the equivalent figures were 0.7% and 60.5%, suggesting that the growth in numbers is not simply down to increased longevity.

7 Statistics are from the NHS, available from <http://www.nhs.uk/Livewell/loseweight/Pages/BodyMassIndex.aspx>. BMI is easily calculated as $weight/(height)^2$ if you operate in metres and kilogrammes; if in pounds and inches, multiply by 703. Note that BMI has been much criticized. It is less useful for very tall or short people or those who are very heavily muscled, and it does not take account of where on the body the fat is; thus apparently slim people may have high levels of fat around their internal organs. However, not every medical practice has the means to do detailed body composition analysis, so BMI is commonly used.

8 The connection between income and obesity is complex. Correlating nation-level data for 2010 from the UN and WHO suggests that greater wealth (GDP per person) is associated with greater BMI, but only in low-income countries, and more for men (r = 0.60) than for women (r = 0.46). In medium- and high-income countries, there is no statistically significant correlation.

9 BMI data were sourced from the WHO, or for older data see Finucane, M. M. *et al.* (2011), 'National, regional, and global trends in body-mass index since 1980: systematic analysis of health examination surveys and epidemiological studies with 960 country-years and 9.1 million participants', *Lancet*, 377, 557–67.

10 Deckersbach, T. *et al.* (2014), 'Pilot randomized trial demonstrating reversal of obesity-related abnormalities in reward system responsivity to food cues with a behavioral intervention', *Nutrition and Diabetes*, 4, e129.

11 Sumithran, P. *et al.* (2011), 'Long-term persistence of hormonal adaptations to weight loss', *New England Journal of Medicine*, 365, 1597–604.

12 Deckers *et al.* (2014) (note 14.11).

13 BMI is influenced by genetic variations—for instance, in the FTO (fat-and-obesity-associated) gene—which have also been linked to Alzheimer's. FTO is thought to interact with ApoE.

14 A figure for the daily calorie intake of 'as little as 400–800 calories/d' is from Schulz, L. C. (2010), 'The Dutch Hunger Winter and the developmental origins of health and disease', *Proceedings of the National Academy of Sciences*, 107, 16757–8. Recommended levels are 2,500 calories for men and 2,000 for women, according to the NHS (<http://www.nhs.uk/chq/pages/1126.aspx?categoryid=51>), with 200 extra per day in the last three months of pregnancy.

15 Autism and attention-deficit-hyperactivity-disorder (ADHD) are among the disorders that have been linked to parental obesity.

16 Qizilbash, N. *et al.* (2015). 'BMI and risk of dementia in two million people over two decades: a retrospective cohort study', *Lancet Diabetes and Endocrinology*, 3, 431–6. Needless to say the article, which unfortunately is not open-access (as of March 2016), attracted considerable comment: SFE Gustafson, D. (2015), 'BMI and dementia: feast or famine for the brain?' in the same issue (no. 6), pages 397–8, and the authors' reply in the following issue, pp. 501–2.

17 This is an example of a controversial phenomenon called the obesity paradox: some studies have observed, in some circumstances, that being overweight is associated with better health than normal weight. What those circumstances may be, how real the effect is, and what it means are not yet clear.

18 Fox, M. *et al.* (2013), 'Maternal breastfeeding history and Alzheimer's disease risk', *Journal of Alzheimer's Disease*, 37, 809–21.

19 Wobst, H. J. *et al.* (2015), 'The green tea polyphenol (−)-epigallocatechin gallate prevents the aggregation of tau protein into toxic oligomers at substoichiometric ratios', *FEBS Letters*, 589, 77–83.

20 For example, a 2013 study found an association of low meat intake with better cognitive health five years later (Titova, O. E. *et al.* (2013), 'Mediterranean diet habits in older individuals: associations with cognitive functioning and brain volumes', *Experimental Gerontology*, 48, 1443–8).

21 Ozawa, M. *et al.* (2014), 'Milk and dairy consumption and risk of dementia in an elderly Japanese population: the Hisayama Study', *Journal of the American Geriatrics Society*, 62, 1224–30. The study sampled 1,081 people aged sixty or older who did not have dementia and followed them up for seventeen years to see how many developed the disease. Of the 303 who did, 166 had Alzheimer's (AD) and ninety-eight had vascular dementia. 'After adjusting for potential confounders, the linear relationship between milk and dairy intake and development of AD remained significant (P for trend = .03)': suggestive perhaps, but by no means conclusive.

22 A 2011 meta-analysis did not find signs of altered iron or zinc levels in Alzheimer's, but copper levels were reduced (Schrag, M. *et al.* (2011), 'Iron, zinc and copper in the Alzheimer's disease brain: a quantitative meta-analysis. Some insight on the influence of citation bias on scientific opinion', *Progress in Neurobiology*, 94, 296–306). The absence of overall changes does not rule out an alteration in transition metal metabolism, given the complexity of these systems. Iron, for example, can be stored in different 'pools' within the brain (e.g. at different sites or bound to different carrier proteins), and imbalances between these could result in, for instance, increased oxidative stress on neurons. The concept of multiple pools is also relevant to other chemicals of interest in Alzheimer's,

such as copper, cholesterol, and Aβ. Note that a more recent study of the iron storage protein ferritin in CSF found higher levels at baseline to be associated with progression to more serious cognitive impairment. Levels of ferritin and brain APOE were also correlated and APOE4 carriers had higher levels of ferritin. See Ayton, S. *et al.* (2015), 'Ferritin levels in the cerebrospinal fluid predict Alzheimer's disease outcomes and are regulated by APOE', *Nature Communications*, 6, 6760.

23 The implication is that meat-eaters would be more likely than vegetarians to develop iron deposits in brain blood vessels as they age, even if both were to consume the same amount of dietary iron.

24 The quotation is from the WHO's information on nutrition, available from <http://www.who.int/nutrition/topics/ida/en/>.

25 Crespo, T. C. *et al.* (2014), 'Genetic and biochemical markers in patients with Alzheimer's disease support a concerted systemic iron homeostasis dysregulation', *Neurobiology of Aging*, 35, 777–85.

26 Both iron and IL-1 can bind to APP mRNA *in vitro* to stimulate production of APP and sAPPα.

27 Some studies have found an anti-oxidant role for Aβ and some see it as increasing oxidative stress. It may, of course, do both, depending on the circumstances.

28 Among the many effects of RAGE activation appears to be the triggering of abnormal cell re-entry into the cell cycle.

29 Fibre slows the digestion of carbohydrates, thereby smoothing out the insulin spikes that are thought to push the body towards type two diabetes. It also binds numerous molecules including fats and cholesterol, soaking them up and carrying them from the body during excretion.

30 SFE Stewart, R. *et al.* (2015), 'Associations between skeletal growth in childhood and cognitive function in mid-life in a 53-year prospective birth cohort study', *PloS One*, 10, e0124163. The study links reduced growth to lower cognitive function at ages fifteen and fifty-three.

31 Katz, D. and S. Meller (2014). 'Can we say what diet is best for health?' *Annual Review of Public Health*, 35, 83–103.

32 Pollan, M. (2008), *In Defense of Food: An Eater's Manifesto* (New York: Penguin).

33 See the Alzheimer's Society website (<http://www.alzheimers.org.uk/site/scripts/documents_info.php?documentID=429>): 'In 2010, the total spent on dementia research was £50.2 million, of which just over £36 million came from government funding and nearly £14 million from charitable funding.' The Society also notes the illogic of this disparity in terms of healthcare costs: 'Comparatively, the combined costs to the UK economy of cancer and heart disease are around the same as dementia, yet the spending on cancer research alone is £521 million a year (Cancer Research UK 2013).'

34 Details of the National Health and Nutrition Examination Survey can be found at the CDC (<http://www.cdc.gov/nchs/nhanes.htm>).

35 Archer, E. *et al.* (2013), 'Validity of U.S. nutritional surveillance: National Health and Nutrition Examination Survey caloric energy intake data, 1971–2010', *PloS One*, 8, e76632.

Chapter 16

1 The study gives statistics for the unfit-dementia association as follows: 'hazard ratio 2.49, 95%, confidence interval 1.87–3.32' (Nyberg, J. *et al.* (2014), 'Cardiovascular and cognitive fitness at age 18 and risk of early-onset dementia', *Brain*, 137, 1514–23).

2 A study of elderly Norwegian men found that those who did most exercise lived longer, and the effects were sizeable: 'Increase in PA [physical activity] was as beneficial as smoking cessation in reducing mortality'—by about 40%. See Holme, I. and S. A. Anderssen (2015), 'Increases in physical activity is as important as smoking cessation for reduction in total mortality in elderly men: 12 years of follow-up of the Oslo II study', *British Journal of Sports Medicine*, 49, 743–8.

3 Some commentators emphasize the oversupply of energy-rich, poor-quality food, arguing that while it supplies more energy than we can use, its lack of essential nutrients, as well as its tastiness, may actually drive us to eat more. They blame Big Food and Big Beverage, and government, for creating an 'obesogenic' environment. Others suggest that modern life has made us slothful, blaming the social structures that make activity and healthy eating difficult. They cite the convenience of Western transport, public and private, the design of cities, pressures on time, the nature of work, and the cultural values which exalt sitting at a desk as economically productive while reducing exercise to the marginal status of 'leisure activity'. Even structures as intangible as a person's beliefs about the causes of obesity may affect their weight: those who blame lack of exercise are more likely to be oversized than those who blame poor diet (McFerran, B. and A. Mukhopadhyay (2013), 'Lay theories of obesity predict actual body mass', *Psychological Science*, 24, 1428–36). Combining these positions is the argument that both gluttony and sloth may be to blame.

  Still others complain of a moral decline, usually somehow linked to the provision of welfare, which has led individuals to abdicate personal responsibility for their health. This claim is often made by food industry representatives. They are correct that you and you alone decide what food you eat and how much exercise you take (usually, for adults). But if you do not have clear information—or cannot get it quickly and easily—can you be blamed for making the wrong decision? And information about food, exercise, and the links between them is far from clear—a state of affairs for which the media, industry, and government all bear responsibility. For example, in the United Kingdom some manufacturers have a 'traffic-light' system which shows at a glance which foods are high in fat, salt, and sugar. Attempts to introduce this easily readable colour coding across the entire market, however, have so far met with resistance from manufacturers and indifference from the media and government.

4 Data are from the WHO report on global health risks cited in note 11.59.

5 The WHO ranking of health risks by mortality in high-income countries is as follows: high blood glucose (0.6 million), physical inactivity (0.6 million), overweight and obesity (0.7 million), high blood pressure (1.4 million), tobacco use (1.5 million).

6 The full guidelines are available from the US government at <http://www.health.gov/paguidelines/guidelines/>.

7 The NHS (<http://www.nhs.uk/Livewell/fitness/Pages/physical-activity-guidelines-for-adults.aspx>) gives further details on what kinds of exercise count as moderate or vigorous.

8 Data are from a 2015 WHO statement on exercise, available from <http://www.who.int/mediacentre/factsheets/fs385/en/>.

9 Gurven, M. *et al.* (2009), 'Inflammation and infection do not promote arterial aging and cardiovascular disease risk factors among lean horticulturalists', *PloS One*, 4, e6590.

Chapter 17

1 Anstey *et al.* (2007). For the full reference see note 10.7.

2 Nicotine activates the nicotinic acetylcholine receptor subtype.

3 Of the forty-three studies reviewed by Cataldo *et al.* (2010), the three cohort studies with industry affiliation were smaller than all but two of the fourteen non-affiliated studies, and nine of the latter were more than twice the size of the largest industry-affiliated study. In total, industry-related studies included 1,290 people; non-affiliated studies included a little over 320,000. For case-control studies, the eight linked to industry averaged more than twice the size of the eighteen non-affiliated studies, and the total sample included was just under 6,000 in both cases. For the full reference see note 10.5.

4 Cohort studies have other problems too. Over time people drop out, and this can cause attrition bias if those who leave are different from those who stay in some relevant aspect (e.g. cardiac health or baseline cognitive function). It can be tricky to obtain representative samples. If possible, participants should be drawn from several sources, not just the nearest care home. As we saw earlier, controlling for covariates is a fraught endeavour, and measurement techniques may change over time. Available knowledge may also change, such that the variables which researchers decided not to record at the study's start may be the ones they end up wishing they had recorded. Sometimes participants may also get better at doing tests when these are repeated.

5 Beecham, G. W. *et al.* (2014), 'Genome-wide association meta-analysis of neuropathologic features of Alzheimer's disease and related dementias', *PLoS Genetics*, 10, e1004606.

6 Ideally, a meta-analysis should allow some assessment to be made of how varied the literature is, whether there is publication bias, and whether there are significant effects that may have been missed, or only hinted at, by individual studies because of their smaller sample sizes.

7 The key to meta-analysis, apart from doing a properly systematic review, is the choices made about which studies are included—decisions which should be reported fully in the write-up. As well as excluding studies without baseline dementia and smoking measures, Anstey and colleagues ruled out any research that didn't have at least two measures of cognitive performance and/or dementia status. They excluded any research with fewer than fifty participants, and they only looked at non-clinical samples—even if the illness in question was apparently unrelated, like HIV infection. They also wrote to the authors of studies with missing data, did a lot of work to get the data they did have into compatible form, and dealt with multiple reports from the same study group.

8 For 'ever/never smokers, relative risk (RR) 0.64, 95% confidence interval (CI) 0.54–0.76'
   (Lee, P. N. (1994), 'Smoking and Alzheimer's disease: a review of the epidemiological
   evidence', *Neuroepidemiology*, 13, 131–44).

9 Cataldo *et al.* (2010) (note 10.5). The study is available from *PubMed* (<http://www.ncbi.
   nlm.nih.gov/pmc/articles/PMC2906761/>) if you wish to compare their selection criteria
   with those of Anstey *et al.* (2007) (note 10.7).

10 The author of Lee (1994) is listed on that paper simply as 'P. N. Lee Statistics and
   Computing Limited, Sutton, UK', but a search of the US Legacy Tobacco Documents
   Library reveals that Peter Lee has worked extensively for the industry.

11 Cataldo *et al.* (2010) (note 10.5) report data as follows (TIA: tobacco industry affiliation;
   CC: case-control study; COH: cohort study):

Non-TIA CC (n = 18)	pooled odds ratio =	0.91 (95% CI 0.75–1.10)
TIA CC (n = 8)	pooled odds ratio =	0.86 (95% CI 0.75–0.98)
Non-TIA COH (n = 14)	pooled relative risk =	1.45 (95% CI 1.16–1.80)
TIA COH (n = 3)	pooled relative risk =	0.60 (95% CI 0.27–1.32).

12 Zhong, G. *et al.* (2015), 'Smoking is associated with an increased risk of dementia: a
   meta-analysis of prospective cohort studies with investigation of potential effect
   modifiers', *PLoS One*, 10, e0118333.

13 Karama, S. *et al.* (2015), 'Cigarette smoking and thinning of the brain's cortex', *Molecular
   Psychiatry*, 20, 778–85. The study did MRI on 504 people in their seventies without
   apparent dementia. Comparisons between ex-smokers and current-smokers (0.56), ex-
   and never-smokers (0.29), and current- and never-smokers (0.81) were all significant with
   a p value < 0.01. The figures in brackets are effect sizes.

14 Alcohol seems to affect particularly subcortical areas such as the hypothalamus and
   cerebellum, hippocampal areas—possibly by affecting neurogenesis—and the prefrontal
   cortex, long associated with impulse control. (Like a clever virus, excessive drinking
   attacks the very systems needed to stop it.)

15 Alcohol may act as a mild stressor, i.e. via hormesis.

16 Anstey, K. J. *et al.* (2009), 'Alcohol consumption as a risk factor for dementia and cognitive
   decline: meta-analysis of prospective studies', *American Journal of Geriatric Psychiatry*, 17,
   542–55; Neafsey, E. J. and M. A. Collins (2011), 'Moderate alcohol consumption and
   cognitive risk', *Neuropsychiatric Disease and Treatment*, 7, 465–84.

17 Neafsey and Collins (2011) (note 16). At the time of this research, the UK government
   classified 'safe' drinking levels as two drinks per day for men, one for women; but in 2016,
   as this book went to press, new proposed guidelines were issued which reduced the level
   to fourteen units per week, ideally spread over time, for both sexes. The review that gave
   rise to the new advice was conducted in 2015 by the Committee on Carcinogenicity
   of Chemicals in Food, Consumer Products and the Environment (CoC) and published
   in 2016.

18 The CoC review cited in the previous note found that 'people who drink even low levels
   of alcohol have a greater risk of getting cancers of the mouth and throat, gullet, and of
   breast cancer in women than people who do not drink alcohol at all. Drinking
   approximately 1.5 units per day (10.5 units per week) or more increases the risk of cancers

of the voice box and large bowel, whilst cancers of the liver and pancreas are more common in people who drink approximately six units per day (forty-two units per week) or more. The risk of getting these cancers increases the more alcohol a person drinks.' The review gives relative risks (RRs) from the studies it assessed. Taking the largest cited RRs for each cancer type gives risk estimates which are highest for head, neck, mouth, and throat cancers (RR between 3.63 and 6.62), and lower for cancers of the larynx (RR = 2.65), liver (RR = 2.07), large bowel (RR = 1.82), female breast, and pancreas (RR = 1.61 and 1.60, respectively).

19 Excessive drinking may go with less healthy eating, and in some cases weight gain—although any link with obesity is complex and not well understood.

20 The Greek word for plant, φυτόν, is usually rendered 'phyton' rather than 'futon'. Phytochemicals are chemicals made by plants, and phytophenols are polyphenols made by plants. Polyphenols are molecules containing more than one phenol ring—a hexagon of six carbon atoms with one hydroxyl group attached.

21 Among the best known, and most-hyped, polyphenols are a group of structurally similar molecules called flavonoids. They offer beauty as well as—possibly—health, since among them are the anthocyanins. These are behind the colour changes of leaves in autumn, and they give colour to many vegetables. Flavonoids in turn include chemicals called flavonols and other, very similar chemicals confusingly called flavanols. Both seem to be beneficial, as are many other phytochemicals, though more research in humans is needed to confirm this.

22 The risk/benefit balance of various soy compounds for cancer, heart disease, menopause, osteoporosis, thyroid function, etc. remains controversial. How the food is processed appears to make a considerable difference. For an introduction to the topic see Harvard University's 'Straight talk about soy', available from <http://www.hsph.harvard.edu/nutritionsource/2014/02/12/straight-talk-about-soy/>.

23 You would have to drink a lot of cups of coffee to overdose on caffeine, but as it is also found in medicines and energy drinks, ingesting high levels of caffeine is easier than one might expect.

24 For example, the phytophenol resveratrol is found in grapes and available as a health supplement despite little evidence of its long-term benefits in humans—except that if they study it they get to go to conferences in Hawaii (SFE <http://resveratrol2014.hawaii-conference.com/>). It appears to prolong the life and vitality of lab rats, and reduce the risk of various diseases, including cancer and diabetes. Large-scale clinical trials in people are awaited.

Chapter 18

1 As for many risk factors, the epidemiological evidence varies greatly in quality and quantity.

2 Note that some authorities refer to arsenic as a metal, some call it a semi-metal and some a metalloid; all agree, however, that large quantities of the stuff are bad for you.

3 Bhatt, D. P. *et al.* (2015), 'A pilot study to assess effects of long-term inhalation of airborne particulate matter on early Alzheimer-like changes in the mouse brain', *PLoS*

One, 10, e0127102. Interestingly, the study did not find an effect on tau protein phosphorylation.

4   Ejaz, S. *et al.* (2014), 'MRI and neuropathological validations of the involvement of air pollutants in cortical selective neuronal loss', *Environmental Science and Pollution Research*, 21, 3351–62.

5   Calderón-Garcidueñas *et al.* (2012) (note 6.11).

6   Chang, K. H. *et al.* (2014), 'Increased risk of dementia in patients exposed to nitrogen dioxide and carbon monoxide: a population-based retrospective cohort study', *PloS One*, 9, e103078.

7   Richardson, J. R. *et al.* (2014), 'Elevated serum pesticide levels and risk for Alzheimer disease', *Journal of the American Medical Association Neurology*, 71, 284–90.

8   Ruder, A. M. *et al.* (2014), 'Mortality among 24,865 workers exposed to polychlorinated biphenyls (PCBs) in three electrical capacitor manufacturing plants: a ten-year update', *International Journal of Hygiene and Environmental Health*, 217, 176–87.

9   For example, a population-based study in Denmark found little effect of living within 50 metres of a power line (Frei, P. *et al.* (2013), 'Residential distance to high-voltage power lines and risk of neurodegenerative diseases: a Danish population-based case-control study', *American Journal of Epidemiology*, 177, 970–8). An earlier twin study found a hint of a relationship between low-frequency electromagnetic field exposure in manual occupations and earlier onset dementia risk (Andel, R. *et al.* (2010), 'Work-related exposure to extremely low-frequency magnetic fields and dementia: results from the population-based study of dementia in Swedish twins', *Journals of Gerontology. Series A, Biological Sciences and Medical Sciences*, 65, 1220–7). And a study in rats reckoned that exposure might actually be beneficial for Alzheimer-like symptoms (Liu, X. *et al.* (2015), 'Improvement of spatial memory disorder and hippocampal damage by exposure to electromagnetic fields in an Alzheimer's disease rat model', *PLoS One*, 10, e0126963).

10 Ionizing radiation, such as X-rays, has sufficient energy to be able to disrupt molecules by interfering with electrons, and is thus a potential source of molecular changes, including DNA mutations.

11 SFE the American Psychological Association's resolution on poverty and socioeconomic status, adopted in 2000, which lays out numerous reasons why poverty is a problem, available from <http://www.apa.org/about/policy/poverty-resolution.aspx>. It has, for instance, been linked to signs of cellular ageing (Park, M. *et al.* (2015), 'Where you live may make you old: the association between perceived poor neighborhood quality and leukocyte telomere length', *PLoS One*, 10, e0128460), and to brain structure: a large neuroimaging study suggests that kids from low-income households have smaller brain surface areas (Noble, K. G. *et al.* (2015), 'Family income, parental education and brain structure in children and adolescents', *Nature Neuroscience*, 18, 773–8).

12 The Avon Longitudinal Study of Parents and Children recruited over 14,000 pregnant women from the Bristol area in 1991–1992 and has studied them and their children ever since, collecting a wide range of biological, social, and psychological data.

13 Children born in Scotland took a test of their cognitive ability at eleven years old. When the archived results of two such cohorts, born in 1921 and 1936, were discovered,

researchers at the University of Edinburgh working on how cognition changes with age realized they had a potential data goldmine, and began tracing the participants. The result was the two now much-studied Lothian Birth Cohorts, source of some fascinating research.

14 Moreover, in cultures where money is coveted and poverty is seen as shameful, financial deprivation can also inflict a sense of being powerless, insecure, and despised which is terribly damaging for any human creature. (Wars have been fought over lesser insults, though only by people who have the means to fight.) The tendency to see others as less than human, which helps the better-off distance themselves from those less fortunate, leads to poorer people being blamed for their situation despite the fact that they lack the money and power to do anything about it. As I argue in my book *Cruelty* (note 2.2), this 'otherization', with its associated feelings of contempt and disgust, is tightly bound up with social power and does an immense amount of harm. Individual variables, like genes, trauma and accident, and personal beliefs and attitudes—such as whether a person feels in control of their destiny or not—are also relevant, of course. But it is hard to feel empowered when you're getting messages from society that you are not in control, never have been, and never will be, because you aren't worthy of it.

15 Kivimäki, M. *et al.* (2014), 'Long working hours, socioeconomic status, and the risk of incident type 2 diabetes: a meta-analysis of published and unpublished data from 222 120 individuals', *Lancet Diabetes and Endocrinology*, 3, 27–34.

16 A systematic review of risk factor research judged the overall quality of evidence to be low (Plassman, B. L. *et al.* (2010), 'Systematic review: factors associated with risk for and possible prevention of cognitive decline in later life', *Annals of Internal Medicine*, 153, 182–93).

17 Qian, W. *et al.* (2014), 'Impact of socioeconomic status on initial clinical presentation to a memory disorders clinic', *International Psychogeriatrics*, 26, 597–603.

18 Goldbourt, U. *et al.* (2007), 'Socioeconomic status in relationship to death of vascular disease and late-life dementia', *Journal of the Neurological Sciences*, 257, 177–81. SES was divided into five categories. For dementia prevalence, the odds ratios for the two lowest categories (2 and 1) relative to the highest (5) were 3.09 (1.83–5.21) and 5.99 (3.50–10.26), respectively. Figures in brackets are 95% confidence intervals.

19 Fischer, C. *et al.* (2009), 'Impact of socioeconomic status on the prevalence of dementia in an inner city memory disorders clinic', *International Psychogeriatrics*, 21, 1096–104.

20 The hazard ratio was 0.49 (Zeki Al Hazzouri, A. *et al.* (2011), 'Life-course socioeconomic position and incidence of dementia and cognitive impairment without dementia in older Mexican Americans: results from the Sacramento Area Latino Study on Aging', *American Journal of Epidemiology*, 173, 1148–58).

21 Fernald, L. C. *et al.* (2008), 'Role of cash in conditional cash transfer programmes for child health, growth, and development: an analysis of Mexico's Oportunidades', *Lancet*, 371, 828–37.

22 Schoeni, R. F. *et al.* (2011), 'The economic value of improving the health of disadvantaged Americans', *American Journal of Preventive Medicine*, 40, S67–72.

23 Taking naps may help to some extent.

24 Statistics are from the UK government's Health and Social Care Information Centre (<http://www.hscic.gov.uk/catalogue/PUB16076/HSE2013-Ch6-sft-wrk.pdf>).

25 Microglial release of cytokines and reactivity to immune stimuli show a circadian rhythm, according to work in rats (Fonken, L. K. *et al.* (2015), 'Microglia inflammatory responses are controlled by an intrinsic circadian clock', *Brain, Behavior, and Immunity*, 45, 171–9).

26 Punjabi, N. M. (2008), 'The epidemiology of adult obstructive sleep apnea', *Proceedings of American Thoracic Society*, 5, 136–43. For a guide to sleep apnoea (the term comes from the Greek for 'no breath'), see the NHS (<http://www.nhs.uk/conditions/Sleep-apnoea/Pages/Introduction.aspx>).

Chapter 19

1 Wang, H.-X. *et al.* (2012), 'Education halves the risk of dementia due to apolipoprotein ε4 allele: a collaborative study from the Swedish Brain Power initiative', *Neurobiology of Aging*, 33, 1007.e1-7.

2 The speech 'All the world's a stage' is from Shakespeare's play *As You Like It*.

3 'The Pythagoreans divided the life of mankind into four ages, that of a child, a lad, a young man, and an old man; and they said that each one of these had its parallel in the changes which take place in the seasons' (Diodorus Siculus (1946), 'Fragments of Book IX', *Library of History*, (Cambridge, MA: Loeb Classical Library: Harvard University Press), IV, 69. The old man, needless to say, was assigned winter. Many later thinkers viewed life as having seven stages, of which the last (age 63+) was marked by failing body and mind. Pythagoras is thought to have been born in 580 BC or thereabouts, Aristotle roughly two centuries later.

4 Demosthenes (1936), 'Against Stephanus', *Private Orations* (Cambridge, MA: Loeb Classical Library: Harvard University Press), II, 14–17.

5 Cicero, M. T. (1923), *De Senectute* (Cambridge, MA: Loeb Classical Library: Harvard University Press). Cicero didn't live long enough to test his hypothesis; he was murdered in his sixties.

6 Not all studies have found an effect of education in delaying Alzheimer's onset. SFE a small study in a low-education sample by de Oliveira, F. F. *et al.* (2014), 'Risk factors for age at onset of dementia due to Alzheimer's disease in a sample of patients with low mean schooling from Sao Paulo, Brazil', *International Journal of Geriatric Psychiatry*, 29, 1033–9.

7 See Murdoch's 2004 entry, by her biographer Peter Conradi, in the *Oxford Dictionary of National Biography*.

8 For example, a large study that took into account a number of possible biases (e.g. attrition), found that education, while strongly associated with cognitive performance at the start (baseline), probably did not influence the rate of decline (Gottesman, R. F. *et al.* (2014), 'Impact of differential attrition on the association of education with cognitive change over 20 years of follow-up', *American Journal of Epidemiology*, 179, 956–66).

9 Some patients do indeed express a 'wish to hasten death', although what they appear to mean by this can vary. Such patients are, however, typically facing severe suffering, such as advanced cancer. It is not clear from the literature whether patients with advanced dementia have such wishes, and if so what they would mean, although earlier in the

disease a raised risk of suicide has been reported. The role of depression also needs to be considered.

10 Gutman, S. A. and V. P. Schindler (2007), 'The neurological basis of occupation', *Occupational Therapy International*, 14, 71–85.

11 Fritsch, T. *et al.* (2005), 'Associations between dementia/mild cognitive impairment and cognitive performance and activity levels in youth', *Journal of American Geriatrics Society*, 53, 1191–6.

12 Deckers *et al.* (2014) (note 14.11).

13 The hazard ratio was 0.74 (Crooks, V. C. *et al.* (2008), 'Social network, cognitive function, and dementia incidence among elderly women', *American Journal of Public Health*, 98, 1221–7). Of course, one's propensity to form large social networks depends on personality as well as opportunity, and personality may affect dementia risk in its own right. Research has suggested, for example, that high neuroticism and anxiety may be linked to an increased risk of dementia, whereas high openness to experience and conscientiousness may be protective.

14 See the *Loneliness and Isolation Evidence Review* by Age UK, available from <http://www .ageuk.org.uk/documents/en-gb/for-professionals/evidence_review_loneliness_and _isolation.pdf?dtrk=true>.

15 The same small study also suggested that those who blamed themselves for their illness got more lonely, emphasizing the role that beliefs about illness can have in making it worse (Barlow, M. A. *et al.* (2015), 'Chronic illness and loneliness in older adulthood: the role of self-protective control strategies', *Health Psychology*, 34, 870–9).

16 Ravona-Springer, R. *et al.* (2013), 'Satisfaction with current status at work and lack of motivation to improve it during midlife is associated with increased risk for dementia in subjects who survived thirty-seven years later', *Journal of Alzheimer's Disease*, 36, 769–80. The odds ratio was 1.96 (controlling for age) and 1.78 (controlling for age and SES). The authors say: 'These results were not attenuated when midlife diabetes, blood pressure values, serum-cholesterol levels, and coronary heart disease were controlled for in the analysis.'

17 Andel, R. *et al.* (2005), 'Complexity of work and risk of Alzheimer's disease: a population-based study of Swedish twins', *Journals of Gerontology. Series B, Psychological Sciences and Social Sciences*, 60, 251–8.

18 Beeri, M. S. *et al.* (2008), 'Religious education and midlife observance are associated with dementia three decades later in Israeli men', *Journal of Clinical Epidemiology*, 61, 1161–8. The odds ratios 'relative to those with exclusively religious education, adjusted for age, area of birth, and socioeconomic status' were 0.49 'for those with mixed education' and 0.76 'for those with secular education'.

19 Explanations suggested by Beeri *et al.* (2008) (note 18) include increased cognitive load (the effort required to reconcile two very different outlooks might have forced men who experienced a mixed education to do more mental work, thereby sharpening their wits) and personality (perhaps parents with different personalities tended to favour different kinds of education).

20 For example, a longitudinal study of over 32,000 US citizens which used objective measures of health as well as asking people how they felt found that people who had

professed a conservative ideology tended to have lower ratings on the objective measure of health—time until death—compared with liberals (Pabayo, R. *et al.* (2015), 'Political party affiliation, political ideology and mortality', *Journal of Epidemiology and Community Health*, 69, 423–31). The authors controlled for a large number of covariates, well beyond the usual sociodemographic data, and their statistical investigation of whether these contributed to the relationship they identified between liberal ideology and longer time to death found that adjusting to take account of measures of happiness and of religious fundamentalism did not alter the relationship, suggesting that something else is responsible for the link (if it is real). Unfortunately many of the covariates were measured only once, at the start of the study, so any variation in them over time would not have been detected.

21 A sizeable meta-analysis in 2014, controlling for numerous factors, found an increased risk of dying with dementia in women who left education early, but not in men (Russ, T. C. *et al.* (2013), 'Socioeconomic status as a risk factor for dementia death: individual participant meta-analysis of 86 508 men and women from the UK', *British Journal of Psychiatry*, 203, 10–17). Cognitive ability includes a range of aptitudes, such as verbal fluency, short-term memory, and attention. It is typically measured with a test battery such as the MMSE, which is short—about ten minutes—and easy to administer. Verbal abilities are thought to be better sustained in ageing than others. A brief test, however, may underestimate decline in patients with nontypical cognitive impairment—e.g. those whose memory is relatively preserved—as well as misjudging people with very high or low intelligence or education.

22 For example, one small but life-long study looked at 268 high-achieving white men, formerly at Harvard University, who were unusually long-lived—'60% of our sample, rather than the expected 20%, survived past their 80th birthday'—and healthy, with fewer dementia risk factors than their less privileged compatriots. The only significant predictors of who would still have intact cognition at ninety were how much exercise they took at age sixty, having a good early bond with their mother, and having a highly educated mum. (Dad had no such impact.) As the authors note, however, 'The fact that we found education and IQ non-significant in part reflects the truncated range of these variables in our study.' By age seventy, death and dropout had reduced the sample size to 196, and comparisons among older men are based on even smaller groups, so the data should be regarded as suggestive rather than conclusive. Despite its disadvantages, however, the study measured far more physical, mental, and social variables, over far longer timescales, than usual. It illustrates the constant need to balance resource limitations, the need for big data, and how much questioning the participants will tolerate. See Vaillant, G. E. *et al.* (2014), 'Antecedents of intact cognition and dementia at age 90 years: a prospective study', *International Journal of Geriatric Psychiatry*, 29, 1278–85.

23 Nyberg *et al.* (2014) (note 16.1).

24 A study, using the same Swedish cohort, of adoption's effects on IQ found significant effects of the adoptive parents' education on the adopted sons' IQs; and these were higher than the IQs of the boys who remained with their biological parents (Kendler, K. S. *et al.* (2015), 'Family environment and the malleability of cognitive ability: a Swedish national home-reared and adopted-away cosibling control study', *Proceedings of the National Academy of Sciences*, 112, 4612–17).

25 Katzman, R. *et al.* (1988), 'Clinical, pathological, and neurochemical changes in dementia: a subgroup with preserved mental status and numerous neocortical plaques', *Annals of Neurology*, 23, 138–44.

26 Katzman *et al.* (1988) (note 25) suggested this, and also observed that the type of cell might be important, noting that larger neurons were relatively spared in individuals with higher reserves. Note also that brain tissue loss could in principle relate to the whole brain or to particular regions which appear to be larger—or more densely connected—in more educated people; specifically, association areas such as the superior temporal and anterior cingulate cortices. A small neuroimaging study (*n* = 36) of healthy elderly people found larger volume and higher metabolism of the anterior cingulate cortex (ACC) with education (Arenaza-Urquijo, E. M. *et al.* (2013), 'Relationships between years of education and gray matter volume, metabolism and functional connectivity in healthy elders', *NeuroImage*, 83, 450–7). Larger insular and superior temporal gyrus volume, and greater ACC connectivity, were also linked to educational attainment. Another study, however, did not find thicker cortex in people with higher education (compared with those without), suggesting that volume of brain tissue may be less relevant than connectivity to cognitive reserve (Pillai, J. A. *et al.* (2012), 'Higher education is not associated with greater cortical thickness in brain areas related to literacy or intelligence in normal aging or mild cognitive impairment', *Journal of Clinical and Experimental Neuropsychology*, 34, 925–35).

27 Here the devilish detail concerns what we mean by connectivity. Brain networks can be measured in many ways, including: *efficiency* (more efficient networks use less energy, and transmit signals faster and with more fidelity); the *complexity* of their pathways (generally, fewer synapses mean faster signalling and less chance of the signal becoming corrupted); *redundancy* and flexibility (these reflect whether networks can keep signalling effectively when parts of them are damaged, or whether the brain can reroute around the damaged area); *dynamic range* (how well networks can ramp up, or tone down, activity in response to increased or decreased stimulation or task difficulty); and *signal-to-noise ratio* (a standard measure of transmission fidelity). As any mobile phone user struggling to hear their caller knows, communication networks lose data because of noise. In the brain, signals are probabilistic and hence very noisy, due to the way synaptic signalling works. An action potential may usually trigger the release of neurotransmitter from a synapse, but not always. Plus, the amount which is released, crosses the synaptic cleft, and activates receptors on a recipient neuron will vary depending on what else is happening in the cleft and in both neurons: how much neurotransmitter the sender cell has available, how efficiently it can recycle neurotransmitter from the cleft, how many receptors are on the recipient cell, and so on.

28 Proxy measures of reserve, such as executive function, may themselves be measured differently in different studies. Meanwhile the synapse-level details of human neurodegeneration are still largely invisible to neuroimaging, so much must be inferred from animal models or post-mortem brains. Animal studies have their problems, and post-mortem human studies are limited by insufficient numbers of donors.

29 For instance, it is not yet known what aspects of life experience matter for reserve. Is it the accumulated collection of established neural pathways instantiating the mass of acquired knowledge, which psychologists call crystallised intelligence? Or is it the ability of those

pathways to send signals efficiently and flexibly, perhaps instantiating that mysterious but vital brain capacity called fluid intelligence?

30 Hartshorne, J. K. and L. T. Germine (2015), 'When does cognitive functioning peak? The asynchronous rise and fall of different cognitive abilities across the life span', *Psychological Science*, 26, 433–43.

Chapter 20

1 An example is Wang, R. *et al.* (2013), 'Metabolic stress modulates Alzheimer's beta-secretase gene transcription via SIRT1-PPARgamma-PGC-1 in neurons', *Cell Metabolism*, 17, 685–94. The study, on mice, linked metabolic stress to increased β-secretase production via effects on the nuclear receptor PPAR-γ and sirtuins. These are molecules associated with ageing, metabolic disease, and Alzheimer's.

2 Genetic disorders also suggest a link between osteoporosis and dementia: a rare condition called Nasu-Hakola disease, for example, seems to cause both (Sahebari, M. *et al.* (2014), 'Nasu-Hakola disease as suspected cause for bone disease and dementia', *Journal of Clinical Rheumatology*, 20, 160–2). Depression can also feature low bone density. With respect to smell, problems with this sensory system have also been linked to other disorders, such as schizophrenia, depression, and Parkinson's disease.

3 I exclude blood group, which a large 2015 study found had no influence on dementia risk, because I don't think it counts as a system. See Vasan, S. K. *et al.* (2015), 'ABO blood group and dementia risk—a Scandinavian record-linkage study', *PLoS One*, 10, e0129115.

4 The literature search used major data sources including *SCOPUS* and *PubMed*, identifying systematic reviews and meta-analyses, where available, and cohort studies otherwise, for dementia or Alzheimer's risk factors. Constraints of time prevented my completing the kind of fully systematic review needed for a meta-analysis, so the data should be considered only roughly indicative. In Table 4:

   Data for ApoE were taken from Corder, E. H. *et al.* (1993), 'Gene dose of apolipoprotein E type 4 allele and the risk of Alzheimer's disease in late onset families', *Science*, 261, 921–3; Farrer, L. A. *et al.* (1997), 'Effects of age, sex, and ethnicity on the association between apolipoprotein E genotype and Alzheimer disease. A meta-analysis. APOE and Alzheimer Disease Meta Analysis Consortium', *Journal of the American Medical Association*, 278, 1349–56; Liu, X. *et al.* (2012), 'ApoE gene polymorphism and vascular dementia in Chinese population: a meta-analysis', *Journal of Neural Transmission*, 119, 387–94; Rubinsztein, D. C. and Easton, D. F. (1999), 'Apolipoprotein E genetic variation and Alzheimer's disease: a meta-analysis', *Dementia and Geriatric Cognitive Disorders*, 10, 199–209; and Wang *et al.* (2012) (note 19.1).

   Data for depression were taken from Davydow, D. S. *et al.* (2013), 'Hospitalization, depression and dementia in community-dwelling older Americans: findings from the National Health and Aging Trends Study', *General Hospital Psychiatry*, 36, 135–41; Diniz *et al.* (2013) (note 14.50); Gao *et al.* (2013) (note 14.51); Ownby, R. L. *et al.* (2006), 'Depression and risk for Alzheimer disease: systematic review, meta-analysis, and metaregression analysis', *Archives of General Psychiatry*, 63, 530–8; and Psaltopoulou, T. *et al.* (2013),

'Mediterranean diet, stroke, cognitive impairment, and depression: a meta-analysis', *Annals of Neurology*, 74, 580–91.

Data for diabetes were taken from Cheng, G. *et al.* (2012), 'Diabetes as a risk factor for dementia and mild cognitive impairment: a meta-analysis of longitudinal studies', *Internal Medicine Journal*, 42, 484–91; Gudala, K. *et al.* (2013), 'Diabetes mellitus and risk of dementia: a meta-analysis of prospective observational studies', *Journal of Diabetes Investigation*, 4, 640–50; Hu, E. A. *et al.* (2013), 'Lifestyles and risk factors associated with adherence to the mediterranean diet: a baseline assessment of the PREDIMED trial', *PLoS One*, 8, e60166; Huang, C. C. *et al.* (2014), 'Diabetes mellitus and the risk of Alzheimer's disease: a nationwide population-based study', *PloS One*, 9, e87095; Lu, F. P. *et al.* (2009), 'Diabetes and the risk of multi-system aging phenotypes: a systematic review and meta-analysis', *PloS One*, 4, e4144; and Profenno, L. A. *et al.* (2010), 'Meta-analysis of Alzheimer's disease risk with obesity, diabetes, and related disorders', *Biological Psychiatry*, 67, 505–12.

Data for high blood pressure were taken from Chang-Quan, H. *et al.* (2011), 'The association of antihypertensive medication use with risk of cognitive decline and dementia: a meta-analysis of longitudinal studies', *International Journal of Clinical Practice*, 65, 1295–305; Guan, J. W. *et al.* (2011), 'No association between hypertension and risk for Alzheimer's disease: a meta-analysis of longitudinal studies', *Journal of Alzheimer's Disease*, 27, 799–807; Huang *et al.* (2014) (see **Data for diabetes**); Johnson, M. L. *et al.* (2012), 'Antihypertensive drug use and the risk of dementia in patients with diabetes mellitus', *Alzheimer's and Dementia*, 8, 437–44; McGuinness, B. *et al.* (2006), 'The effects of blood pressure lowering on development of cognitive impairment and dementia in patients without apparent prior cerebrovascular disease', *Cochrane Database of Systematic Reviews*, CD004034; Power, M. C. *et al.* (2011), 'The association between blood pressure and incident Alzheimer disease: a systematic review and meta-analysis', *Epidemiology*, 22, 646–59; and Sharp, S. I. *et al.* (2011), 'Hypertension is a potential risk factor for vascular dementia: systematic review', *International Journal of Geriatric Psychiatry*, 26, 661–9.

Data for prior cancer were taken from Ma, L. L. *et al.* (2014), 'Association between cancer and Alzheimer's disease: systematic review and meta-analysis', *Journal of Alzheimer's Disease*, 42, 565–73; Roe, C. M. *et al.* (2010), 'Cancer linked to Alzheimer disease but not vascular dementia', *Neurology*, 74, 106–12; and Sofi, F. *et al.* (2008), 'Adherence to Mediterranean diet and health status: meta-analysis', *British Medical Journal*, 337, a1344.

Data for diet were taken from Li, F. J. *et al.* (2012), 'Dietary intakes of vitamin E, vitamin C, and β-carotene and risk of Alzheimer's disease: a meta-analysis', *Journal of Alzheimer's Disease*, 31, 253–8; Psaltopoulou *et al.* (2013) (see **Data for depression**); Singh, B. *et al.* (2014), 'Association of Mediterranean diet with mild cognitive impairment and Alzheimer's disease: a systematic review and meta-analysis', *Journal of Alzheimer's Disease*, 39, 271–82; and Sofi *et al.* (2008) (see **Data for prior cancer**).

Data for coffee drinking were taken from Barranco Quintana, J. L. *et al.* (2007), 'Alzheimer's disease and coffee: a quantitative review', *Neurological Research*, 29, 91–5.

Data for alcohol drinking were taken from Anstey *et al.* (2009) (note 17.16); Neafsey and Collins (2011) (note 17.16); and Peters, R. *et al.* (2008), 'Alcohol, dementia and cognitive decline in the elderly: a systematic review', *Age and Ageing*, 37, 505–12.

Data for BMI were taken from Anstey, K. J. *et al.* (2011), 'Body mass index in midlife and late-life as a risk factor for dementia: a meta-analysis of prospective studies', *Obesity Reviews*, 12, e426–37; Beydoun, M. A. *et al.* (2008), 'Obesity and central obesity as risk factors for incident dementia and its subtypes: a systematic review and meta-analysis', *Obesity Reviews*, 9, 204–18; Hu *et al.* (2013) (see **Data for diabetes**); Profenno *et al.* (2010) (see **Diabetes data**); and Ravona-Springer, R. *et al.* (2013), 'Body weight variability in midlife and risk for dementia in old age', *Neurology*, 80, 1677–83.

    Data for fitness were taken from Aarsland, D. *et al.* (2010), 'Is physical activity a potential preventive factor for vascular dementia? A systematic review', *Aging and Mental Health*, 14, 386–95; DeFina, L. F. *et al.* (2013), 'The association between midlife cardiorespiratory fitness levels and later-life dementia: a cohort study', *Annals of Internal Medicine*, 158, 162–8; Fritsch *et al.* (2005) (note 19.11); and Kulmala, J. *et al.* (2014), 'Association between mid-to- late life physical fitness and dementia: evidence from the CAIDE study', *Journal of Internal Medicine*, 276, 296–307.

    Data for smoking were taken from Anstey *et al.* (2007) (note 10.7); Cataldo *et al.* (2010) (note 10.5), and Chen (2012) (note 10.6).

    Data for education were taken from Caamano-Isorna, F. *et al.* (2006), 'Education and dementia: a meta-analytic study', *Neuroepidemiology*, 26, 226–32; De Ronchi, D. *et al.* (2005), 'Occurrence of cognitive impairment and dementia after the age of 60: a population-based study from northern Italy', *Dementia and Geriatric Cognitive Disorders*, 19, 97–105; Meng, X. and D'Arcy, C. (2012), 'Education and dementia in the context of the cognitive reserve hypothesis: a systematic review with meta-analyses and qualitative analyses', *PloS One*, 7, e38268; and Wang *et al.* (2012) (note 19.1).

    Data for SES were taken from Zeki Al Hazzouri *et al.* (2011) (note 18.20) and Goldbourt *et al.* (2007) (note 18.18).

Part 3

1 The quotation is from MIT's translation of *On The Sacred Disease* (<http://classics.mit.edu/ Hippocrates/sacred.html>), attributed to Hippocrates (see note 12.6). The full quotation is as follows: 'Since, then, the brain, as being the primary seat of sense and of the spirits, perceives whatever occurs in the body, if any change more powerful than usual take place in the air, owing to the seasons, the brain becomes changed by the state of the air. For, on this account, the brain first perceives, because, I say, all the most acute, most powerful, and most deadly diseases, and those which are most difficult to be understood by the inexperienced, fall upon the brain.' It nicely captures the mix of brilliance and baffling wrongness of ancient Greek scientific and medical thinking, seen through modern eyes.

Chapter 21

1 Hardy and Higgins (1992) (note 6.12). Neurofibrillary tangles are what I have called tau tangles.
2 Herrup, K. (2015), 'The case for rejecting the amyloid cascade hypothesis', *Nature Neuroscience*, 18, 794–9.

3 Herrup (2015) (note 2). The factors listed are (1) amyloid; (2) tau; (3) autophagy and/or lysosomes; (4) calcium homeostasis (excitotoxicity); (5) cell cycle regulation; (6) inflammation; (7) genes; (8) oxidative stress; (9) DNA damage; (10) mitochondria; (11) senescence; (12) glucose; and (13) 'a general metabolic compromise'.

4 Hardy, J. (2009), 'The amyloid hypothesis for Alzheimer's disease: a critical reappraisal', *Journal of Neurochemistry*, 110, 1129–34. Turn the page after reading Herrup's piece in *Nature Neuroscience*, and you will find one by Erik Musiek and David Holtzman on the same topic (Musiek, E. S. and D. M. Holtzman (2015), 'Three dimensions of the amyloid hypothesis: time, space and 'wingmen'', *Nature Neuroscience*, 18, 800–6). They advocate revising the cascade hypothesis to state that Aβ 'acts primarily as a trigger of other downstream processes'—e.g. inflammation, oxidative stress, tau accumulation—and that these are what lead to neurodegeneration. If so, higher levels of Aβ production should start the process of neurodegeneration earlier—as indeed appears to be the case in familial Alzheimer's. But if Aβ is the only cause, higher levels of the protein should also mean the degeneration takes hold faster in familial cases, and this doesn't seem to happen. On this view, Aβ is a necessary prelude to Alzheimer's, but it may not by itself be sufficient for the disease to take hold; other causes are needed. The authors contrast this with cerebral amyloid angiopathy, where they think Aβ is enough to cause the damage to blood vessels.

5 A 2014 study suggests that microglia respond to Aβ fibrils but not to oligomers (Ferrera, D. *et al.* (2014), 'Resting microglia react to Aβ42 fibrils but do not detect oligomers or oligomer-induced neuronal damage', *Neurobiology of Aging*, 35, 2444–57).

6 The innate immune mechanisms involved in wound healing—from which amyloid may have derived—'preceded the evolution of the inducible combinatorial immune responses characteristic of jawed vertebrates' (i.e. the adaptive immune system we know today). So say Finch, C. E. and J. J. Marchalonis (1996), 'Evolutionary perspectives on amyloid and inflammatory features of Alzheimer disease', *Neurobiology of Aging*, 17, 809–15.

7 Adaptive immune reactions (involving B and T lymphocytes) seem to be a less prominent feature of Alzheimer's than in 'classic' neuroinflammatory disorders like encephalitis, where they play a key role (Heppner *et al.* 2015) (note 13.1); but c.f. Marsh, S.E. *et al.* (2016), 'The adaptive immune system restrains Alzheimer's disease pathogenesis by modulating microglial function', *Proceedings of the National Academy of Sciences*, 113, E1316–25.

8 Oligodendrocytes and endothelial cells also seem to interact with complement, suggesting that the brain's wiring (myelin) and its borders (the blood–brain barrier) could also be affected by complement activation (Heppner *et al.* 2015) (note 13.1).

9 Such molecules include the chemokines fractalkine and CD200. Fractalkine is expressed by neurons and binds to microglial receptors. CD200 sits on neuronal cell membranes and physically locks to its receptor on microglia. Both CD200 and fractalkine can damp down microglial activation. Both have been linked genetically to Alzheimer's, and both are decreased in ageing brains.

10 Mouse models of diffuse axonal injury show that APP levels peak a day after the injury and then slowly decline. Sham-injured animals did not show the same effect, strongly suggesting that the injury caused the changes in APP.

11 Magnoni, S. and D. L. Brody (2010), 'New perspectives on amyloid-beta dynamics after acute brain injury: moving between experimental approaches and studies in the human brain', *Archives of Neurology*, 67, 1068–73.

12 Sutphen, C. L. *et al.* (2015), 'Longitudinal cerebrospinal fluid biomarker changes in preclinical Alzheimer disease during middle age', *Journal of the American Medical Association Neurology*, 72, 1029–42. The researchers note that the apparent lag between falling CSF amyloid levels and brain plaque detection could be a problem with methods, since the neuroimaging technique used does not register all forms of amyloid, or even all forms of amyloid plaque. (It detects compact plaques made of fibrils, but some plaques are diffuse and do not show up on these scans.)

13 As we saw earlier, there is also debate about how the high levels of Aβ come about in sporadic Alzheimer's, with some researchers proposing lower Aβ clearance, rather than increased production, as the key factor.

14 As a study of another mainly late-life disease, breast cancer, remarks: 'It is likely that very few genetic diseases affecting women late in life fail to affect at least some pre-menopausal individuals leading to selection where one might otherwise anticipate none' (Pavard, S. and C. J. Metcalf (2007), 'Negative selection on BRCA1 susceptibility alleles sheds light on the population genetics of late-onset diseases and aging theory', *PloS One*, 2, e1206).

15 It is sometimes argued that because pre-industrial societies, past and present, have much lower average life expectancies than highly developed ones, therefore few people in the former lived to an age where the risk of dementia became significant. This does not take account, however, of the fact that one of the biggest factors reducing life expectancy is child and maternal mortality. In other words, the average is brought down not by adult deaths, but by large losses in the first few years. Those who survive childhood have a decent chance of making it to old age.

16 Hubel, D. H. (1979), 'The brain', *Scientific American*, 241, 44–52.

17 I am not in the business of naming and shaming the worst offenders, but (like most UK scientists in my experience) I would cite the *Daily Mail* as an egregious example of how not to do science communication.

18 The quotation is from Terry, R. D. (1996), 'The pathogenesis of Alzheimer disease: an alternative to the amyloid hypothesis', *Journal of Neuropathology and Experimental Neurology*, 55, 1023–5.

19 Willem, M. *et al.* (2015), 'η-Secretase processing of APP inhibits neuronal activity in the hippocampus', *Nature*, 526, 443–7.

20 Amyloid plaques, for example, were long thought to be tough, fibrous end-stages of Alzheimer's disease, but oligomers—presumed to be an earlier stage—have been found even in advanced diseases, and under certain conditions smaller pieces of amyloid can dissolve back into solution. Animal and cell culture studies are also susceptible to methodological problems. For example, cell studies of neurons have often been done in a lab environment where the oxygen content is much higher than in the brain, and amounts of Aβ used are not always physiological.

21 Technical problems bedevil other parts of the field as well, such as the genetics of sporadic Alzheimer's. In any disease, linkage to specific genes provides important clues to the

underlying mechanisms, allowing research to concentrate on likely suspects. However, commonly used methods like genome-wide association studies have their problems. For example, they are not good at picking up small effects—so if dementia is death by a thousand cuts, some of the genetic knives may be missed because the slashes they make are too small to be detected. Even for larger effects, studies to date have found it extremely difficult to obtain consistent results for genes other than ApoE. This may be because Alzheimer's has complex environmental causes, or involves many genes of small effect, or is many diseases. But for a hypothesis so reliant on gene-based data from rare familial cases, the genetic evidence for sporadic Alzheimer's is disappointing to date, apart from ApoE.

22 This discussion draws heavily on a recent review: Smith, A. M. and M. Dragunow (2014), 'The human side of microglia', *Trends in Neurosciences*, 37, 125–35.

23 Microglia from aborted tissue may also be immature, since the tissues are normally obtained from first-trimester embryos; in any case, even late foetal microglia are immunologically different from adult ones. How quickly the tissue is extracted, and shipped from source to supplier, can affect the cells' later behaviour in the lab.

24 Immune function varies greatly across species, in ways that are not fully understood.

25 Questions are taken from the Alzheimer's Association's brief 'cognitive assessment toolkit', available from <http://www.alz.org/documents_custom/the cognitive assessment toolkit copy_v1.pdf>.

26 Cohen, R. M. *et al.* (2013), 'A transgenic Alzheimer rat with plaques, tau pathology, behavioral impairment, oligomeric abeta, and frank neuronal loss', *Journal of Neuroscience*, 33, 6245–56.

27 Beck, M. *et al.* (1997), 'Amyloid precursor protein in guinea pigs—complete cDNA sequence and alternative splicing', *Biochimica et Biophysica Acta*, 1351, 17–21.

28 Johnstone, E. M. *et al.* (1991), 'Conservation of the sequence of the Alzheimer's disease amyloid peptide in dog, polar bear and five other mammals by cross-species polymerase chain reaction analysis', *Brain Research. Molecular Brain Research*, 10, 299–305. Guinea pigs' vitamin C metabolism is similar to humans' and 'they are the only small animal model that closely mimics human lipoprotein and cholesterol metabolism' (Sharman, M. J. *et al.* (2013), 'The guinea pig as a model for sporadic Alzheimer's disease (AD): the impact of cholesterol intake on expression of AD-related genes', *PLoS One*, 8, e66235).

29 For an example, see the discussion of a form of dementia due to tauopathy in Kawakami, I. *et al.* (2014), 'Tau accumulation in the nucleus accumbens in tangle-predominant dementia', *Acta Neuropathologica Communications*, 2, 40.

30 If amyloid triggers the process, some researchers think tau may be the chief executioner. Musiek and Holtzman (2015) (note 4) grant abnormal tau this status. Tau has been described by another researcher, George Bloom, as the bullet to Aβ's trigger (Bloom, G. S. (2014), 'Amyloid-beta and tau: the trigger and bullet in Alzheimer disease pathogenesis', *Journal of the American Medical Association Neurology*, 71, 505–8). Musiek and Holtzman do not however exclude other proteins such as α-synuclein and TDP-43, and they argue that other changes such as inflammation and oxidative stress follow. Tau tangles can be present without either amyloid deposits or cognitive dysfunction, but Musiek and Holtzman argue that what matters is the severity of the problem. Early on abnormal tau

is seen in subcortex and limbic cortex, but in cases where it has spread widely through cortex, amyloid is also present (Braak, H. and E. Braak (1991), 'Neuropathological stageing of Alzheimer-related changes', *Acta Neuropathologica*, 82, 239–59). Human brains where tau has reached this far show neurodegeneration, although not all forms of degeneration require tau.

31 Musiek and Holtzman (2015) (note 4).

32 Inevitably recent research on cultured neurons suggests a more complex picture, finding that $A\beta_{42}$ can disrupt the cytoskeleton and cause growing neurites (young axons and dendrites) to retract.

33 Braak and Braak (1991) (note 30). How one prompts the other is not clear, since amyloid and tau build up at different times in different parts of the brain. But research on mice and macaques suggests that $A\beta$ oligomers can diffuse through brain tissue, so perhaps they are involved. And the timing difference might be due to protein building up slowly, doing little damage until some threshold quantity has been produced.

34 More advanced stages go with more advanced clinical symptoms. See Braak and Braak (1991) (note 30), which was based on a sample of eighty-three brains, later expanded to 2,661 (Braak and Braak 1997) (note 5.73). The 1997 paper describes its raw materials as 'nonselected autopsy cases' from four pathology departments at three German universities; i.e. these were not people chosen for signs of dementia. Note that I have once again simplified. The spread of proteins like tau and amyloid in human brains is variable, complex, and not yet fully understood; and the idea that it follows standard patterns is not proven. For a lucid review of the challenges involved, see Walsh, D. M. and Selkoe, D. J. (2016), 'A critical appraisal of the pathogenic protein spread hypothesis of neurodegeneration', *Nature Reviews Neuroscience*, 17, 251–60.

35 'The end-stage of amyloid accumulation is characterized by a fairly constant distribution pattern of the pathological material. In contrast, early stages exhibit considerable inter-individual variation' (Braak and Braak 1991) (note 30).

36 'Neither amyloid deposits nor neurofibrillary changes [tau tangles] necessarily accompany old age', according to Braak and Braak (1997) (note 5.73), who studied 2,661 brains from people aged twenty-five to ninety-five. They found that the presence of tau without detectable amyloid (36%) was more common than amyloid without tau (about 1.5%). Across all ages, just under 42% had both pathologies; just under 21% had neither. In the youngest third (aged twenty-five–fifty) and the oldest third (aged seventy and over), the proportions of tau only and amyloid only were similar, but the proportion with both pathologies rose from about 4% in the youngest to almost 64% in the oldest group. Once past seventy, only about 3% had no signs of either amyloid or tau.

37 One research group has found deposition of both tau and $A\beta$ already well underway in children living in a highly polluted environment (SFE Calderón-Garcidueñas, L. *et al.* (2012), 'Neuroinflammation, hyperphosphorylated tau, diffuse amyloid plaques, and down-regulation of the cellular prion protein in air pollution exposed children and young adults', *Journal of Alzheimer's Disease*, 28, 93–107). The Braak group, in a study of forty-two people aged four to twenty-nine, found evidence of tau changes 'before puberty or in early young adulthood' (Braak, H. and K. Del Tredici (2011), 'The pathological process underlying Alzheimer's disease in individuals under thirty', *Acta Neuropathologica*, 121,

171–81). These changes began subcortically—particularly in the locus coeruleus, source of noradrenaline. They did not, however, find amyloid deposits, except in one person who had Down's syndrome.

38 Wang, L. *et al.* (2015), 'Spatially distinct atrophy is linked to beta-amyloid and tau in preclinical Alzheimer disease', *Neurology*, 84, 1254–60.

39 Note that the Braaks were looking at solid amyloid deposits, not oligomers; and people whose brains end up in university pathology departments are not representative of the general population. Nonetheless, this and other evidence—e.g. that cognitive decline need not be accompanied by large amounts of amyloid deposits, or *vice versa*—has led some researchers to argue that Aβ is not the initial cause of the disease (such as Drachman, D. A. (2014), 'The amyloid hypothesis, time to move on: amyloid is the downstream result, not cause, of Alzheimer's disease', *Alzheimer's and Dementia*, 10, 372–80).

40 Cash, A. D. *et al.* (2003), 'Microtubule reduction in Alzheimer's disease and aging is independent of tau filament formation', *American Journal of Pathology*, 162, 1623–7.

41 For a clinical guide to CJD see the NHS (<http://www.nhs.uk/conditions/Creutzfeldt-Jakob-disease/pages/introduction.aspx>). For information about kuru see the NIH (<http://www.ninds.nih.gov/disorders/kuru/kuru.htm>).

42 See Brown, P. *et al.* (2012), 'Iatrogenic Creutzfeldt-Jakob disease, final assessment', *Emerging Infectious Diseases*, 18, 901–7, which lists the sources of the prion infection which caused CJD as mainly 'contaminated growth hormone (226 cases) and dura mater grafts (228 cases) derived from human cadavers with undiagnosed CJD infections; a small number of additional cases are caused by neurosurgical instrument contamination, corneal grafts, gonadotrophic hormone, and secondary infection with variant CJD transmitted by transfusion of blood products'.

43 A fascinating finding from genetic studies of prion diseases is that in carriers, a variation in the prion protein (PrP) of just one amino acid 'can cause two distinct diseases that target different brain regions' (Walsh and Selkoe, 2016) (note 34). If the amino acid is valine, familial CJD results; if it is methionine, the mutation leads to fatal familial insomnia, in which sleep loss (usually beginning in middle age) progresses to ataxia, dementia, and death within a few years. The brain pathology is also distinct, affecting primarily cortex in fCJD and thalamus in FFI. As Walsh and Selkoe remark, 'The fact that two different non-pathogenic PrP variants [in carriers] that are present in all neurons can dictate the specific populations of neurons that are affected by a mutant PrP molecule that is also present in all neurons suggests that the site of origin and initial form of misfolded PrP is mediated by factors present in certain neurons that make these neurons more vulnerable to misfolding of particular PrP structures.'

44 'A novel PrP variant, G127V, was under positive evolutionary selection during the epidemic of kuru—an acquired prion disease epidemic of the Fore population in Papua New Guinea—and appeared to provide strong protection against disease in the heterozygous state' (Asante, E. A. *et al.* (2015), 'A naturally occurring variant of the human prion protein completely prevents prion disease', *Nature*, 522, 478–81). Not all prion proteins are harmful. Some are useful cellular machines. (Growth, proliferation, cell adhesion, and immune function are among the suggested roles for normal prion proteins.)

45 A 2015 paper estimates the 'age-adjusted incidence per million person-years' of CJD at 1.5, or less; the comparable figure for Alzheimer's is 2,589 (de Pedro-Cuesta, J. *et al.* (2015), 'Comparative incidence of conformational, neurodegenerative disorders', *PloS One*, 10, e0137342). Even among those at the highest risk of CJD due to past medical procedures, the prevalence of the disease is thought to be between about 1% and 10% (Brown *et al.* 2012) (note 42).

46 I say 'like viruses', but it is not yet fully understood how prions spread, and especially what happens, when, and where in order for the process to start—that is, for aggregation-prone forms of the protein to begin aggregating. Nor is it yet clear which aggregates are toxic. For a recent review of the templating hypothesis see Brettschneider, J. *et al.* (2015), 'Spreading of pathology in neurodegenerative diseases: a focus on human studies', *Nature Reviews Neuroscience*, 16, 109–20. For a critique see Walsh and Selkoe (2016) (note 34).

47 The earliest study I have found suggesting that Aβ may be transmissible is Baker, H. F. *et al.* (1994), 'Induction of beta (A4)-amyloid in primates by injection of Alzheimer's disease brain homogenate. Comparison with transmission of spongiform encephalopathy', *Molecular Neurobiology*, 8, 25–39.

48 SFE Johnstone *et al.* (1991) (note 28); also Animal Aid's website (<http://animalaid.org .uk/h/n/YOUTH/farming/1957/>) gives slaughter ages and natural lifespans. The cheapest meat cuts tend to be from older animals. Genetic analysis has found that pig, sheep, and cow do have the human-like form of Aβ, so could in principle form amyloid deposits. Rats do not, but so far the idea of roast rat has not proved popular. (An intriguing aside: the animal species known to develop amyloid deposits—like dogs, bears, chimpanzees, and humans—eat much more meat than rodents do.)

49 Jaunmuktane, Z. *et al.* (2015), 'Evidence for human transmission of amyloid-β pathology and cerebral amyloid angiopathy', *Nature*, 525, 247–50. This use of growth hormone was discontinued in the 1980s.

50 Demonstrating that Alzheimer's could spread by person-to-person transmission, in rare iatrogenic cases, is one thing. Demonstrating that this is a major cause of sporadic, late-onset Alzheimer's is another. If the disease process really does begin in midlife or earlier, as the amyloid hypothesis implies, determining causality would be a formidable technical challenge for an infection with an incubation period of perhaps four decades. (Kuru, for comparison, incubates for around twenty-five to thirty years; and kuru's cause was far easier to identify.)

51 The clinical trial, of the chemotherapy drug doxycycline, was abandoned due to lack of effect (Haïk, S. *et al.* (2014), 'Doxycycline in Creutzfeldt-Jakob disease: a phase 2, randomised, double-blind, placebo-controlled trial', *Lancet Neurology*, 13, 150–8). Survival time data are for thirty-nine patients with neuropathologically confirmed CJD, of whom nine survived beyond one year (see Table 3). The average quoted is the mean for both treated and placebo patients (8.6 months); the median is even lower (5.9 months).

52 Walsh and Selkoe (2016) (note 34) note other questions raised by the analogy with prions. For instance, although Aβ and prion protein can be secreted from cells, tau and α-synuclein are not thought to use the same mechanism, so how do they get out of cells (and indeed back in again)? One possibility is that they leave cells via exosomes, small vesicles shed into the extracellular space. Another is that they use tunnelling nanotubes,

which are tiny membrane bridges between cells; or they might leak out into synapses during neurotransmission. Alternatively, toxic aggregates may not spread directly between cells, but instead may cause other changes in one cell, which then affect its neighbours. A second issue is which forms of the protein are toxic and which are responsible for the spread. A third is what sets the process going; and there is also the related question of why some cells are more vulnerable than others to changes in proteins found in all of them. The pattern of damage is not so stereotyped as to mean that all brains with Alzheimer's decline in the same way, but neither is it random.

53 TAR (transactive response) DNA-binding protein of 43 kDa interacts with both DNA and RNA to regulate protein building. In post-mortem elderly human brains a study found TDP-43 in areas of high neuronal loss such as the hippocampus and entorhinal cortex (Uryu, K. *et al.* (2008), 'Concomitant TAR-DNA-binding protein 43 pathology is present in Alzheimer disease and corticobasal degeneration but not in other tauopathies', *Journal of Neuropathology and Experimental Neurology*, 67, 555–64). Thus Alzheimer's, and probably other dementias too, may involve multiple protein problems, just as changes in Aβ are not unique to Alzheimer's.

54 Pearce, M. M. *et al.* (2015), 'Prion-like transmission of neuronal huntingtin aggregates to phagocytic glia in the Drosophila brain', *Nature Communications*, 6, 6768.

55 Determining the exact subtype may require neuropathological analysis—and that is not easy even if the brain is available, because brains often don't fit the tidy theoretical categories. Future research will no doubt uncover more aggregating proteins with important roles in normal and diseased cells. For example, cofilin and actin, two proteins involved in the cytoskeleton, have been shown to aggregate into filaments called rods in response to oxidative stress, pro-inflammatory cytokines, or Aβ, using a mechanism which involves the prion protein (Walsh, K. P. *et al.* (2014), 'Amyloid-β and proinflammatory cytokines utilize a prion protein-dependent pathway to activate NADPH oxidase and induce cofilin-actin rods in hippocampal neurons', *PLoS One*, 9, e95995).

Chapter 22

1 Free radical scavengers used to treat stroke have also shown promise in animal models of neurodegeneration (Jiao, S.-S. *et al.* (2015), 'Edaravone alleviates Alzheimer's disease-type pathologies and cognitive deficits', *Proceedings of the National Academy of Sciences*, 112, 5225–30).

2 SFE Griebel, G. *et al.* (2012), 'SAR110894, a potent histamine H(3)-receptor antagonist, displays procognitive effects in rodents', *Pharmacology, Biochemistry, and Behavior*, 102, 203–14. The paper suggests that blocking histamine receptors might be a treatment avenue worth exploring.

3 ACAT1 (Acyl-CoA:cholesterol acyltransferase 1) blocks cholesterol by esterifying it, i.e. replacing a hydrogen atom with a fatty acid. Of ten lipid molecules whose levels were found to differ in the blood of Alzheimer patients and controls, six were esters of cholesterol (Proitsi, P. *et al.* (2015), 'Plasma lipidomics analysis finds long chain cholesteryl esters to be associated with Alzheimer's disease', *Translational Psychiatry*, 5, e494).

4 Cholesterol has also been shown to regulate levels of APLP-1 in neurons.

5 For example, brain cholesterol is metabolized to oxysterols, and these activate nuclear receptors called liver X receptors. These are 'crucial for cholesterol homeostasis' and have recently been shown to be involved in myelination (Meffre, D. *et al.* (2015), 'Liver X receptors alpha and beta promote myelination and remyelination in the cerebellum', *Proceedings of the National Academy of Sciences*, 112, 7587–92).

6 The patent 'Delivery, use and therapeutic applications of the crispr-cas systems and compositions for targeting disorders and diseases using particle delivery components' (WO 2015089419 A2) was filed at the end of 2014 by researchers at MIT.

Chapter 23

1 This is a fair point but somewhat cowardly, so here are two suggestions for fund raising. First, research suggests that paying top executives enormous amounts doesn't guarantee excellent performance, but does inflict social harms by boosting inequality, so how about disincentivizing this behaviour with a specific 'research investment' tax on the highest earners and/or the companies who pay them so generously? Secondly, how about a tax on junk food and sugary drinks—extending beyond that proposed by the UK Chancellor of the Exchequer in his March 2016 Budget? Surely that should boost the budget for understanding brain disorders?

2 Gandy, S. (2012), 'Lifelong management of amyloid-beta metabolism to prevent Alzheimer's disease', *New England Journal of Medicine*, 367, 864–6. The calculation of time-to-onset is possible because in families with mutations causing Alzheimer's the age of onset tends to be similar across generations, giving sufferers some estimate of how long they've got.

Chapter 24

1 Extract from Tom Lehrer (©1959), 'The Elements'. Used by permission.

2 Hall, D. A. *et al.* (2005), 'PRNP H187R mutation associated with neuropsychiatric disorders in childhood and dementia', *Neurology*, 64, 1304–6.

3 Insel, T. R. and B. N. Cuthbert (2015), 'Brain disorders? Precisely', *Science*, 348, 499–500. For an example of this approach with respect to cognitive decline, see Ngandu, T. *et al.* (2015), 'A 2 year multidomain intervention of diet, exercise, cognitive training, and vascular risk monitoring versus control to prevent cognitive decline in at-risk elderly people (FINGER): a randomised controlled trial', *Lancet*, 385, 2255–63.

4 One of the most common, and surely most preventable, traumas inflicted on children is sexual abuse. If I ever became dictator of Britain, top of my to-do list would be a thorough review of the childcare system and funding for a major research programme into paedophilia's causes and treatments. (How else are we going to eradicate it? Neither demonizing paedophiles nor locking them up has solved the problem.) I would also change the law to ensure that anyone convicted of such offences had a sizeable chunk of their assets removed and given to a NHS fund to help abuse survivors. And I'd set up an annual, high-profile, generous prize for the best social worker.

5 One age-unfriendly aspect of modern life is its growing complexity. Existence as a process of negotiation between citizens and 'authorities' (corporations, governments) requires considerable cognitive capacity, from school exams to filling in tax returns—and the latter, unlike the former, do not recede as you get older. Fearsome bureaucracy makes societies much less dementia-friendly than they could be. Our increasing dependence on computers has also made life harder for many elderly people, and it has not yet brought many rewards to dementia care. There are hopes that technology can be used to make life easier for patients and their carers, but translating assistive technologies from theory to practice is not proving easy.

Further Reading

The Internet has made many databases of biological information available and easily searchable. (Most of the references given here can quickly be found using search engines; where the link is to a subsection of a large website, hyperlinks are given.) Among the research resources that I found particularly helpful in preparing *The Fragile Brain* are the following:

- Georgia State University's *Hyperphysics* website, biology section (<http://hyperphysics.phy-astr.gsu.edu/hbase/biology/biocon.html>) is a lucid guide to processes such as glycolysis and the TCA cycle;
- For in-depth, often highly technical information about particular genes, molecules, or topics, search for NIH's NCBI *Gene*, *PubChem*, or *PubMed*;
- *ChemWiki* at the University of California, Davis is more accessible than *PubChem*;
- For data on fats, try the *AOCS Lipid Library* from the American Oil Chemists' Society;
- the *Kyoto Encyclopaedia of Genes and Genomes (KEGG)* has diagrams of biochemical pathways (and much else);
- the journal *Nature's SciTable* is clearly written and informative;
- For a lucid guide to microbes, see *Microbiology online*;
- For elderly but still useful introductions to immunology and biochemistry, *PubMed*'s ebooks include Janeway, C. A. *et al.* (2001), *Immunobiology: The Immune System in Health and Disease,* 5th edn (New York: Garland Science), available from http://www.ncbi.nlm.nih.gov/books/NBK10757/; and Berg, J. M. *et al.* (2002), *Biochemistry,* 5th edn (New York: W. H. Freeman), available from <http://www.ncbi.nlm.nih.gov/books/NBK21154/>;
- For a specific topic in neuroscience, try searching *Nature Reviews Neuroscience,* which publishes such high-quality, well-written pieces about hot topics that its place as the number one neuroscience journal is no surprise. For example, see the supportive and critical reviews about the templating hypothesis of

neurodegeneration that I cite in the notes to Chapter 21: Brettschneider *et al.* (2015) and Walsh and Selkoe (2016).

For those seeking clinical information, the NHS, patient.co.uk, and the Centers for Disease Control and Prevention (CDC) offer clear guides to many medical conditions as well as to UK and US recommendations for healthy living. I recommend starting with one of these, especially if you would prefer to have your information in a plainer English than scientists tend to provide. For dementia, the NIH's National Institute of Aging, AlzForum, and the charities listed under 'Organizations' at the front of this book are good starting points. They also have a lot of information about the main scientific hypotheses, biochemistry and neuroscience, recent new findings, and so on.

Abbreviations

Aβ	amyloid-beta protein
ACTH	adrenocorticotrophic hormone, involved in the release of stress hormones
AD	Alzheimer's disease
ALS	amyotrophic lateral sclerosis, a form of motor neuron disease
ApoE	apolipoprotein E, a fat-transporting protein and one of the biggest risk factors for Alzheimer's disease
APP	amyloid precursor protein
ATP	adenosine trisphosphate, an energy-storing molecule
BDNF	brain-derived neurotrophic factor
BMI	body mass index, which measures weight in relation to height
CDC	the United States government's Centers for Disease Control and Prevention
CJD	Creutzfeldt-Jakob disease
CNS	central nervous system: the brain and spinal cord
CSF	cerebrospinal fluid
CVOs	circumventricular organs
DAMPs	danger-associated molecular patterns: molecules which indicate cellular ill health
DHA	docosahexaenoic acid, an omega-3 fatty acid
EPA	eicosapentaenoic acid, an omega-3 fatty acid
ER	endoplasmic reticulum
GABA	gamma-amino-butyric acid, the brain's major inhibitory neurotransmitter
HDL	high-density lipoprotein, sometimes called good cholesterol
HIV	human immunodeficiency virus
HPA	hypothalamic-pituitary-adrenal; the HPA axis regulates the body's response to stress
HSV	herpes simplex virus

In vitro and *in vivo*	these Latin terms refer to biological experiments done 'in glass'—e.g. on cultured cells or brain slices—or 'in the living thing' (usually meaning non-human animals, although technically a research fMRI scan on a patient is also done *in vivo*)
ISF	interstitial fluid
LDL/oxLDL	low-density lipoprotein/oxidized low-density lipoprotein, sometimes called bad cholesterol
LPS	lipopolysaccharide, a toxin associated with bacteria which stimulates a potent immune response
MHC	major histocompatibility complex, a set of molecules which help immune cells recognize and destroy pathogens
(f)MRI	(functional) magnetic resonance imaging, a form of neuroimaging
NFκB	nuclear factor kappa beta, an important transcription factor and regulator of inflammation-related genes
NGF	nerve growth factor
NHS	the United Kingdom's National Health Service
NIH	the United States National Institutes of Health
NMDAR	n-methyl-d-aspartate receptor, a type of glutamate receptor particularly involved in learning, memory, and excitotoxicity
ONS	the United Kingdom government's Office for National Statistics
PAMPs	pathogen-associated molecular patterns: molecules on pathogen surfaces that the immune system has evolved to recognize as danger signals
PET	positron emission tomography, a form of neuroimaging
PubMed	a database of scientific articles, containing well over twenty-four million items as of September 2015, many of which are fully accessible
ROS	reactive oxygen species, oxygen-containing molecules such as hydrogen peroxide which can cause oxidative stress
SES	socioeconomic status—roughly, how rich/poor you are and your place in society
SFE	see, for example
SNS	sympathetic nervous system
TBI	traumatic brain injury
TNFα	tumour necrosis factor alpha, a potent pro-inflammatory cytokine
WHO	the World Health Organization

Publisher's Acknowledgements

We are grateful for permission to include the following copyright material in this book.

Extracts from Tony Harrison (2002), 'The Mother of the Muses', in *The Gaze of the Gorgon* (Newcastle-upon-Tyne: Bloodaxe Books). With permission from Faber and Faber Ltd.

Extract from Hughes, T. F. and M. Ganguli (2009), 'Modifiable midlife risk factors for late-life cognitive impairment and dementia', *Current Psychiatry Reviews*, 5, 73–92. With permission.

'We know there is virtually no disorder of the CNS . . .' extract reprinted by permission from Macmillan Publishers Ltd: Heppner, F. L., Ransohoff, R. M., and Becher, B. (2015), 'Immune attack: the role of inflammation in Alzheimer disease', *Nature Reviews Neuroscience*, 16, 358–72.

Extract from Rainulf A. Stelzmann, H. Norman Schnitzlein and F. Reed Murtagh (1995), 'An English translation of Alzheimer's 1907 paper, "Über eine eigenartige Erkankung der Hirnrinde"', *Clinical Anatomy*, 8, 429–31. © Wiley Periodicals, Inc.

Extract from Tom Lehrer (©1959), 'The Elements'. Used by permission.

The publisher and author have made every effort to trace and contact all copyright holders before publication. If notified, the publisher will be pleased to rectify any errors or omissions at the earliest opportunity.

Index

Endnotes are referenced by chapter (e.g. n.5.43 refers to endnote 43 of Chapter 5) and are given after text entries.

SOCIAL

Why our brains are wired to connect

Matthew D. Lieberman

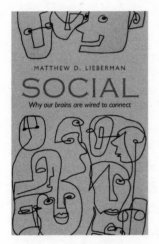

978-0-19-964504-6 | Hardback | £18.99

"This isn't just fascinating for its own sake. Lieberman has a social and political purpose."

Julian Baggini, **Financial Times**

"SOCIAL is the book I've been waiting for: a brilliant and beautiful exploration of how and why we are wired together, by one of the field's most prescient pioneers."

Daniel Gilbert, Harvard University

Why are we influenced by the behaviour of complete strangers? Why does the brain register similar pleasure when I perceive something as 'fair' or when I eat chocolate? Why can we be so profoundly hurt by bereavement? The young discipline of 'social cognitive neuroscience' has been exploring this fascinating interface between brain science and human behaviour since the late 1990s.

THE BRAIN SUPREMACY

Notes from the frontiers of neuroscience

Kathleen Taylor

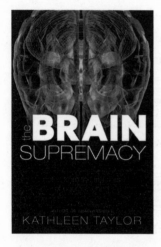

978-0-19-968385-7 | Paperback | £12.99

"This is a thoughtful guide to a rapidly advancing field and its implications."

Network Review

In recent years funding and effort is being poured into brain research. We are entering the era of the brain supremacy. What will the new science mean for us, as individuals, consumers, parents and citizens? Should we be excited, or alarmed, by the remarkable promises of drugs that can boost our brain power, ever more subtle marketing techniques, even machines that can read minds?

The Brain Supremacy is a lucid and rational guide to this exciting new world. Using recent examples from the scientific literature and the media, it explores the science behind the hype. Looking to the future, the book sets current neuroscience in its social and ethical context, as an increasingly important influence on how all of us live our lives.

THE BRAIN

A Very Short Introduction

Michael O'Shea

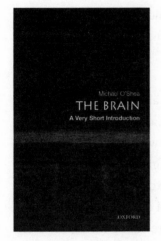

978-0-19-285392-9 | Paperback | £7.99

How does the brain work? How different is a human brain from other creatures' brains? Is the human brain still evolving?

Michael O'Shea provides a non-technical introduction to the main issues and findings in current brain research, and gives a sense of how neuroscience addresses questions about the relationship between the brain and the mind. He tackles subjects such as brain processes, perception, memory, motor control and the causes of 'altered mental states'. A final section discusses possible future developments in neuroscience, touching on artificial intelligence, gene therapy, the importance of the Human Genome Project, drugs by design, and transplants.